Perhalopyridines: Synthesis and Synthetic Utility

Authored by

Reza Ranjbar-Karimi

&

Alireza Poorfreidoni

Department of Chemistry, Faculty of Science
Vali-e-Asr University of Rafsanjan
Islamic Republic of Iran

Perhalopyridines: Synthesis and Synthetic Utility

Authors: Reza Ranjbar-Karimi and Alireza Poorfreidoni

ISBN (Online): 978-981-14-7379-1

ISBN (Print): 978-981-14-7377-7

ISBN (Paperback): 978-981-14-7378-4

need for a court order if at any point you breach any terms of this License Agreement. In no event will any delay or failure by Bentham Science Publishers in enforcing your compliance with this License Agreement constitute a waiver of any of its rights.

3. You acknowledge that you have read this License Agreement, and agree to be bound by its terms and conditions. To the extent that any other terms and conditions presented on any website of Bentham Science Publishers conflict with, or are inconsistent with, the terms and conditions set out in this License Agreement, you acknowledge that the terms and conditions set out in this License Agreement shall prevail.

Bentham Science Publishers Pte. Ltd.
80 Robinson Road #02-00
Singapore 068898
Singapore
Email: subscriptions@benthamscience.net

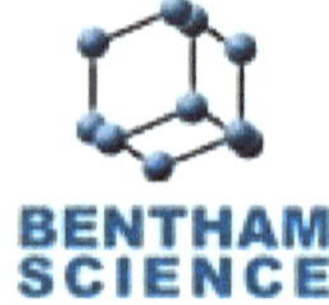

CONTENTS

PREFACE i
   CONSENT FOR PUBLICATION i
   CONFLICT OF INTEREST i
   ACKNOWLEDGEMENTS i

FOREWORD ii

ABBREVIATIONS iii

CHAPTER 1 PROPERTIES OF PERHALOPYRIDINES 1
   1. PHYSICAL AND CHEMICAL PROPERTIES 1
   2. SPECTROSCOPY 2
   3. REACTIONS 3
   REFERENCES 5

CHAPTER 2 PERFLUOROPYRIDINES 8
   1. INTRODUCTION 8
   2. SYNTHESIS OF PENTAFLUOROPYRIDINE 9
   3. REACTION MECHANISM 10
   4. REACTION OF PENTAFLUOROPYRIDINE WITH VARIOUS MONO DENTATE NUCLEOPHILES 12
      4.1. Reaction of S-centered Nucleophile with Pentafluoropyridine 12
      4.2. Reaction of O-centered Nucleophile with Pentafluoropyridine 17
      4.3. Reaction of C-centered Nucleophile with Pentafluoropyridine 22
      4.4. Reaction of N-centered Nucleophile with Pentafluoropyridine 32
      4.5. Reaction of Pentafluoropyridine 3 with Halogenating Reagents (Cl, Br, I) 51
      4.6. Reduction of Perfluorinated Pyridines 56
   5. REACTION OF PERFLUOROPYRIDINES WITH VARIOUS MULTIDENTATE NUCLEOPHILES 59
      5.1. Synthesis of Perfluorinated Heterocyles 59
      5.2. Synthesis of Fluorinated Ring-fused Heterocyles 76
   6. ORGANOMETALLIC COMPOUNDS OF PERFLUORO- HETEROAROMATICS 94
   7. PHOTOCHEMICAL REACTIONS OF FLUORINATED PYRIDINES 109
   8. COPOLYMERIZATION OF PENTAFLUOROPYRIDINE 121
   9. THE PENTAFLUOROPYRIDINE CATION C5F5N+ 122
   10. SALTS OF PERFLUOROPYRIDINE 122
   11. SYNTHESIS OF MACROCYCLIC COMPOUNDS FROM POLYFLUOROPYRIDINES 123
   12. PENTAFLUOROPYRIDINE IN MEDICINAL CHEMISTRY AND BIOCHEMISTRY 129
   REFERENCES 135

CHAPTER 3 PERCHLOROPYRIDINES 152
   1. INTRODUCTION 152
   2. SYNTHESIS OF PENTACHLOROPYRIDINE 153
      2.1. By Straight Chlorination 153
      2.2. By Ring-closing Method 154
      2.3. Synthesis of Pentachloropyridine-1-15N-2,6-13C2 154
   3. NUCLEOPHILIC REACTIONS OF PERCHLOROPYRIDINES 155
      3.1. Reaction of Pentachloropyridine with Various Mono Dentate Nucleophiles 155
         3.1.1. Reaction of N-centered Nucleophile with Pentachloropyridine 156
         3.1.2. Reaction of S-centered Nucleophile with Pentachloropyridine 172
         3.1.3. Reaction of C-centered Nucleophile with Perchloropyridines 184

3.2. Reaction of Perchloropyridines with Bidentate Nucleophiles 184
4. CROSS-COUPLING REACTIONS OF PERCHLOROPYRIDINES 192
5. BROMINATION OF PENTACHLOROPYRIDINE 195
6. OXIDATION OF POLYCHLOROPYRIDINES 196
7. REDUCTION OF POLYCHLOROPYRIDINES 200
8. ALKYLATION OF POLYCHLOROPYRIDINES 201
9. PHOTOCHEMICAL REACTIONS OF POLYCHLOROPYRIDINES 203
10. ORGANOMETALLIC REAGENTS OF PERCHLOROPYRIDINE 205
REFERENCES 210

CHAPTER 4 PERBROMOPYRIDINES 219
1. SYNTHESIS OF PENTABROMOPYRIDINE 219
2. NUCLEOPHILIC REACTIONS OF PENTABROMOPYRIDINE 220
2.1. Reaction of O-centered Nucleophile with Pentabromopyridine 220
2.2. Reaction of N-centered Nucleophile with Pentabromopyridine 221
2.3. Reaction of S-centered Nucleophile with Pentabromopyridine 225
3. ORGANOMETALIC REAGENT OF POLYBROMOPYRIDINES 228
4. SALTS OF PENTABROMOPYRIDINE 229
5. OXIDATION OF PENTABROMOPYRIDINE 229
6. PHOTOCHEMICAL REACTIONS OF PENTABROMOPYRIDINE 229
7. SYNTHESIS AND REACTIONS OF 2,4,6-TRIBROMO-3,5-DIFLUOROPYRIDINE 230
8. SYNTHESIS AND REACTIONS OF 3,5-DIBROMO-2,6-DICHLOROPYRIDINE 233
REFERENCES 234

SUBJECT INDEX 236

PREFACE

The heterocyclic ring is found in half of known compounds and most of these compounds have possessed an aromatic heterocyclic ring. Heteroaromatic compounds were found in a great number of metabolism products, pest-controlling agents, dyeing agents, flavors and commercial synthetic compounds such as drugs. Heterocyclic systems have broad applications especially in pharmaceutical chemistry and this accelerated the discovery and development of the chemistry of heterocycles. Heteroaromatic compounds have broad chemistry and numerous investigations have been carried out for synthetic methods of heteroaromatic derivatives to continuous development and applications of these systems. Perhalogenated pyridines are an attractive group of heteroaromatics that play an important role in organic chemistry, biochemistry, and pharmaceutical chemistry. These compounds have great interesting chemistry because of their reactivity toward nucleophilic attack. Therefore, they have become unique scaffolds for the construction of other heterocyclic and macrocyclic compounds. So far, there has been extensive research on perhalopyridine compounds. Some of the books published in the heterocyclic chemistry area have been cited for the synthesis, their reactions and their applications. For example, in "Fluorinated heterocyclic compounds: synthesis, chemistry, and applications" (Edited by Petrov, Viacheslav A. 2009), a brief summary of perfluoropyridine has been gathered or in "Pyridine and Its Derivatives" (Edited by R. A. Abramovitch 2009), some aspect about pentafluoro- and pentachloropyridine are briefly mentioned. Recently, we published a review article concerning "Utility of pentachloropyridine in organic synthesis" in the journal of the Iranian chemical society. In this book, we tried to focus on perhalopyridine including perfluoropyridine, perchloropyridine, perbromopyridine, so that readers can easily get to know the chemistry of these compounds. I would like to thank my coworker, Dr. Alireza Poorfreidoni, who helped me complete this book. I wish to thank those that reviewed the book and provided helpful suggestions. Finally, I have to thank my wife, Fatemeh SayyedBagheri, and my children, Javad, Mohadeseh, Ali, and Zahra, for putting up with me during manuscript preparation. I would also like to thank Bentham Science for the opportunity to publish this book. I have no conflicts of interest in relation to this book.

CONSENT FOR PUBLICATION

Not applicable.

CONFLICT OF INTEREST

The authors declare no conflict of interest, financial or otherwise.

ACKNOWLEDGEMENTS

Declared none.

Reza Ranjbar-Karimi
Department of Chemistry, Faculty of Science
Vali-e-Asr University of Rafsanjan
Islamic Republic of Iran

ii

FOREWORD

This book highlights all aspects of the synthetic reactions and various applications of perhalopyridines. Halogenated pyridines can be used as interesting starting materials in a wide range of organic synthesis and/or synthetic organic methodologies. Substituted pyridine compounds are used generally as starting materials in the nucleophilic substitution reactions. Also, they have important features of various medicinal agents. Due to synthetic difficulties in the synthesis of the highly substituted pyridine derivatives from pyridine itself, perhalopyridines have special importance in this regard. The author, Prof. Reza Ranjbar-Karimi, has attracted many outstanding contributions to emphasize regio- and chemoselectivity of perhalopyridines toward various nucleophiles. I think that this book will be a very valuable source of information for every chemist in the area of heterocyclic chemistry and a useful document in the area of synthetic/medicinal chemistry.

Mohammad Ali Zolfigol
Bu-Ali Sina University
Hamadan
Iran

Abbreviations

1,4-CHD 1,4-Cyclohexadiene

AChE Acetylcholinesterase

AE Addition-Elimination

ANRORC Addition of the Nucleophile, Ring Opening, and Ring Closure

BDC Benzodichalcogenophene

BINOL 1,1′-Binaphthyl-2,2′-diol

COD 1,5-Cyclooctadiene

Cp Cyclopentadienyl

DBU 1,8-Diazabicyclo[5.4. 0]undec-7-ene

DCE 1,2-Dichlroethane

DIBAL Diisobutylaluminium Hydride

DIPEA Diisopropylethylamine

DLP Lauroyl Peroxide

DMAD Dimethyl Acetylenedicarboxylate

DMEU 1,3-dimethyl-2-imidazolidinone

DMF N,N-Dimethylformamide

DMI 1,3-dimethylimidazolidin-2-one

DMSO Dimethyl Sulfoxide

DNA Deoxyribonucleic Acid

DPPA Diphenyl Phosphorazidate

EA Elimination-Addition

HDF Hydrodefluorination

HOMO Highest Occupied Molecular Orbital

LDA Lithium diisopropylamide

MAs Meldrum's Acids

NHCs N-heterocyclic Carbenes

OLEDs Organic Light-Emitting Diodes

PET Photoinduced Electron Transfer

PFC Perfluorocarbone

$S_{RN}1$ Unimolecular Radical Nucleophilic Substitution

TBHS Tetrabutylammonium hydrogen sulfate

TFA Trifluoroacetic Acid

TFAA Trifluoroacetic Anhydride THF: Tetrahydrofuran

TMG 1,1,3,3-Tetramethylguanidine

TMSCl Trimethylsilyl chloride

Vis/NIR Visible/Near Infra-Red

CHAPTER 1

Properties of Perhalopyridines

Abstract: The introduction of halogen atoms on the pyridine ring causes significant changes in its properties. Halogens reduced basicity of pyridine ring as well as dipole moment. The presence of dense halogen atoms renders a higher density of perhalopyridines than pyridine. Fluorine atoms cause a low-field shift of pyridine carbons than chlorine and bromine atoms. Perhalopyridines are mainly involved in nucleophilic substitution reactions due to the electron-withdrawing nature of halogens while perfluoropyridines are more active than others.

Keywords: ^{13}C-NMR spectrum, ^{19}F-NMR spectrum, Activating Effect, Addition-Elimination Mechanism, Basicity, Chemical Shifts, Density, Dipole Moment, Intermolecular Forces, IR spectrum, Meisenheimer Intermediate, Nucleophilic Substitution, Pentabromopyridine, Pentachloropyridine, Pentafluoropyridine, Raman Analysis, Shielding Effect, Spectroscopy, Steric Factors, UV-Vis Spectrum.

1. PHYSICAL AND CHEMICAL PROPERTIES

Pentafluoropyridine is a colorless, mobile and almost odorless liquid with boiling point 83-84 °C. Replacement of a C-F group by N in fluorocarbons has little effect on the boiling point (C_6F_6 has b. p. 81 °C) [1]. The boiling point pentafluoropyridine is lower than the corresponding hydrocarbon (pyridine; bp 115 °C), and this attributed to the much lower intermolecular forces and the very low basicity of pentafluoropyridine. Fluorine atoms ortho to ring nitrogen have a major influence on low basicity of the system and superacids are required to protonate pentafluoropyridine [1, 2]. Its reaction with hydrogen chloride not converted to hydrochloride form, but react with hot aqueous solution of sodium hydroxide and formed 2,3,5,6-tetrafluoro-4-hydroxypyridine in 58% yield. 40% aqueous solution of sodium hydroxide converted completely pentafluoropyridine to ammonia, carbonate, fluoride ions and 3,5,6-trifluoro-2,4-dihydroxypyridine (20% yield) in 12 h [3]. Replacement of C-F groups by C-Cl in leaded to increasing intramolecular forces and basicity of system, thus pentachloropyridine has more intermolecular forces and basicity in comparison with pentafluoro-pyridine [4, 5]. It is methylated by methyl fluorosulphonate and give the

Reza Ranjbar-Karimi & Alireza Poorfreidoni

corresponding *N*-methylpyridinium fluorosulphonate [6]. Also, it converted to tetrachloro-2-hydroxypyridine on treatment with a mixture of acetic acid and concentrated sulphuric acid [6]. Similar to pentachloropyridine, pentabromo-pyridine methylated on treatment with methyl fluorosulphonate [7].

The dipole moment (μ) of pentafluoropyridine is 1.26 D [8, 9], which is lower than pyridine (2.24 D [8], 2.26 D [9]). Fluorine atoms on pyridine ring (especially para fluorine) have major effect on decreasing dipole moment of pyridine. Also, it has lower dipole moment than pentachloropyridine (1.53 D) and pentabromo-pyridine (2.01 D) due to lower electron affinity of Cl and Br atoms than F atom [8]. Presence of five dense fluorine atoms on pentafluoropyridine render more density of system (1.540 g/cm^3) than pyridine (0.987 g/cm^3) (Fig. **1-1**) [9].

Fig. (1-1). Dipole moment values of pyridine and pentahalpoyridines.

2. SPECTROSCOPY

Aromatic character of pentafluoropyridine has been shown by its spectroscopy properties. IR and Raman analysis confirmed plannering of pentafluoropyridine. IR spectrum of pentafluoropyridine has been shown strong bands at 980, 1075 and 1081 cm^{-1} attributed to stretching vibrations of C-F bonds and three strong bands at 1497, 1529, 1645 cm^{-1} for pyridine ring. UV-Vis spectrum of pentafluoro-pyridine has been shown a type B absorption band at 256 μm [3]. In ^{19}F-NMR spectrum of pentafluoropyridine, the resonances of the *ortho, meta* and *para* fluorines located at δ = -86.72, -160.1 and -132.82 ppm, respectively [10]. In ^{13}C-NMR spectroscopy, carbons of pentafluoropyridine appear to multiplets because of the presence of fluorine atoms. In ^{13}C-NMR spectrum (CDCl$_3$, 22.635 MHz) of pentafluoropyridine, C$_{(3,5)}$, C$_{(2,6)}$ and C$_{(4)}$ appeared at δ = 134.3, 144.8 and 150.3 ppm, respectively [10]. A comparison of chemical shifts of pentachloropyridine carbons with that for pentafluoropyridine indicates that the chlorine atom at 2-position lead to a low-field shift, while at 3- and 4-positions has a shielding effect (Table **1-1**) [10]. In contrast with chlorine atom, bromine atom at 2-position has shielding effect as well as 3- and 4-positions in comparison between pentabromopyridine and pentafluoropyridine (Table **1-1**) [11].

Table 1-1. Spectroscopic properties of pentahalopyridines.

^{13}C-NMR	$C_{2,6}$	$C_{3,5}$	C_4
$C_5F_5N^a$	144.8	134.3	150.3
$C_5Cl_5N^a$	146.8^a	129.9	144.9
$C_5Br_5N^b$	141.2	127^b	140.4^b

[a] 22.635 MHz, CDCl$_3$
[b] 75 MHz, DMSO-d$_6$

3. REACTIONS

Pentahalopyridines and their derivatives are very active toward aromatic nucleophilic substitution reactions due to presence of halogen atoms on pyridine ring and their nucleophilic substitution reactions have been used widely in organic synthesis. Substitution reactions carried out *via* various mechanisms. Aromatic nucleophilic substitution reactions proceed frequently *via* two steps addition-elimination mechanism (AE mechanism) [12 - 14]; but, EA [15 - 17], SN (ANRORC) [18], $S_{RN}1$ [19 - 21] mechanisms are also observed. 3-position of pyridine ring is inert toward nucleophilic attack, unless, elimination-addition mechanism acts by amide ions or metallic catalysts [22]. In general, 2- and 4-positions of pyridine ring are most activated sites toward nucleophilic attack due to the stabilizing influence of the ring nitrogen atom in the transition state [23 - 25]. Nucleophilic substitution reactions in these systems followed from bimolecular addition-elimination mechanism *via* meisenheimer intermediate (Scheme **1-1**) [26, 27].

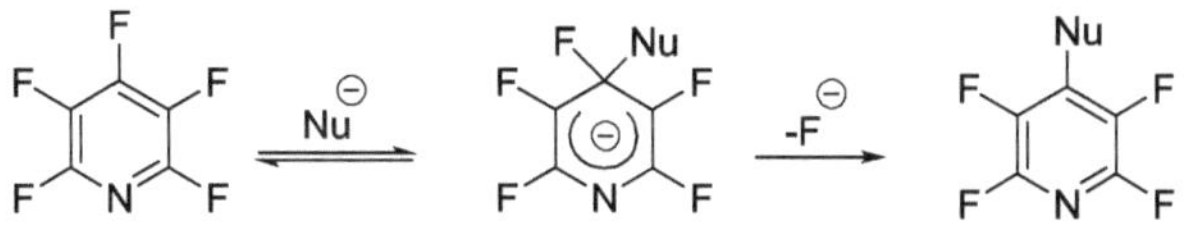

Scheme 1-1. Meisenheimer intermediate in pentafluoropyridine **2**.

A comparison between these compounds, pentafluoropyridine **2** is more activated system than pentachloropyridine **3** and pentabromopyridine **4** in nucleophilic substitution reactions because of high activating effect of fluorine atom than chlorine and bromine atoms. Furthermore, order reactivity toward nucleophilic attack in pentafluoropyridine is 4 > 2 >> 3 (Scheme **1-2**) [28 - 30], while it for pentachloropyridine is changed depending on nature of solvent and nucleophile

[31, 32]. Pentachloropyridine **3** reacted with nucleophiles at both 2- and 4-position of pyridine. Heron, steric factors are important. The large nucleophiles gave more ratio of substitution at 2-position because of less steric hindrance at 2-position than 4-position (Scheme **1-3**) [33]. Similarly, pentabromopyridine **4** with large nucleophiles reacted at 2-position and with small nucleophiles reacted at 4-position (Scheme **1-4**) [34].

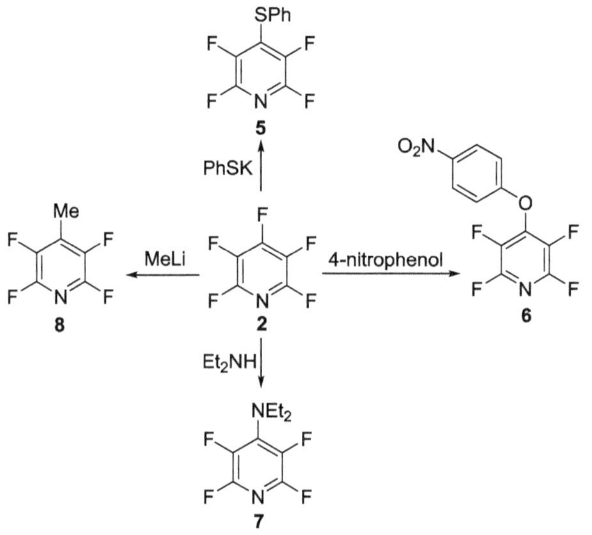

Scheme 1-2. Reaction of *N*-, *S*-, *O*- and *C*-centered nucleophiles with pentafluoropyridine **2**.

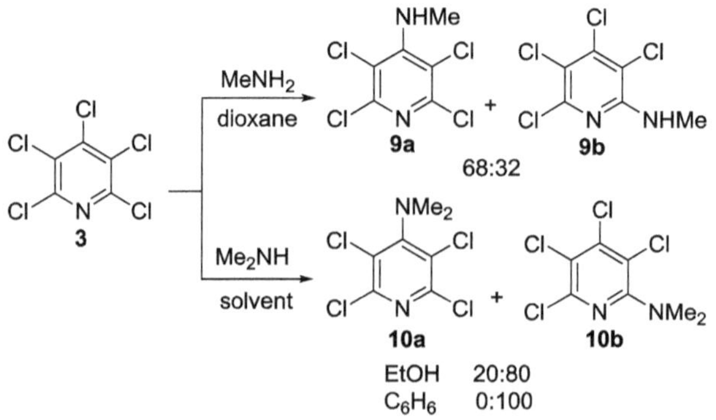

Scheme 1-3. Dependence of pentachloropyridine reactions to reaction condition.

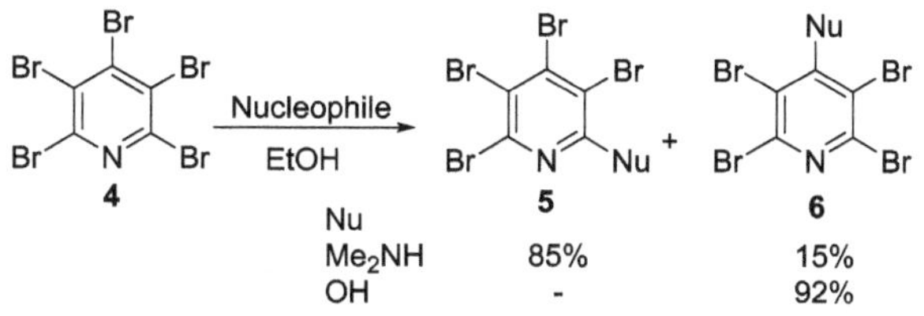

Nu	5	6
Me$_2$NH	85%	15%
OH	-	92%

Scheme 1-4. Dependence of pentabromopyridine reactions to reaction condition.

REFERENCES

[1] Banks, R.E.; Ginsberg, A.E.; Haszeldine, R.N. *338. Heterocyclic polyfluoro-compounds. Part I. Pentafluoropyridine. Journal of the Chemical Society*; Resumed, **1961**, pp. 1740-1743.

[2] Burdon, J.; Gilman, D.J.; Patrick, C.R.; Stacey, M.; Tatlow, J.C. Pentafluoropyridine. *Nature,* **1960**, *186*, 231.
[http://dx.doi.org/10.1038/186231a0]

[3] Banks, R. E.; Burgess, J. E.; Cheng, W. M.; Haszeldine, R. N. Heterocyclic polyfluoro-compounds. Part IV. Nucleophilic substitution in pentafluoropyridine: the preparation and properties of some 4-substituted 2,3,5,6-tetrafluoropyridines. *Journal of the Chemical Society (Resumed),* **1965**, *1*(0), 575-581.

[4] den Hertog, H.J.; Schogt, J.C.M.; de Bruyn, J.; de Klerk, A. The chloropyridines. *Recl. Trav. Chim. Pays Bas,* **1950**, *69*(6), 673-699.
[http://dx.doi.org/10.1002/recl.19500690604]

[5] Joshi, A.V.; Baidossi, M.; Qafisheh, N.; Chachashvili, E.; Sasson, Y. Mild electrophilic halogenation of chloropyridines using CCl4 or C2Cl6 under basic phase transfer conditions. *Tetrahedron Lett.,* **2004**, *45*(26), 5061-5063.
[http://dx.doi.org/10.1016/j.tetlet.2004.04.177]

[6] Suschitzky, H., Ed. *Polychloroaromatic compounds*; Plenum Press: London, New York, **1974**.

[7] Ager, E.; Suschitzky, H. Reactions of polyhalogenopyridines with methyl fluorosulphonate. *J. Fluor. Chem.,* **1973**, *3*(2), 230-232.
[http://dx.doi.org/10.1016/S0022-1139(00)84167-6]

[8] Kisilenko, A.A.; Zeikan', A.A.; Vdovenko, S.I.; Kukhar', V.P. Calculation of the electronic structure and dipole moments of 4-substituted tetrabromopyridines. *Chem. Heterocycl. Compd.,* **1981**, *17*(7), 684-689.
[http://dx.doi.org/10.1007/BF00506036]

[9] Xu, S.; Jonas, J. 13C NMR Relaxation Studies of Pyridine and Pentafluoropyridine Liquids Confined to Nanopores of Porous Silica Glasses. *J. Phys. Chem.,* **1996**, *100*(40), 16242-16246.
[http://dx.doi.org/10.1021/jp960769r]

[10] Chambers, R.D.; Matthews, R.S.; Kenneth, W.; Musgrave, R.; Urben, P.G. Polyhaloheterocyclic compounds. Part XXXI—carbon-13 NMR spectra as a structural probe for polychloroaromatic compounds. *Org. Magnet. Reson.,* **1980**, *13*(5), 363-367.
[http://dx.doi.org/10.1002/mrc.1270130514]

[11] Pomarański, P.; Roszkowski, P.; Maurin, J.K.; Budzianowski, A.; Czarnocki, Z. Convenient synthesis of selected meta- and ortho-substituted pentaarylpyridines *via* the Suzuki-Miyaura cross-coupling

reaction. *Tetrahedron Lett.,* **2017**, *58*(5), 462-465.
[http://dx.doi.org/10.1016/j.tetlet.2016.12.064]

[12]   Weissberger, A. E. C. T., The Chemistry of Heterocyclic Compounds. *Pyridine and its Derivatives,* 4th
ed; Wiley-Interscience: New York, **1974/1975**, Vol. 14, .

[13]   Spitzner, D. *Methoden der Organischen Chemie*; Thieme: Stuttgart, Germany, **1994**, E7b, .

[14]   Spitzner, D. Product Class 1: Pyridines.*Six-Membered Hetarenes with One Nitrogen or Phosphorus Atom*; Thieme: Stuttgart, Germany, **2004**, Vol. 15, .

[15]   Hoffmann, R.W. *Dehydrobenzene and Cycloalkynes*; Verlag Chemie: Weinheim, **1967**.

[16]   Kauffmann, T.; Wirthwein, R. Fortschritte auf dem Hetarin-Gebiet. *Angew. Chem.,* **1971**, *83*(1), 21-34.
[http://dx.doi.org/10.1002/ange.19710830104]

[17]   Reinecke, M.G. Hetarynes. *Tetrahedron,* **1982**, *38*(4), 427-498.
[http://dx.doi.org/10.1016/0040-4020(82)80092-6]

[18]   De Bie, D.A.; Geurtsen, B.; Berg, I.E.; Van der Plas, H.C. A mechanistic study on the amination of 2-chloro-3, 5-dinitropyridine with liquid ammonia. *J. Org. Chem.,* **1986**, *51*(16), 3209-3211.
[http://dx.doi.org/10.1021/jo00366a027]

[19]   McGill, C.K.; Rappa, A. Advances in the Chichibabin Reaction.*Adv. Heterocycl. Chem*; Katritzky, A.R., Ed.; Academic Press, **1988**, Vol. 44, pp. 1-79.

[20]   Boy, P.; Combellas, C.; Thiebault, A. Synthesis of 4-(Trifluoromethylpyridyl) phenol Derivatives. *Synlett,* **1991**, *1991*(12), 923-924.
[http://dx.doi.org/10.1055/s-1991-20925]

[21]   Beugelmans, R.; Chastanet, J. SRN1 reactions of chlorotrifluoromethyl pyridines with naphtholate, phenolate and malonate anions. *Tetrahedron,* **1993**, *49*(36), 7883-7890.
[http://dx.doi.org/10.1016/S0040-4020(01)88013-3]

[22]   Schmidt, A.; Mordhorst, T.; Nieger, M. Heteroarenium salts in synthesis. Highly functionalized tetra- and pentasubstituted pyridines. *Tetrahedron,* **2006**, *62*(8), 1667-1674.
[http://dx.doi.org/10.1016/j.tet.2005.11.065]

[23]   Smart, B.E. Fluorine substituent effects (on bioactivity). *J. Fluor. Chem.,* **2001**, *109*(1), 3-11.
[http://dx.doi.org/10.1016/S0022-1139(01)00375-X]

[24]   Halpern, D.F. *G. G. V., Chemistry of Organic Fluorine Compounds II*; American Chemical Society: Washington, **1995**.

[25]   Welch, J.T. Tetrahedron report number 221: Advances in the preparation of biologically active organofluorine compounds. *Tetrahedron,* **1987**, *43*(14), 3123-3197.
[http://dx.doi.org/10.1016/S0040-4020(01)90286-8]

[26]   Brooke, G.M. The preparation and properties of polyfluoro aromatic and heteroaromatic compounds. *J. Fluor. Chem.,* **1997**, *86*(1), 1-76.
[http://dx.doi.org/10.1016/S0022-1139(97)00006-7]

[27]   Chambers, R.D.; Sargent, C.R. Polyfluoroheteroaromatic Compounds. *Adv. Heterocycl. Chem*; Katritzky, A.R.; Boulton, A.J., Eds.; Academic Press, **1981**, Vol. 28, pp. 1-71.

[28]   Cartwright, M.W.; Sandford, G.; Bousbaa, J.; Yufit, D.S.; Howard, J.A.; Christopher, J.A.; Miller, D.D. Imidazopyridine and pyrimidinopyridine systems from perfluorinated pyridine derivatives. *Tetrahedron,* **2007**, *63*(30), 7027-7035.
[http://dx.doi.org/10.1016/j.tet.2007.05.016]

[29]   Sandford, G.; Slater, R.; Yufit, D.S.; Howard, J.A.; Vong, A. Tetrahydropyrido[3,4-b]pyrazine scaffolds from pentafluoropyridine. *J. Org. Chem.,* **2005**, *70*(18), 7208-7216.
[http://dx.doi.org/10.1021/jo0508696] [PMID: 16122239]

[30] Sandford, G.; Slater, R.; Yufit, D.S.; Howard, J.A.; Vong, A. Pyrido [3, 2-b][1, 4] oxazine and pyrido [2, 3-b][1, 4] benzoxazine systems from tetrafluoropyridine derivatives. *J. Fluor. Chem.*, **2014**, *167*, 91-95.
[http://dx.doi.org/10.1016/j.jfluchem.2014.05.003]

[31] Roberts, S.; Suschitzky, H. Nucleophilic reactions of pentachloropyridine 1-oxide and pentachloropyrine. *Chem. Commun. (Camb.)*, **1967**, (17), 893-894.

[32] Roberts, S.; Suschitzky, H. Polychloroaromatic compounds. Part I. Oxidation of pentachloropyridine and its NN-disubstituted amino-derivatives with peroxyacids. *J. Chem. Soc. C: Organ.*, **1968**, 1537-1541.

[33] Flowers, W.T.; Haszeldine, R.N.; Majid, S.A. Synthesis and reactions of pentachloropyridine. *Tetrahedron Lett.*, **1967**, *8*(26), 2503-2505.
[http://dx.doi.org/10.1016/S0040-4039(00)90842-6]

[34] Collins, I.; Suschitzky, H. Polyhalogeno-aromatic compounds. Part XIV. Nucleophilic substitution and peroxy-acid oxidation of pentabromopyridine and some of its NN-dialkylamino- and bis-(NN-dialkylamino)-derivatives. *J. Chem. Soc. C: Organ.*, **1970**, *1*(11), 1523-1530.

CHAPTER 2

Perfluoropyridines

Abstract: Fluorine atom has unique properties and has a great interest in organic chemistry and pharmaceuticals. Insertion of fluorine atoms on pyridines induces significant properties to the pyridine ring. The introduction of fluorine atoms on pyridine is carried out by the fluorination of pyridine or pentachloropyridine. The withdrawing nature of these atoms is mainly responsible for the high reactivity of perfluoropyridines toward nucleophilic attack. Therefore, perfluoropyridines are a significant starting material for the synthesis of other substituted pyridines, ring-fused systems as well as macrocyclic compounds *via* reaction with various monodentate and bidentate nucleophiles, whereas the nature of nucleophile, reaction condition, and solvent have a basic role in the regiochemistry of the reactions. Furthermore, these compounds could participate in organometallic reactions by the reaction of halogen atom with metals and organometallic reagents. Additionally, they underwent hydrodefluorination in photochemical reactions in the presence of catalysts.

Keywords: Bidentate Nucleophile, Continuous Flow Processes, Copolymers, Hard–Hard Interaction Principle, Hydrodefluorination, Macrocycle, Medicinal Chemistry, Meisenheimer Intermediate, Monodentate Nucleophile, *N*-Methylated Pyridinium, Nucleophilic Substitution, Organometallic Perfluoroheteroaromatics, Pentafluoropyridine, Pentafluoropyridine Cation, Photochemical Reaction, Polyhaloheterocyls, Radical Addition, Regioselectivity, Ring-Fused, Tetrafluoropyridine.

1. INTRODUCTION

Chemistry of fluorinated heterocyclic compounds is rapidly progressing. In the last decade, checking of fluorine chemistry international conferences has shown close to 40 percent of presented papers containing heterocyclic compounds due to high and diverse biological activity of fluorinated heterocyclic compounds. Also, fluorinated heterocyclic systems used in dielectrics, liquid crystals, High temperature lubricants, complexones and extragents. About 10% of the total commercial drugs currently used for the medical treatment are containing fluorine atom. Over 50 years, large number fluorinated medicinal and agrochemical compounds have been discovered and attracted considerable interest toward development of fluorinated compounds have been existed. The strong interest to

Reza Ranjbar-Karimi & Alireza Poorfreidoni

fluorinated systems arose from unique biological properties of fluorine. Also, development fluorine chemistry fluorination technology accelerated due to availability of the fluorinated synthetic blocks, the broadly reliable fluorination technology, the effective fluorinating reagents [1].

2. SYNTHESIS OF PENTAFLUOROPYRIDINE

For first time, pentafluoropyridine **3** was prepared in low yield from electrochemical fluorination of pyridine **1** and following elimination of fluorine (Scheme **2-1**) [2].

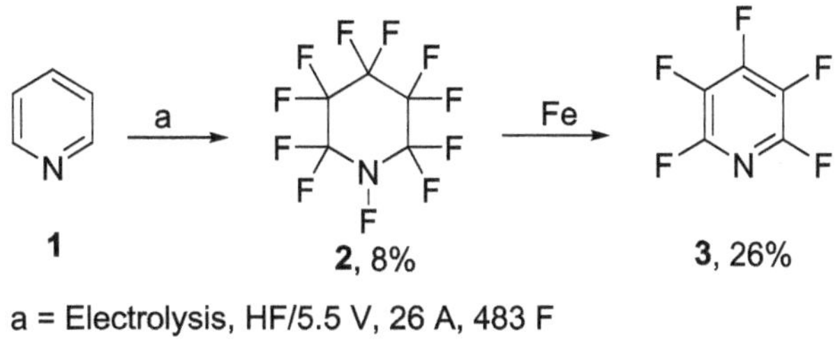

Scheme 2-1. Synthesis of pentafluoropyridine **3** by electrochemical methods.

Standard method for synthesis of pentafluoropyridine **3** is halogen exchange of perchlorinated systems with KF in autoclave at high temperature (Scheme **2-2**) [3].

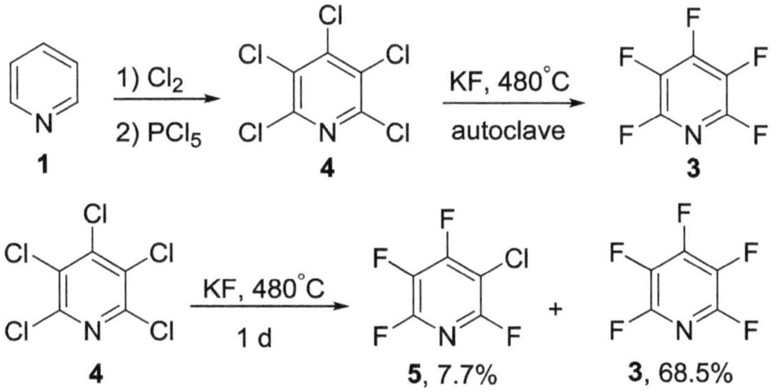

Scheme 2-2. Synthesis of pentafluoropyridine **3** by halogen exchange method.

Fluorination of pyridine over caesium tetrafluorocobaltate (III) at 300-400°C gave pentafluoropyridine **3** and a mixture of other products (Scheme **2-3**) [4].

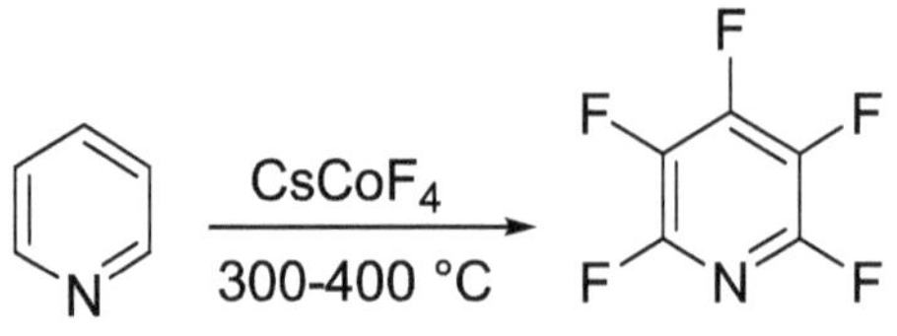

Scheme 2-3. Synthesis of pentafluoropyridine **3** by direct fluorination of pyridine.

3. REACTION MECHANISM

Pyridine is not very active aromatic electrophilic substitution, but active toward nucleophilic attack [5]. Density of electronic cloud in pyridine follows the sequence 4 > 2 > 3; therefore, it is expect to follow order reactivity 4 > 2 >> 3 toward nucleophilic attack [6]. Nucleophilic substitution reactions in *N*-heterocyclic systems followed from bimolecular addition-elimination mechanism *via* meisenheimer intermediate (Scheme **2-4**) [7, 8]. Nevertheless, some reactions carried out *via* elimination-addition mechanism when starting materials are inactive and nucleophile is very basic [9, 10].

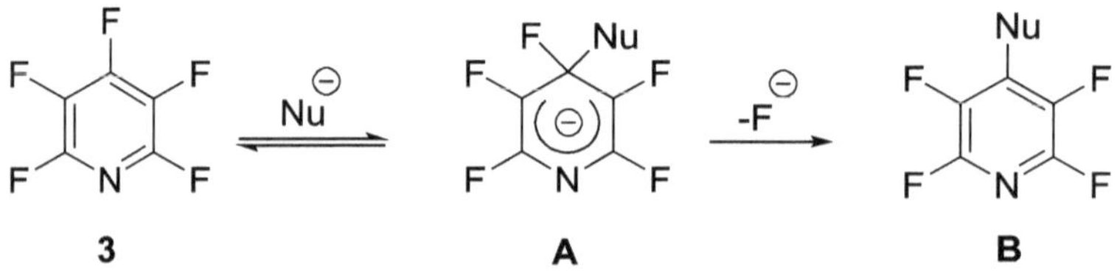

Scheme 2-4. Addition nucleophile mechanism to pentafluoropyridine **3**.

Polyhaloheterocyls are more active systems than corresponding benzoied compounds toward aromatic nucleophilic substitution. Activating effect of aza group is similar to nitro group effect in aromatic systems and active *ortho* and *para* positions [9, 11]. Halogen substitution act as a good activating group because of the effect of electron induced withdrawing as well as a good leaving group. Polychloro- and polyfluoroaromatic compounds become easily undergo nucleophilic substitution reactions toward various nucleophiles [12 - 14].

Chemistry of pentafluoropyridine affected by reaction with nucleophile species due to presence of electronegative atoms of fluorine that activate the ring toward nucleophilic attack. Ring nitrogen have dominant effect on activation of *ortho* and *para* positions because of stabilizing negative charge produced in intermediate. Also, fluorine atom has important role on regioselectivity of nucleophilic substitution. Fluorine atoms located at *ortho* and *meta* positions of attacking situation hav high activating effect while *para* fluorine atom has inactivating effect. Inactivating effect of *para* fluorine has been explained by stabling carbanion. In planner carbanions such as meisenheimer intermediate have been existed maximum repulsion between free couple electron on fluorine atom and negative charge, therefore generally is inactivating. *Meta* fluorine atoms stabilized negative charge by using inductive effect. It is expected *meta* fluorine atoms act similar to *para* fluorine atom if carbanion stability considered, but this has been experimentally violated by kinetic measurements, heron electron density of C-F bond is more reduced by induced withdrawing effect (Fig. **2-1**) [1].

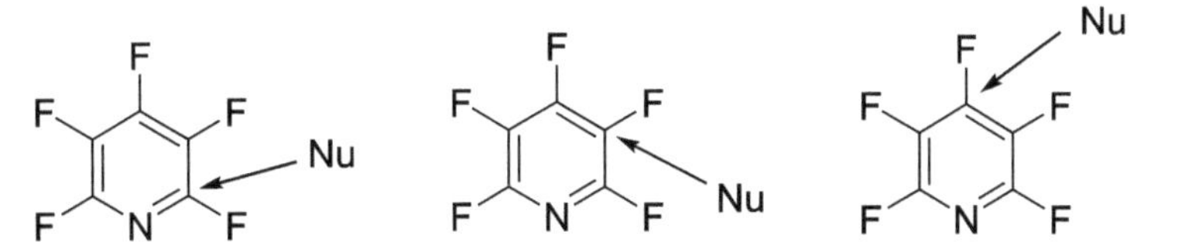

Fig. (2-1). Effects of fluorine and nitrogen atoms on aromatic nucleophilic substitution precess.

Therefore, reaction of pentafluoropyridine **3** with nucleophiles carried out regioselectivity at 4-position of pyridine ring [7, 8]. Nevertheless, keto-oxime salts had high ratio of substitution at 2–position of pyridine ring due to leading effect of complex formed between ring nitrogen and salt (Scheme **2-5**) [15].

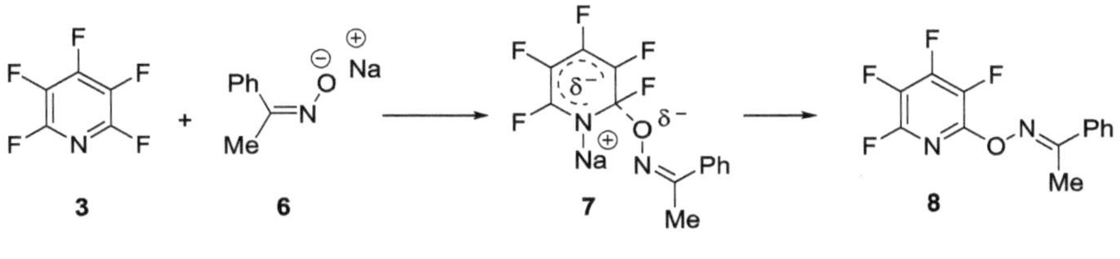

Scheme 2-5. Reaction of keto-oxime with pentafluoropyridine **3**.

4. REACTION OF PENTAFLUOROPYRIDINE WITH VARIOUS MONO DENTATE NUCLEOPHILES

Formation of monosubstituted fluoropyridine derivatives carried out *via* nucleophilic replacement of fluorine atom by various nucleophiles. Chambers and co-workers in 1964 and banks *et al.* in 1965 have reported synthesis of some 4-substituted tetrafluoropyridines by using nucleophilic substitution on pentafluoropyridine (Scheme **2-6**) [16, 17].

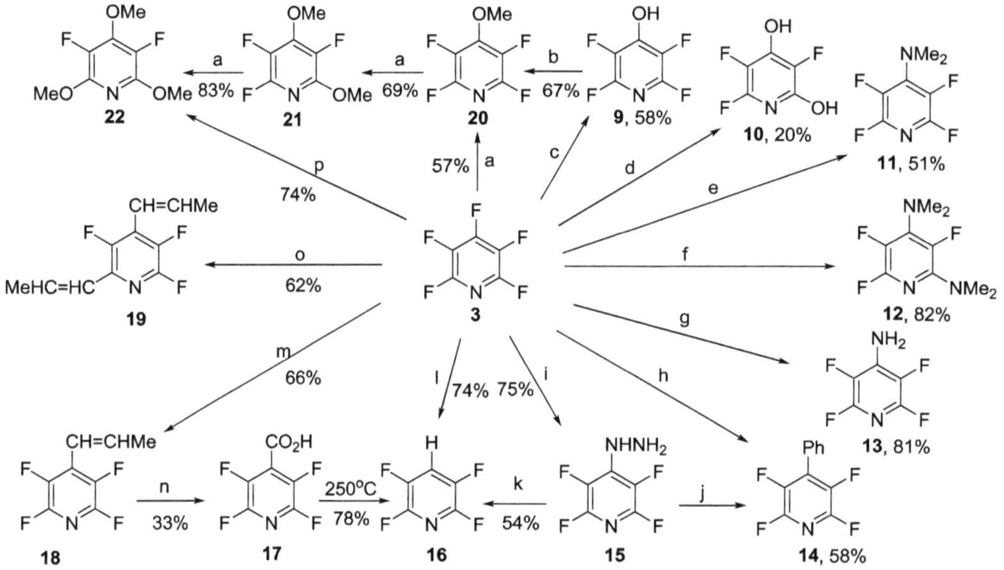

a) NaOMe; b) CH_2N_2; c) aq. NaOH; d) 40% NaOH; e) Me_2NH; f) excess of Me_2NH; g) NH_3; h) PhLi, Et_2O; i) N_2H_2; j) C_6H_6-$CaCl_2$; k) aq.$CuSO_4$; l) $LiAlH_4$; m) MeCH=CHLi; n) HNO_3; o) excess of MeCH=CHLi; p) excess of NaOMe

Scheme 2-6. Reaction of pentafluoropyridine **3** with various necleophiles.

4.1. Reaction of S-centered Nucleophile with Pentafluoropyridine

Reaction of sulfur nucleophiles with pentafluoropyridine **3** has been carried out dominantly at 4-position of pyridine ring (Scheme **2-7**). There is no to attack of oxygen in reaction of SO_3^{2-} and $PhSO_2^-$ with pentafluoropyridine [18].

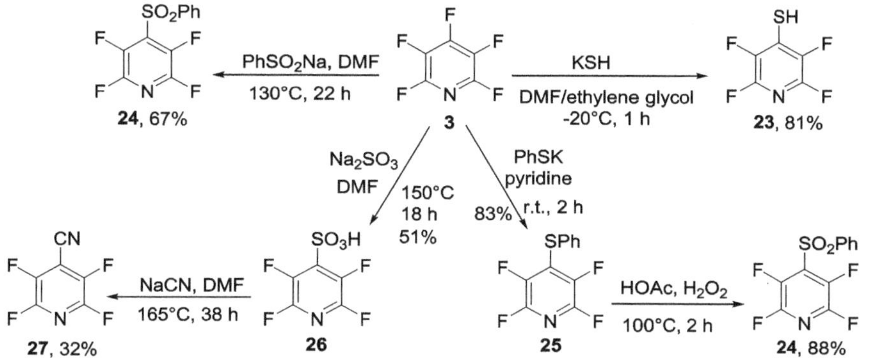

Scheme 2-7. Reaction of pentafluoropyridine **3** with sulfur nucleophiles.

Tetrafluoropyridine-4-thiol **23** can be acts as nucleophile and attacks electrophilic species (Scheme **2-8**) [18].

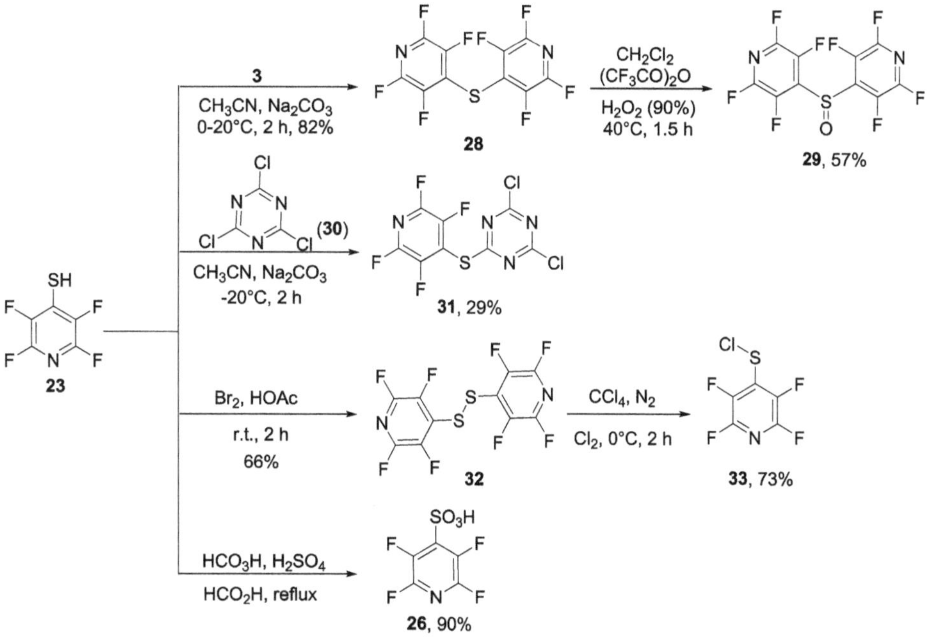

Scheme 2-8. Reactions of tetrafluoropyridine-4-thiol **23**.

Perfluoroalkylation of compounds **23** has been carried out in the presence of bisperfluoroalkyl carboxylates of divalent xenon (Scheme **2-9**) [19].

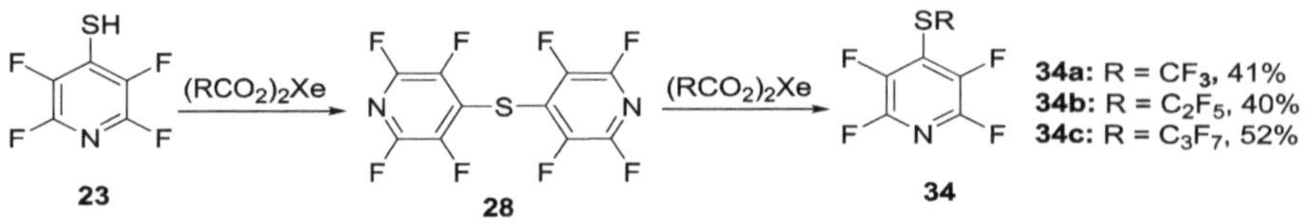

Scheme 2-9. Synthesis of 4-(perfluoroalkylthio)tetrafluoropyridines **24**.

It has been specified that pentafluoroalkylthio group is more resistant than corresponding perchloropyridine toward replacement. Fluorine of 2-position replaced in the presence of *N* and *O*-centered nucleophiles with maintaining of pentafluoroalkylthio group (Scheme **2-10**) [19, 20].

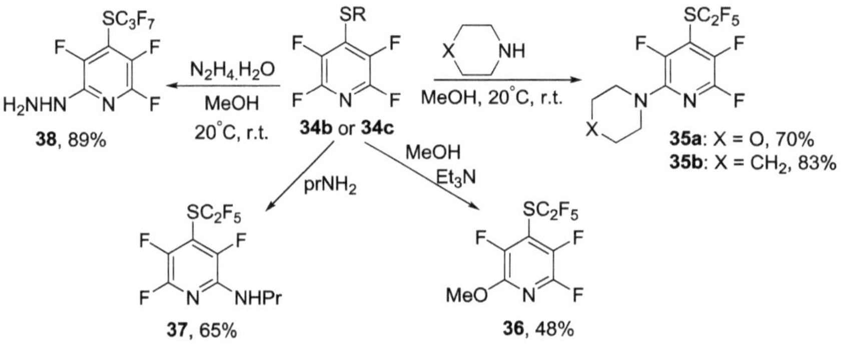

Scheme 2-10. Reactions of 4-thioalkyltetrafluoropyridines **34b,c**.

Compound **34b** tolerated complex conversions in methanolic solution [19]. Formation of **36**, **39**, **40** and **41** takes placed with replacement of methoxy and methanethiolate groups while formation of **42**, **43** and **44** have been explained by complex replacement and oxidation-reduction process (Scheme **2-11**).

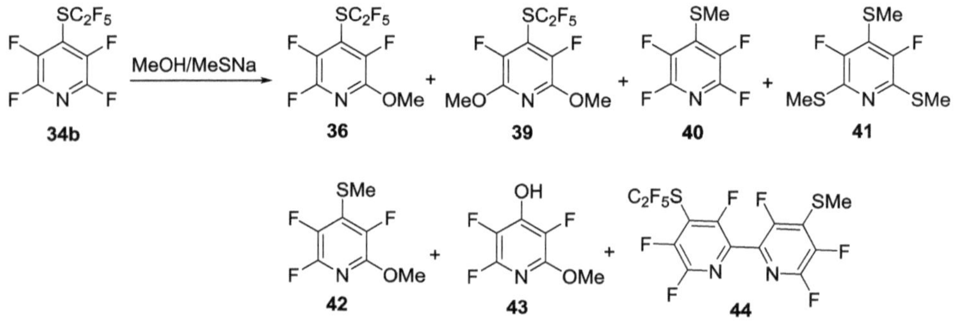

Scheme 2-11. Reaction of **34b** with methanolic solution of sodium methanethiolate.

Tetrafluoropyridine-substituted dithiocarbamic acid ester **47** has been successfully synthesized *via* one–pot two–step sequential reaction of dibenzylamine, carbon disulfide and pentafluoropyridine (Scheme **2-12**) [21].

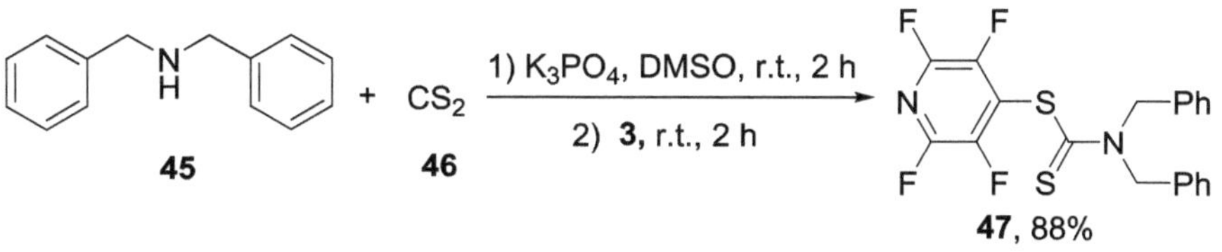

Scheme 2-12. synthesis of perfluoropyridin-4-yl dibenzylcarbamodithioate **47**.

Persulfurated aromatics are very interesting compounds in chemistry due to their attractive physical organic properties [22]. Persulfurated nitrogen-heteroaromatics are rare, for instance, MacNicol and co-workers [23] have reported persulfuration of pentafluoropyridine. Pentakis(isopropylthio)- and pentakis(methylthio)-pyridine were prepared on the reaction of pentafluoropyridine with excess sodium isopropanethiolate and methanethiolate, respectively (Scheme **2-13**). Another study has described preparations of pentakis((arylthio)pyridines **49a** and **49b** and from reaction of arylthiolates and pentafluoropyridine in 1,3-dimethylimidazolidin-2-one (DMI) at room temperature and evaluated in clathrate formation [24] and in electroreduction [25], Also, benzothienopyridines **50a** and **50b** were obtained as side products (Scheme **2-14**) [24].

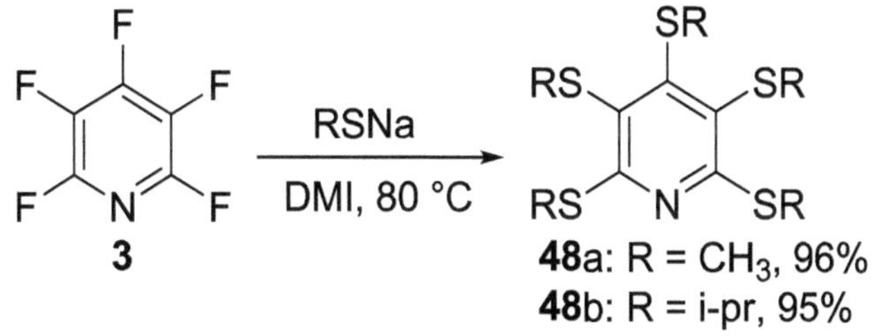

Scheme 2-13. Synthesis of persulfurated pyridine derivatives **48**.

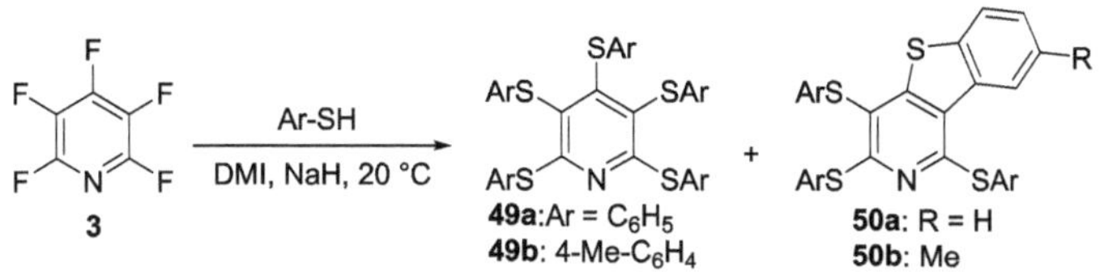

Scheme 2-14. Reaction of arylthiolates **49** with pentafluoropyridine **3**.

Pentafluoropyridine **3** has been reacted with excess PhSNa in the presence of 1,3-dimethyl-2-imidazolidinone (DMEU) as solvent and produced pentakis (phenylthio)pyridine in near near quantitative yield (Scheme **2-15**) [24].

excess PhSNa
DMEU, r.t., 6 d
3
49a, 100%

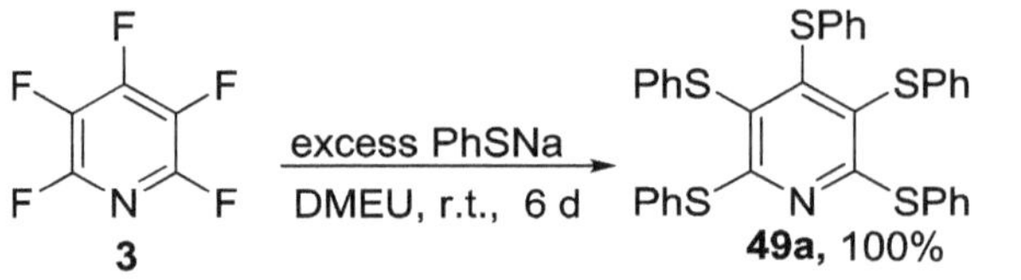

Scheme 2-15. Synthesis of pentakis(phenylthio)pyridine **49a**.

CF_3S^- anion, generated from reaction of CsF with $(CF_3S)_2C{=}S$, has been reacted successfully with pentafluoropyridine **3** and gave 2,3,5,6-tetrafluoro-4-trifluoromethylthiopyridine **34a** arising replacement at 4-position of pyridine ring (Scheme **2-16**) [26]. This compound on reaction with CF_3S^- anion produced 2,4,6-trimethoxy-3,5-bis(trifluoromethylthio)pyridine **52** and mixture of other products (Scheme **2-17**). The reaction of compound **34a** with potassium thiophenolate and potassium phenolate led to a substitution of fluorines and the CF_3S group with the PhS or PhO substituents (Scheme **2-17**). Oxidation of **34a** with CrO_3/H_2SO_4 gave corresponding sulphonyl **57** (Scheme **2-17**).

CsF, CH3CN
-15 °C
3
51
34a, 73%

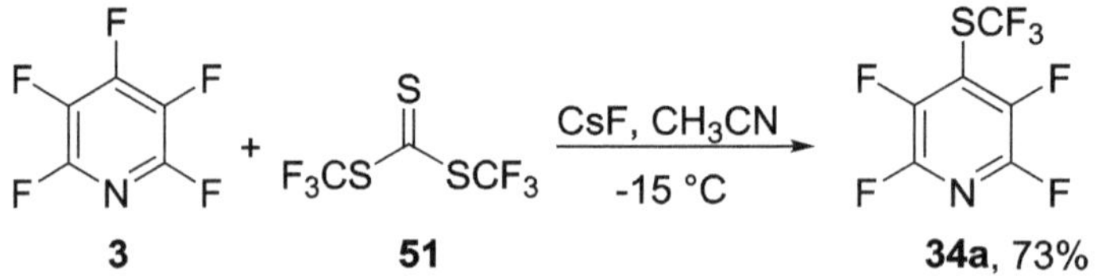

Scheme 2-16. Synthesis of 2,3,5,6-tetrafluoro-4-trifluoromethylthiopyridine **34a**.

57, 80%
52, 66%
34a
56
55
54
25, 39%
53
overall yield 77% with ratio 56:55:54, 90:5:5
a) (CF3S)2C=S, CsF, sulpholane, 108 °C, 36 h; b) PhSK, CH3CN, r.t., 15 min; c) PhOK, CH3CN, r.t.; d) CrO3, H2SO4, 30 °C, 30 min.

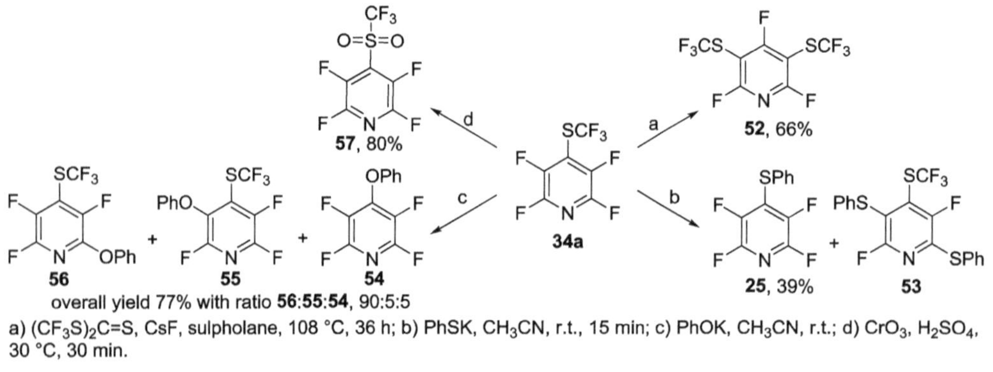

Scheme 2-17. Reactions of 2,3,5,6-tetrafluoro-4-trifluoromethylthiopyridine **34a**.

Selective sulfonylation of pentafluoropyridine **3** has been carried out under a green and mild condition using proline-based surfactant Fl-750-M on reaction various sulfonate salts **58** (Scheme **2-18**) [27]. In comparison with current method for sulfonylation of pentafluoropyridine, this micellar medium provides a region for high solubility of sulfonates and reaction was carried out at water without using DMF.

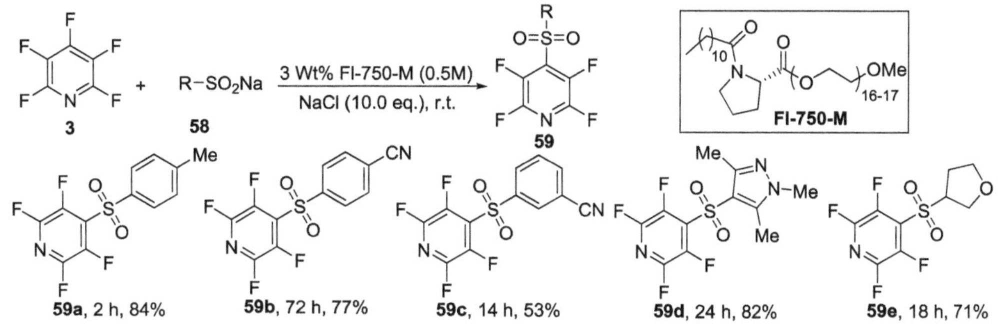

Scheme 2-18. Sulfonylation of pentafluoropyridine **3** under micellar medium.

4.2. Reaction of O-centered Nucleophile with Pentafluoropyridine

Reaction of pentafluorophenolb **60a** and 4-nitrophenol **60b** with pentafluoropyridine **3** have produced mixture of products in the presence of KF and 18-crown-6 (Scheme **2-19**). Whiles reaction of heptafluoro-2-naphthol and heptafluoro-1-naphthol have produced monosubstituted products (Scheme **2-20**). In addition, reaction of pentafluoropytridine **3** with phenol **60e** and 4-methylphenol **60f** gave disubstituted products (Scheme **2-21**). In these reaction, determinant factor is power basic of aroxides in acetonitrile [28].

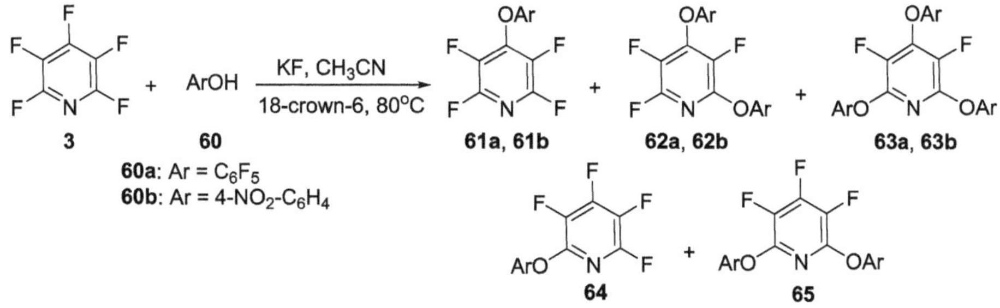

Scheme 2-19. Reaction of aroxides **60** with pentafluoropyridine **3** in the presennce of crown ether.

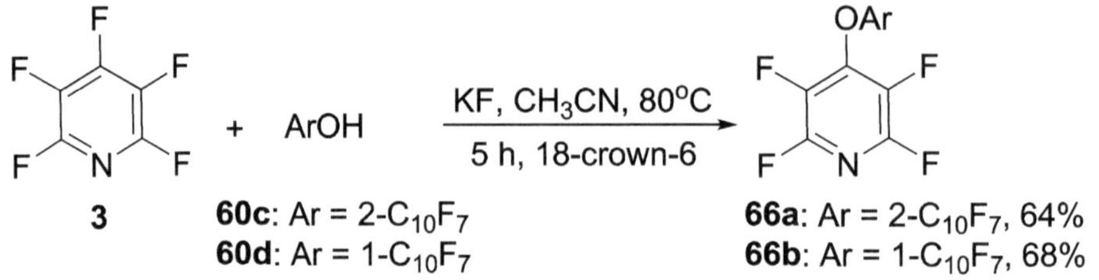

$$3 + ArOH \xrightarrow[\text{5 h, 18-crown-6}]{\text{KF, CH}_3\text{CN, 80°C}} 66$$

3

60c: Ar = 2-$C_{10}F_7$
60d: Ar = 1-$C_{10}F_7$

66a: Ar = 2-$C_{10}F_7$, 64%
66b: Ar = 1-$C_{10}F_7$, 68%

Scheme 2-20. Reaction of perfluoronaphthols **60** with pentafluoropyridine **3**.

3

60e: Ar = Ph
60f: Ar = 4-CH_3-C_6H_4

54, Ar = Ph, 60%
67, Ar = 4-CH_3-C_6H_4, 89%

62b, Ar = Ph, **6%**
68, Ar = 4-CH_3-C_6H_4, 1%

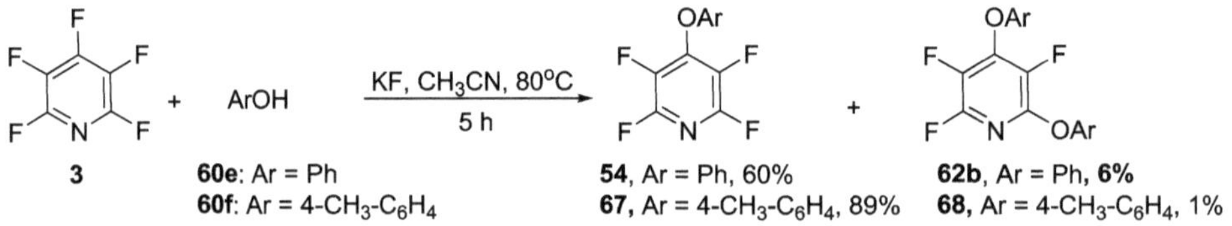

Scheme 2-21. Reaction of aroxides **60** with pentafluoropyridine **3**.

Reaction of pentafluoropyridine **3** with 4-nitrophenol produced 4-(4--nitrophenoxy)-2,3,5,6-tetrafluoropyridine **61b**, while in excess amount of 4-nitrophenol gave trisubstituted difluoropyridine **63b** (Scheme **2-22**) [29].

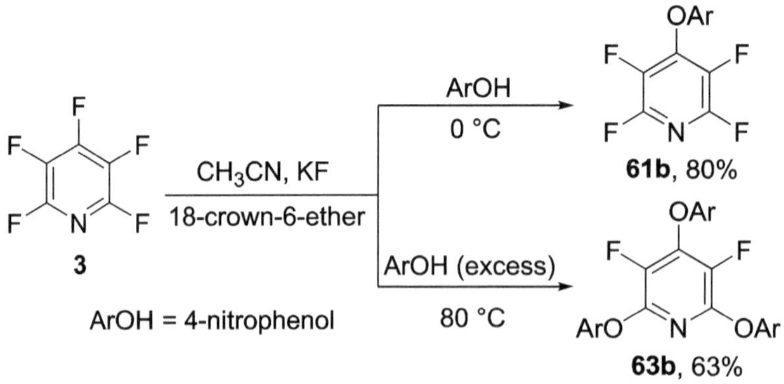

3

ArOH = 4-nitrophenol

CH$_3$CN, KF
18-crown-6-ether

ArOH
0 °C

61b, 80%

ArOH (excess)
80 °C

63b, 63%

Scheme 2-22. Reaction of pentafluoropyridine **3** with 4-nitrophenol.

Potassium *t*-butoxide in THF is reactive towards polyfluoroaromatic compounds, which gave mixture of di- and tri-substituted products (Scheme **2-23**) [30].

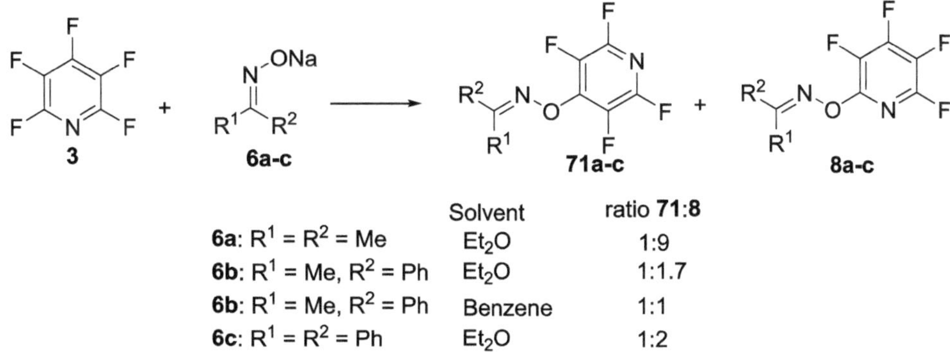

Scheme 2-23. Reaction of pentafluoropyridine **3** with KO-Bu^t.

Reaction of pentafluoropyridine **3** with ketoximes **6a-c** have been investigated by Banks and co-workers (Scheme **2-24**) [31]. Nucleophilic reaction of an equimolar amount of sodium salt of acetone oxime **6a** with pentafluoropyridine **3** in diethyl have been carried out at both 2- and 4-positions of pentafluoropyridine with ratio 1:9, respectively. Under identical conditions, the oximate **6b** gave the corresponding *o*-tetrafluoropyridyl derivatives **71b** and **8b** in 30 and 52% (isolated yield), respectively. With using of benzene instead of diethyl ether at 20 °C, the ratio 1:1.7 converted to 1:1. Similarly, the sodium salt of benzophenone oxime on reaction with pentafluoropyridine yielded mixture of 2- and 4-substituted products in ratio 1:2, respectively.

The *ortho* orientation of nucleophilic attack oximate anion to pentafluoropyridine have been explained by formation of the resonance-stabilized A-complex (Scheme **2-25**). Also, the ratio 2-substitution to 4-substitution have been affected by solvation of the sodium cation.

	Solvent	ratio **71:8**
6a: R^1 = R^2 = Me	Et$_2$O	1:9
6b: R^1 = Me, R^2 = Ph	Et$_2$O	1:1.7
6b: R^1 = Me, R^2 = Ph	Benzene	1:1
6c: R^1 = R^2 = Ph	Et$_2$O	1:2

Scheme 2-24. Reaction of pentafluoropyridine **3** with ketoximes **6a-c**.

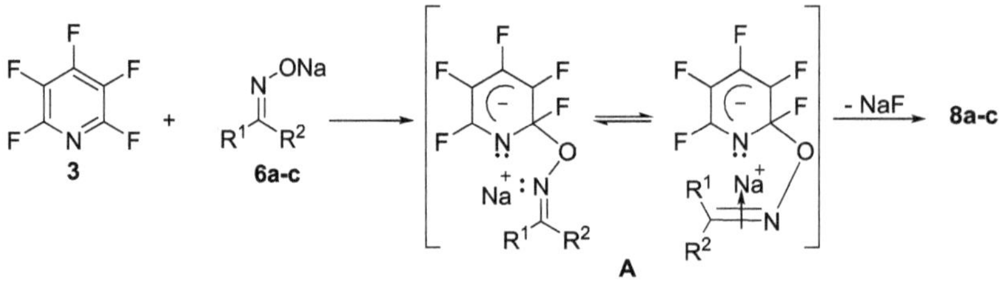

Scheme 2-25. Proposed mechanism for substitution of oximes **6a-c** at 2-position of pentafluoropyridine **3**.

O-heteroarylation of anomeric hydroxyl group **72a** and **72b** have been carried out directly by pentafluoropyridine **3** and β products obtained (Scheme **2-26**) [32]. Reaction of anomeric hydroxyl group with pentafluoropyridine produced *O*-glycopyranosyl in high yield. Also, reaction of pentafluoropyridine with unprotected glucose **72c** generated exclusively *O*-(β-D-glycopyranosyl) derivative (Scheme **2-26**) [32].

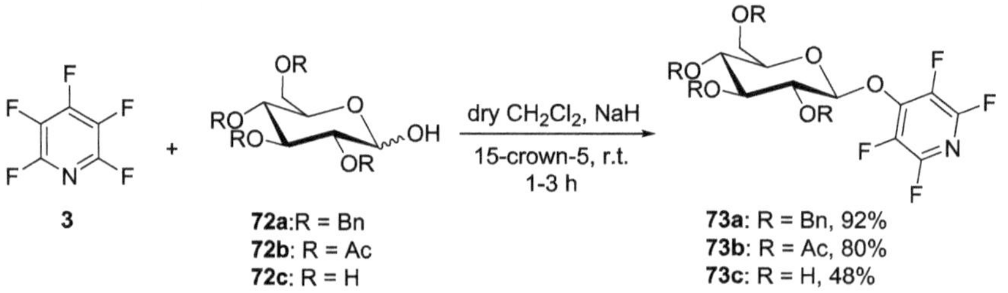

Scheme 2-26. Reaction of pentafluoropyridine **3** with anomeric OH group.

O-glycosylic derivatives in the presence of trimethylsilyl trifluoromethane-sulphonate and glycoside acceptors converted to disaccharide derivatives [32]. Compound **73a** in reaction with **74** produced only α-isomer **75** (Scheme **2-27**). However, compound **73b** in the presence of **74** produced exclusively β-isomer **76** (Scheme **2-28**).

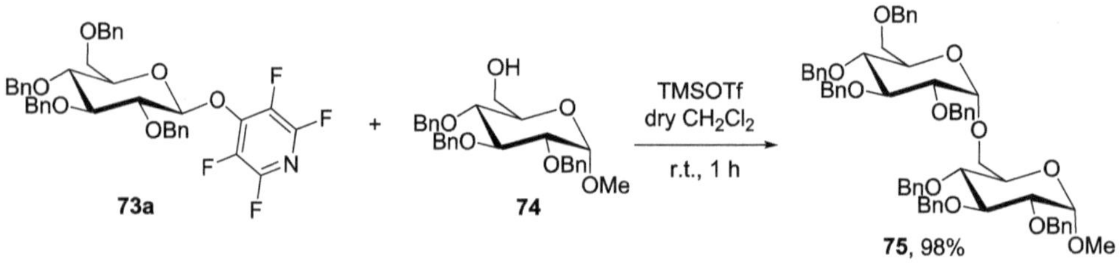

Scheme 2-27. Synthesis of disaccharides **75**.

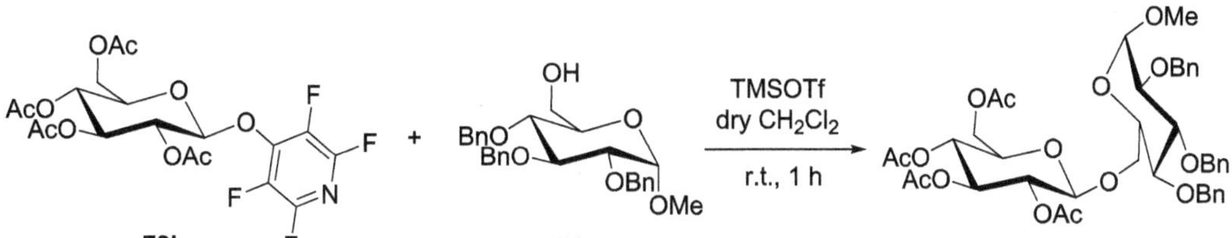

Scheme 2-28. Synthesis of disaccharides **76**.

The sodium salt $(CF_3)_2NO\text{-}Na$ **79** {from $(CF_3)_2NOH$ + NaH in Et_2O} and $(CF_3)_2NOH\text{-}CsF$ **77** are bis(trifluoromethyl)amino-oxylating agents that used for the synthesis of bis(trifluoromethyl)amino-oxy fluouropyridines. Their treatment with perfluoropyridines afforded some $(CF_3)_2NO$-substituded perfluoropyridins (Schemes **2-29** to **2-32**) [33].

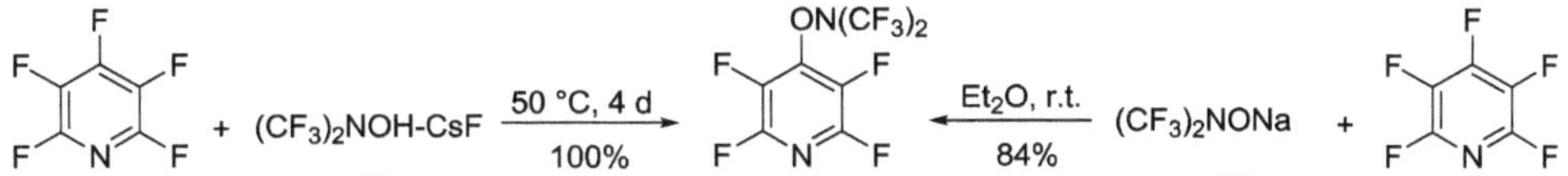

Scheme 2-29. Synthesis of 4-$(CF_3)_2NO$-tetrafluoropyridine **78**.

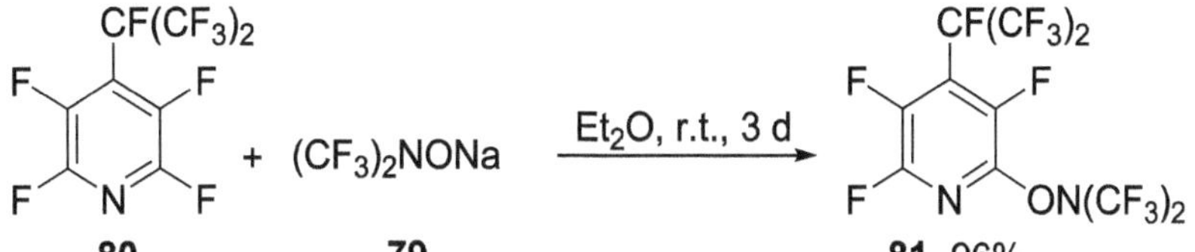

Scheme 2-30. Synthesis of 2,4-di($(CF_3)_2NO$) trifluoropyridine **81**.

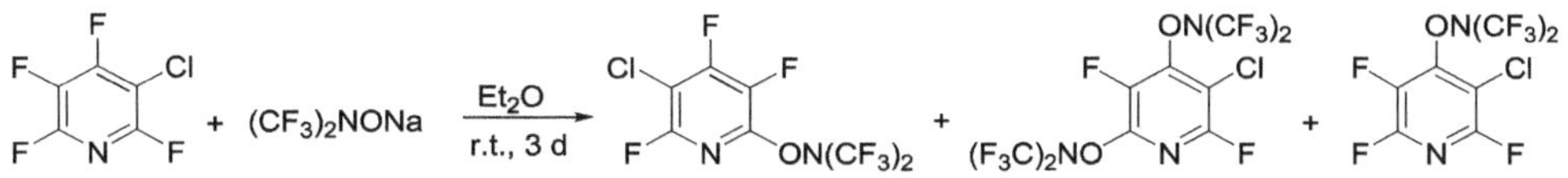

Scheme 2-31. Reaction of $(CF_3)_2NONa$ **79** with 3-chloro-2,4,5,6-tetrafluoropyridine **5**.

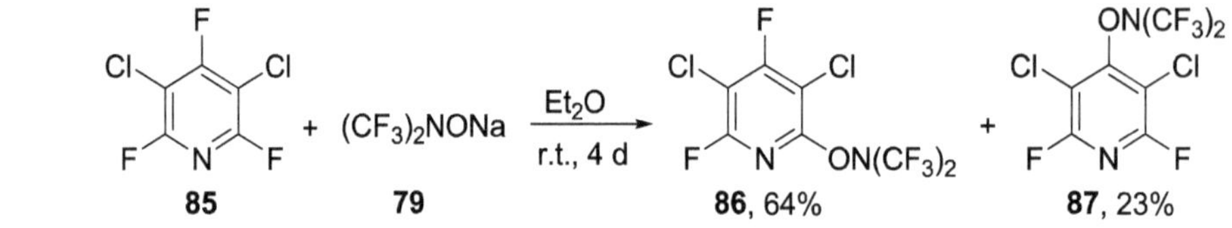

Scheme 2-32. Reaction of $(CF_3)_2NONa$ **79** with 3,5-dichloro-2,4,6-trifluoropyridine **85**.

4.3. Reaction of C-centered Nucleophile with Pentafluoropyridine

Reaction of fluoride ion with fluoro-olfines produced carbanions that can be reacted with fluorinated aromatic systems by replacement of fluorine atom. For example, anions derived from reaction of acetylene and olfine derivatives with cesium fluoride reacted with pentafluoropyridine **3** and produced a mixture of products (Schemes **2-33** and **2-34**) [34, 35].

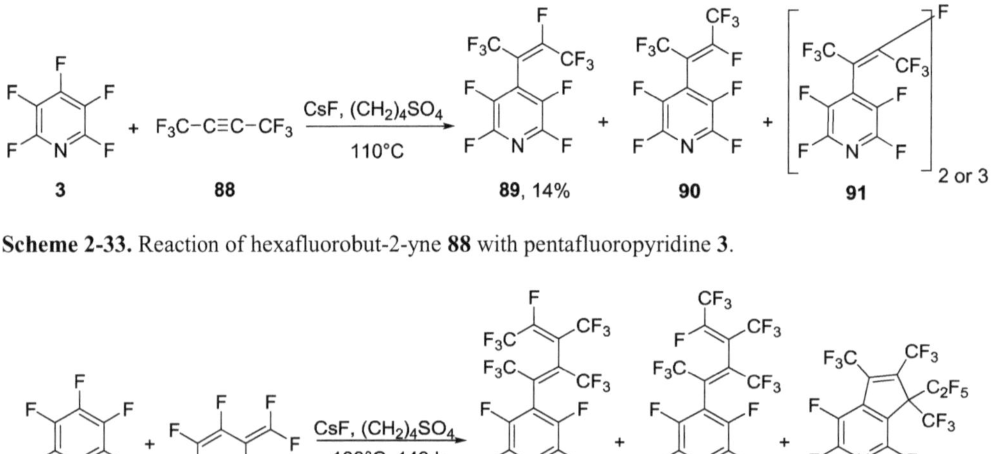

Scheme 2-33. Reaction of hexafluorobut-2-yne **88** with pentafluoropyridine **3**.

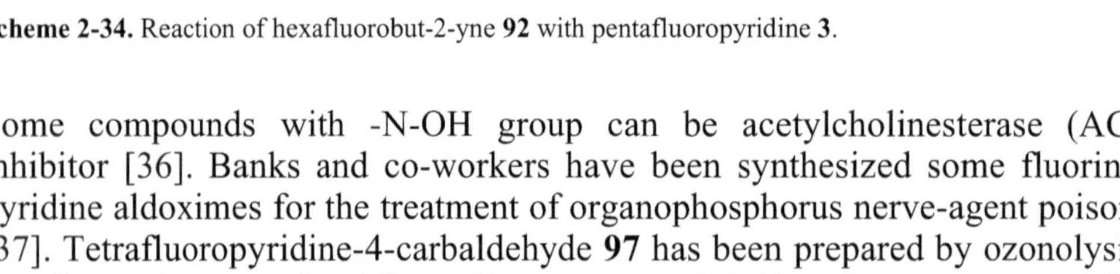

Scheme 2-34. Reaction of hexafluorobut-2-yne **92** with pentafluoropyridine **3**.

Some compounds with -N-OH group can be acetylcholinesterase (AChE) inhibitor [36]. Banks and co-workers have been synthesized some fluorinated pyridine aldoximes for the treatment of organophosphorus nerve-agent poisoning [37]. Tetrafluoropyridine-4-carbaldehyde **97** has been prepared by ozonolysis of tetrafluoro-4-propenylpyridine **18** or raney Ni-Al of tetrafluoropyridine--carbonitrile (Sheme 2-35). Reaction of carbaldehyde **97** with hydroxylamine produced corresponding aldoxime. In similar manner, 2,3,5,6-tetrafluoro-

4-methylpyridine **99** converted to perfluoropyridine 2-aldoxime **102** (Scheme **2-36**).

Scheme 2-35. Synthesis of tetrafluoropyridine-4-aldoxime **98**.

Scheme 2-36. Synthesis of tetrafluoropyridine-2-aldoxime **102**.

Furthermore, tetrafluoropyridine-4-carbonitrile **27** was obtained by fluorination of tetrachloropyridine-4-carbonitrile **104** with KF (Scheme **2-37**) [38]. Nitrile **27** on treatment with conc. H_2SO_4 converted to corresponding acid **17** [38]. Aldehyde **97** carried out common reactions of aldehydes such as reaction with hydroxylamine, 2,4-dinitrophenylhydrazine, aniline, phenylmagnesium iodide and oxygen (Scheme **2-38**) [38].

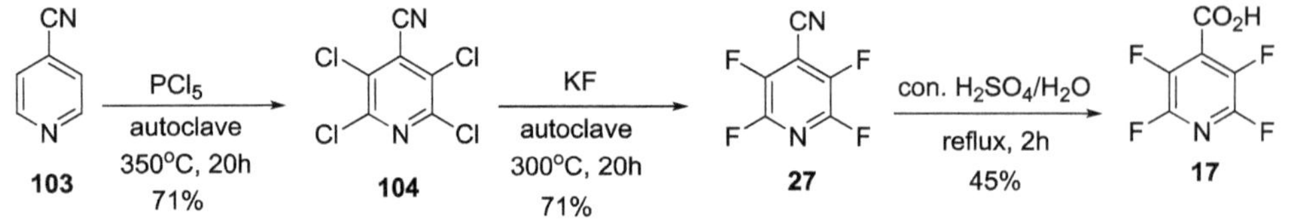

Scheme 2-37. Synthesis of tetrafluoropyridine-4-carboxylic acid **17**.

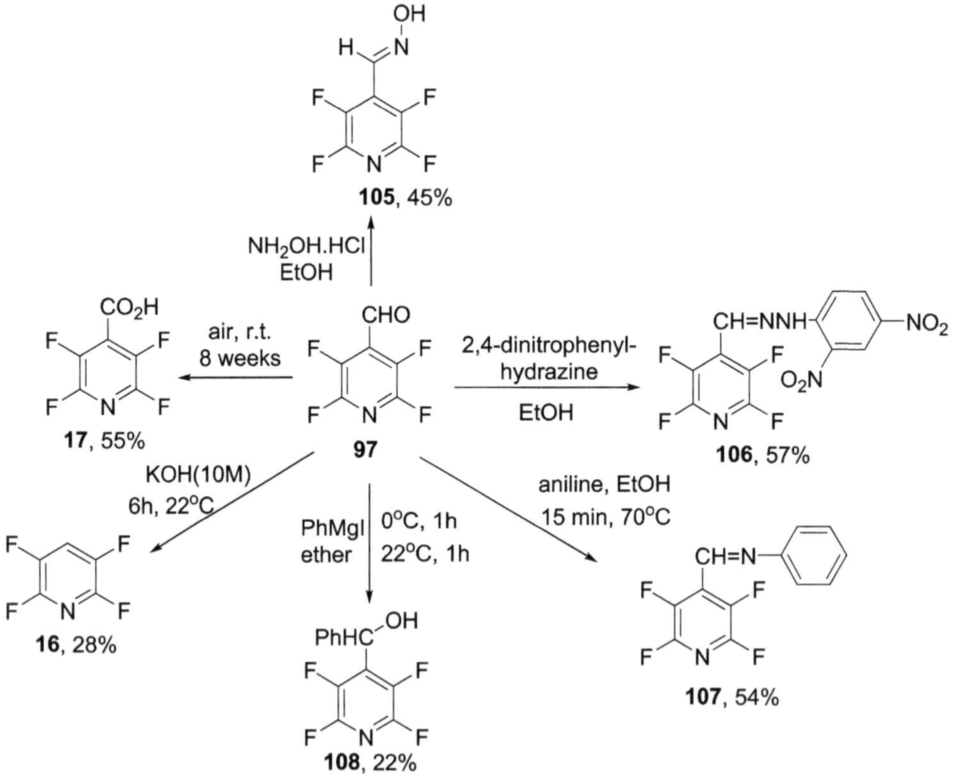

Scheme 2-38. Some reactions of tetrafluoropyridine-4-carbaldehyde **97**.

Substitution reactions of perfluorinated heteroaromatics with *C*-centered nucleophiles are less common and limited to reactions of alkyl, vinyl and phenyl lithium derivatives and perfluorinated anions [7]. Stable perfluoropyridyl carbanion **119** have been synthesized and isolated by reaction of pentafluoropyridine **3** with nitromethane (Scheme **2-39**) [39].

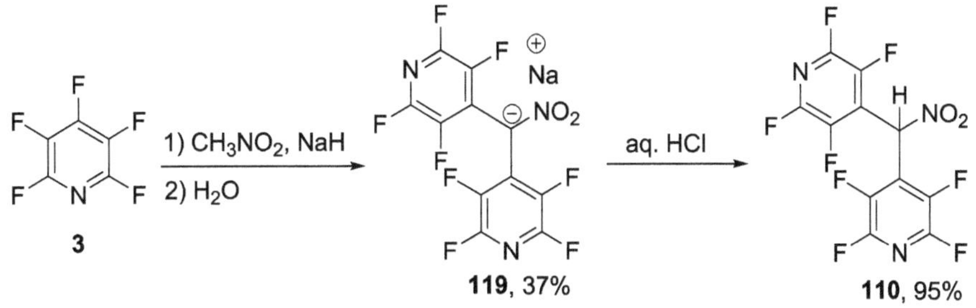

Scheme 2-39. Synthesis of perfluoropyridyl carbanion **119**.

It is emphasized the need to short, regioselective, high yields and flexible methods for synthesis of multifunctional heteroaromatic systems. Polyfluorinated heteroaromatic compounds have been used for synthesis of multisubstituted heteroaromatics [40]. Pentafluoropyridine **3** is an efficient perfluorinated structural system for synthesis of these compounds due to the replacement of every five fluorine atoms by nucleophiles and have been obtained a wide range of polysubstituted systems from its nucleophilic reactions. Various synthetic methods have been reported for preparation of pyridine derivatives with five different substituents using pentafluoropyridine [31]. Champers *et al.* [41] have represented synthesis of ring-fused and multifunctional bispyridine systems. Perfluoroalkylation of pentafluoropyridine **3** by hexafluoropropene produced compound **80** that in following converted to compound **111** on treatment with methylamine (Scheme **2-40**). Compound **111** could be used as a precursor for synthesis of bispyridine systems. Proton elimination of **111** by BuLi and attack of formed anion to compound **80** produced bispyridine **112** (Scheme **2-40**). Fluorine atoms of compound **112** can easily replace by nucleophiles (Scheme **2-41**).

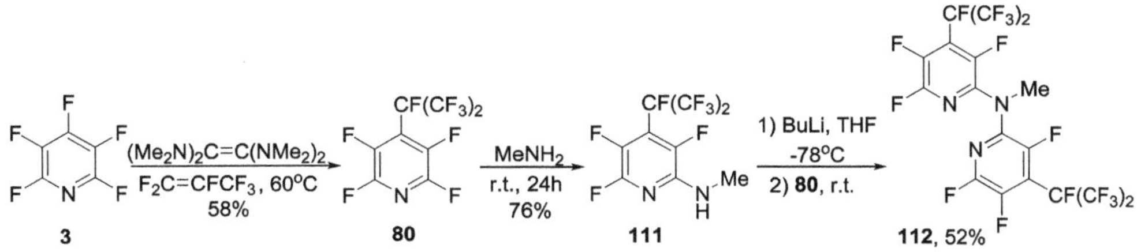

Scheme 2-40. Synthesis of bi-perfluoropyridine **112**.

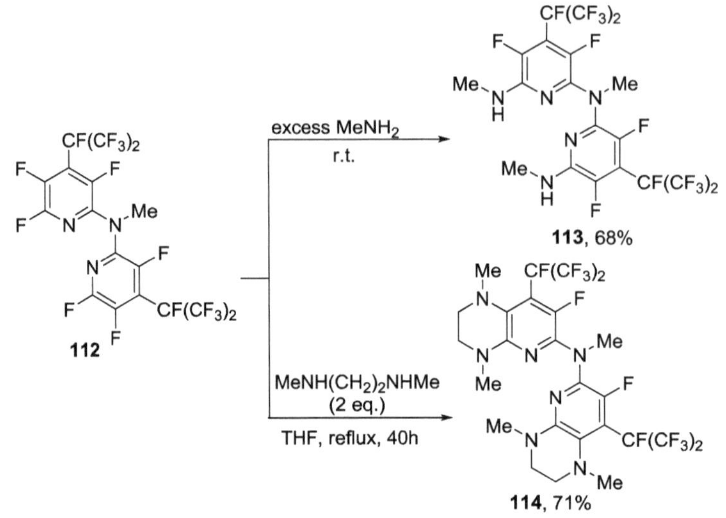
excess $MeNH_2$
r.t.
$MeNH(CH_2)_2NHMe$
(2 eq.)
THF, reflux, 40h
112
113, 68%
114, 71%

Scheme 2-41. Nucleophilic reactions of bi-perfluoropyridine **112**.

Perfluoro-4-isopropylpyridine **80** reacted selectively at the 2-position of pyridine ring with *O*, *C* and *N*-centered nucleophiles and produced multisubstituted perfluoropyridine derivatives (Schemes **2-42**, **2-43** and **2-44**) [42].

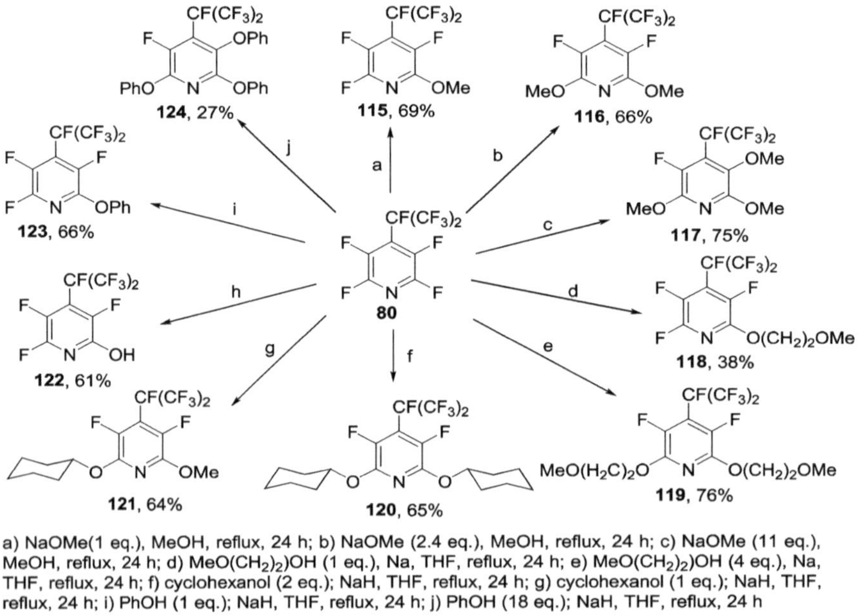
124, 27%
115, 69%
116, 66%
123, 66%
117, 75%
80
122, 61%
118, 38%
121, 64%
120, 65%
119, 76%
a) NaOMe(1 eq.), MeOH, reflux, 24 h; b) NaOMe (2.4 eq.), MeOH, reflux, 24 h; c) NaOMe (11 eq.), MeOH, reflux, 24 h; d) MeO(CH2)2)OH (1 eq.), Na, THF, reflux, 24 h; e) MeO(CH2)2)OH (4 eq.), Na, THF, reflux, 24 h; f) cyclohexanol (2 eq.); NaH, THF, reflux, 24 h; g) cyclohexanol (1 eq.); NaH, THF, reflux, 24 h; i) PhOH (1 eq.); NaH, THF, reflux, 24 h; j) PhOH (18 eq.); NaH, THF, reflux, 24 h

Scheme 2-42. Reaction of tetrafluoro-4-isopropyl pyridine **80** with *O*-centered nucleophiles.

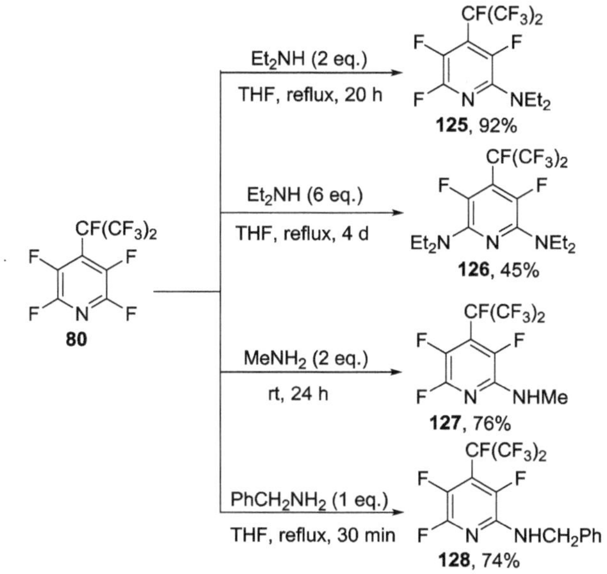

Scheme 2-43. Reaction of tetrafluoro-4-isopropylpyridine **80** with *N*-centered nucleophiles.

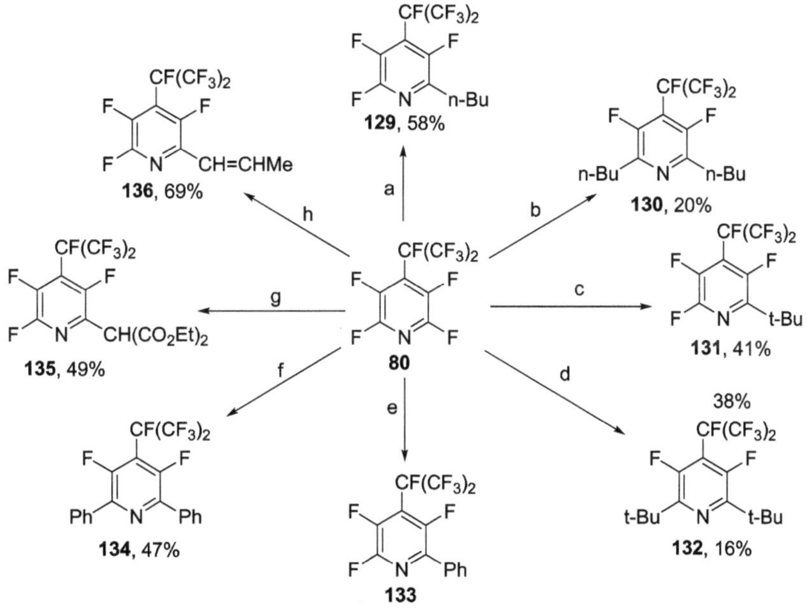

a) n-BuLi (1 eq.), Et$_2$O, -78°C, 45 min; b) n-BuLi (2 eq.), Et$_2$O, -78°C, 45 min; c) t-BuMgCl (1 eq.), THF, -15°C, 5 h; d) t-BuLi (2 eq.), Et$_2$O, -41°C, 30 min; e) PhMgCl (1 eq.), THF, reflux, 24 h; f) PhMgBr (2 eq.); THF, reflux, 24 h; g) CH$_2$(CO$_2$Et)$_2$, NaH, THF, r.t., 5 h; h) CH$_3$CH=CHMgBr, THF, reflux, 20 h.

Scheme 2-44. Reaction of tetrafluoro-4-isopropylpyridine **80** with *C*-centered nucleophiles.

Bromination of tetrafluoro-4-isopropylpyridine **80** has been proceeded at the 2- and 6-positions of pyridine by heating with hydrogen bromide and aluminium tribromide in an autoclave [43]. The subsequent reaction of **137** with *n*-butyl lithium afforded the lithio derivative **138**, which in the presence of one equivalent of the heterocycle **80** gave 2,2′-bipyridyl derivative **139**. This is very reactive towards nucleophiles and on heating with sodium methoxide formed product **140** *via* substitution the *ortho* fluorine atom (Scheme **2-45**).

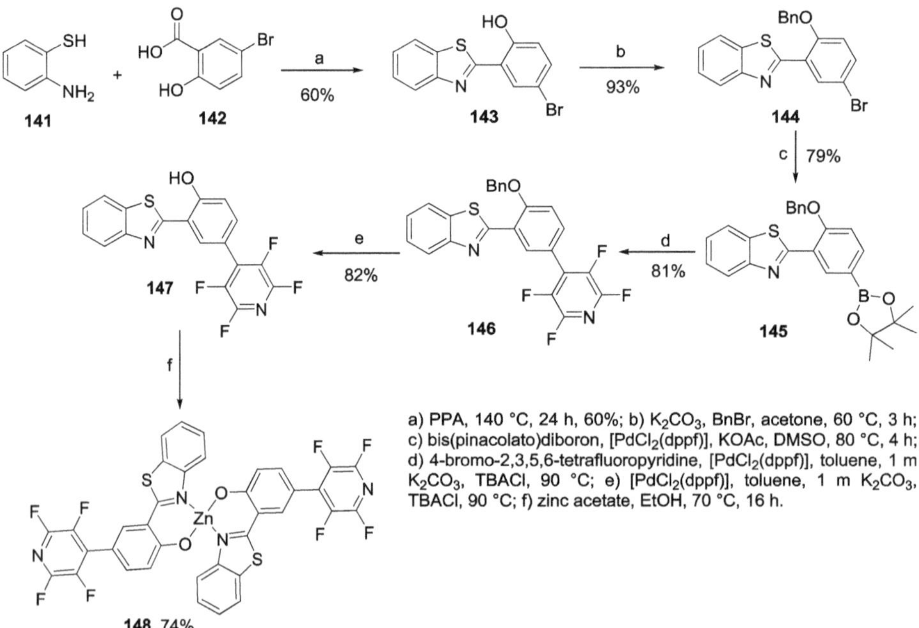

a) AlBr$_3$ (2.2 equiv.), HBr (2.2 equiv.), 160 °C, 48 h.
b) n-BuLi (1.2 equiv.), THF, -78 °C.
c) **80**, -78 °C to r.t.
d) NaOMe, MeOH, reflux, 24h.

Scheme 2-45. Synthesis of perfluoroisopropyl-2,2′-bipyridyl derivatives **140**.

a) PPA, 140 °C, 24 h, 60%; b) K$_2$CO$_3$, BnBr, acetone, 60 °C, 3 h;
c) bis(pinacolato)diboron, [PdCl$_2$(dppf)], KOAc, DMSO, 80 °C, 4 h;
d) 4-bromo-2,3,5,6-tetrafluoropyridine, [PdCl$_2$(dppf)], toluene, 1 m K$_2$CO$_3$, TBACl, 90 °C; e) [PdCl$_2$(dppf)], toluene, 1 m K$_2$CO$_3$, TBACl, 90 °C; f) zinc acetate, EtOH, 70 °C, 16 h.

Scheme 2-46. Synthesis of bis{2-[2-hydroxy-5-(perfluoropyridine) phenyl]benzothiazolato]zinc (II) **148**.

bis[2-(2-hydroxyphenyl)benzothiazolato]zinc (II) (Znb$_2$) has good electron mobility and can be used in OLEDs [44], or as buffer layers in organic solar cells. Zinc complexes **148** produced by reaction of ligand **147** with zinc acetate in ethanol (Scheme **2-46**). UV/Vis absorption spectra shown shifts in the maximum absorption of complexe **148** to the blue shift. The electronic properties of the perfluoropyridyl group attached to the 2-phenylbenzothiazole ligand of Znb$_2$ derivative change the HOMO energy levels. The oxidation process for Complexe **148** with blue shifted emission became more difficult [45].

The reaction of pentafluoropyridine and 3,5-dichlorotrifluoropyridine with enamines at boiling benzene led to formation of pyridylenamines from nucleophilic attack of enamaine *via* C site (Scheme **2-47**) [46].

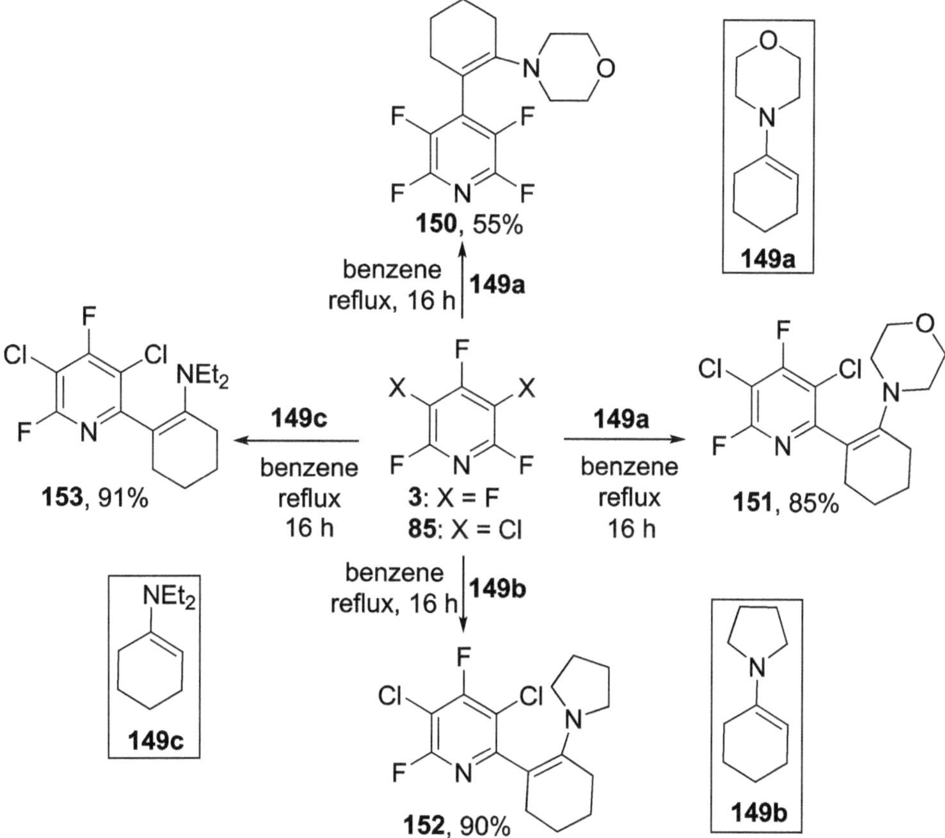

Scheme **2-47**. Synthesis of pyridylenamines **150-153**.

C-F bond activation of pentafluoropyridine **3** has been widely investigated on reaction with transition metals, NHCs and mesoionic carbenes [47 - 56]. Reaction of CAAC **154** with C_5F_5N in hexanes yielded compound **155** resulting insertion into the *para* C-F bond pyridine ring [57]. The iminium-pyridyl adduct $[156]^+$ has been isolated after fluoride abstraction from **155** by Me_3SiX, while its reduction with magnesium gave CAAC-pyridyl radical $[157]^{\cdot}$ (Scheme **2-48**).

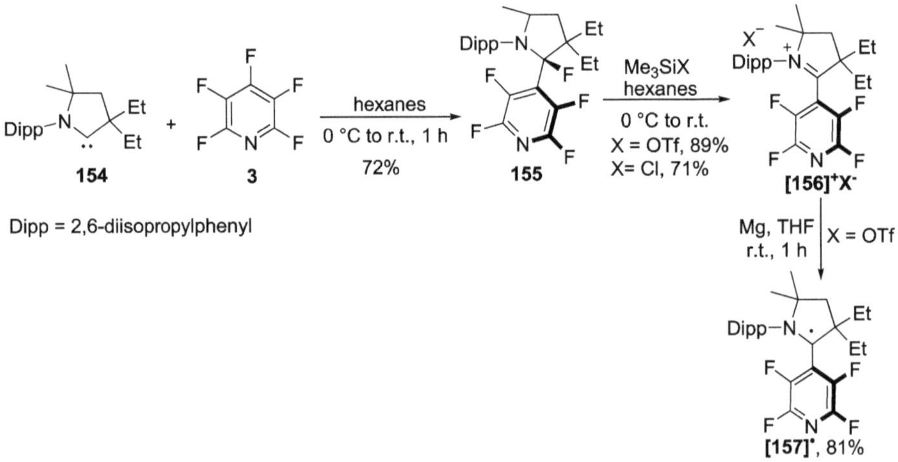

Scheme 2-48. Synthesis of CAAC-tetrafluoropyridyl radical.

Reaction of pentafluoropyridine with tetrafluoroethylene in autoclave has been produced pentakis(pentafluoroethyl)pyridine **151** at 14% yield and mixture of other products (Scheme **2-49**) [58].

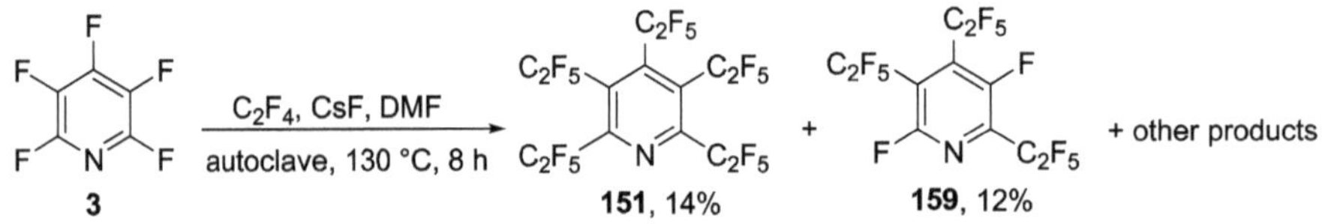

Scheme 2-49. Reaction of pentafluoropyridine **3** with tetrafluoroethylene.

A series of tetrafluoropyridynyl substituted acetylene amino acid conjugates have been synthesized in order to comprising a DNA cleaving moiety which contains an aryl alkyne group and a polyfunctional pH-regulated DNA-binding moiety which contains at least one or two amino groups (Fig. **2-2**) [59].

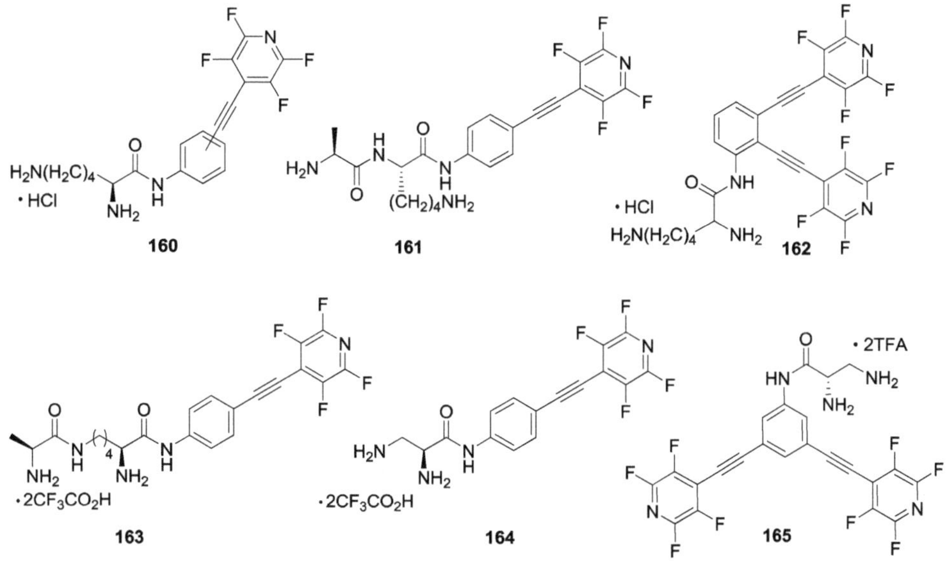

Fig. (2-2). Tetrafluoropyridynyl substituted acetylene amino acid conjugates.

Three isomeric aryl-tetrafluoropyridyl alkynes with amide and lysine substituents in different positions (*o-*, *m-*, and *p-*) have been synthesized in several steps from nitrobenzenes **166** (Scheme **2-50**) [60]. The three isomeric lysine conjugates cleaved DNA with different efficiencies consistent with the alkylating ability of the respective acetamides. The significant protecting effect of the hydroxyl radical and singlet oxygen scavengers to DNA cleavage has been shown only with m-lysine conjugate. All three isomeric lysine conjugates inhibited human melanoma cell growth under photoactivation [60].

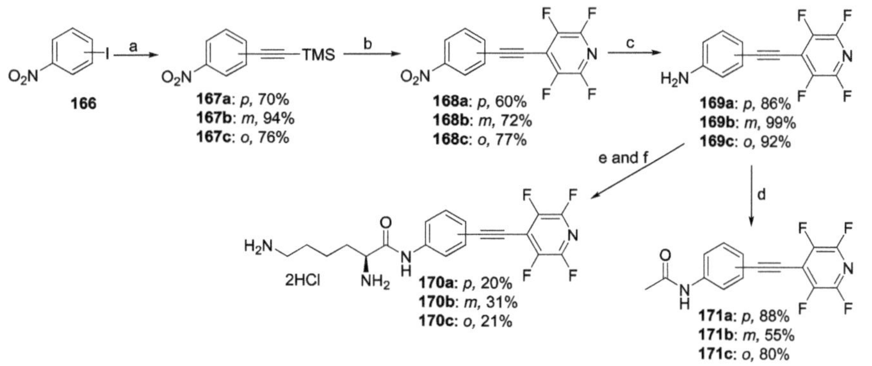

a) $PdCl_2(PPh_3)_2$, CuI, HCCSiMe$_3$/Et$_3$N, rt; b) CsF, pentfluoropyridine/DMF; c) SnCl$_2$, EtOH, reflux; d) $(CH_3CO)_2O$, Et$_3$N/CH$_2$Cl$_2$; e) POCl$_3$, Boc-Lys(Boc)-OH/pyridine; f) HCl(g)/MeOH.

Scheme 2-50. Synthesis of amido-substituted monoacetylenes and lysine conjugates.

Pentafluoropyridine underwent direct arylation *via* reaction with aryl sulfonates using Pd catalysts [61]. Its reaction with phenyl triflate carried out by Pd(OAc)$_2$/MePhos as catalyst, whereas the reaction with hindered 2,4,6-trimethylphenyl triflate done using Pd(OAc)$_2$/RuPhos (Scheme **2-51**).

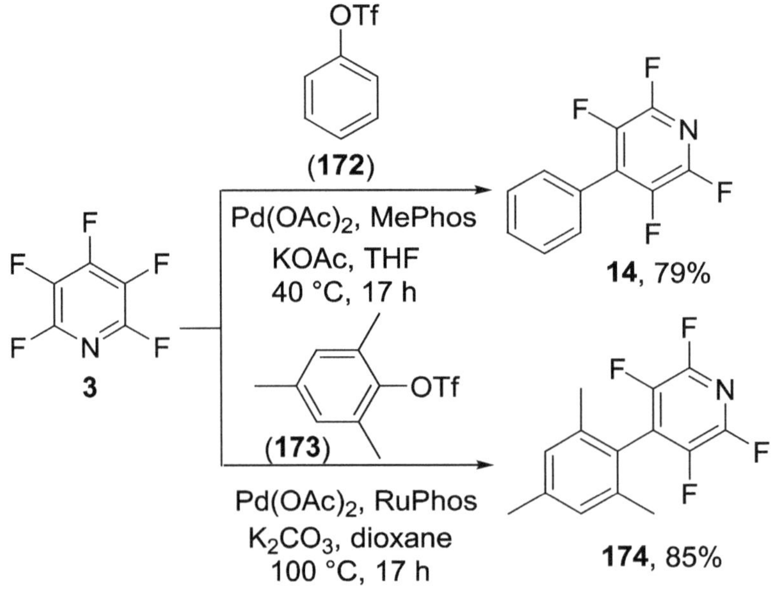

Scheme 2-51. Direct arylation of pentafluoropyridine **3** with aryl sulfonates.

4.4. Reaction of N-centered Nucleophile with Pentafluoropyridine

4-Aminotetrafluoropyridine **13** is a weak base that is prepared easily by reaction between aqueous solution of ammonia and pentafluoropyridine [16, 17]. Amino group of **13** as a nucleophile has been reacted with anhydrides and benzoyl chlorides to produce various *N*-(perfluoropyridin-4-yl) amides **175** and **176**. It has also been reacted with with di-*tert*-butyl dicarbonate which yielded *tert*-butyl (perfluoropyridin-4-yl)carbamate **177** (Scheme **2-52**) [62].

Diazotization of 4-aminotetrafluoropyridine **13** is so difficult that only 4-bromotetrafluoropyridine **178** was obtained from its diazotization (Scheme **2-53**) [63]. Its oxidation to nitro derivate is difficult but it can be oxidized with peroxytrifluoroacetic acid in reflux for 22 hours (Scheme **2-53**) [63].

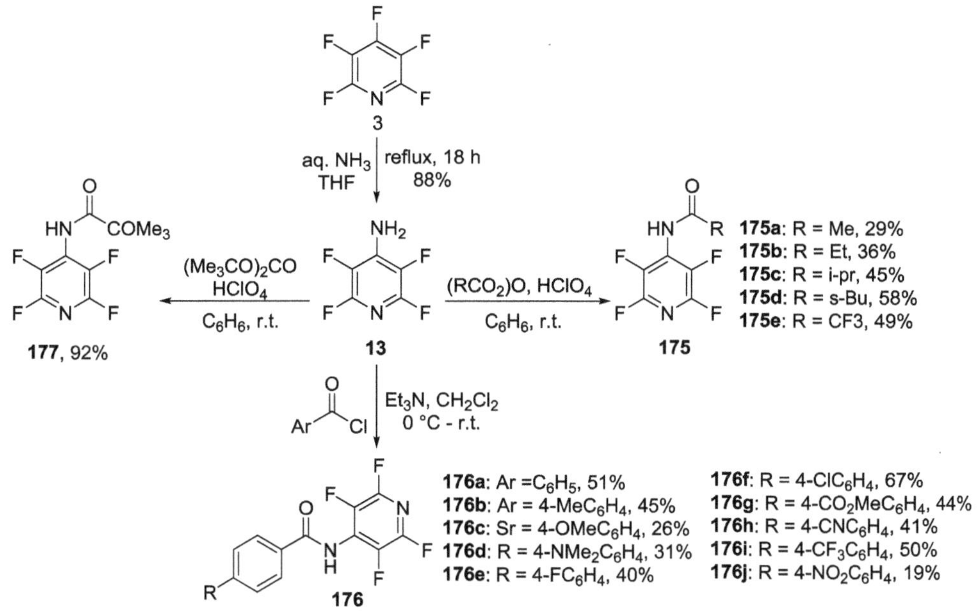

Scheme 2-52. Reaction of 2,3,5,6-tetrafluoropyridin-4-amine **13** with various electrophiles.

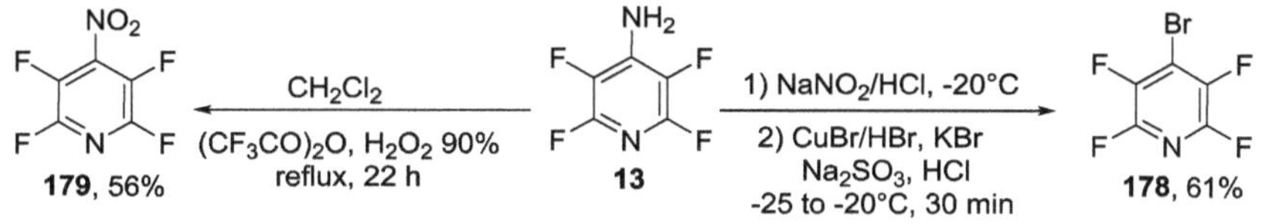

Scheme 2-53. Synthesis of 4-aminotetrafluoropyridine and its conversion to 4-bromo and 4-nitrotetrafluoropyridine.

4-Bromotetrafluoropyridine **178** is a useful building block that can complete versatility of pentafluoropyridine. Presence of bromine in pyridine ring led to more synthesis possibilities. 4-bromotetrafluoropyridine produced 4,4′-octafluorobipyridine **180** using copper powder in sealed tube in 230°C or in DMF at reflux condition (Scheme **2-54**) [63]. Also, compound **180** was obtained by reaction of pentafluoropyridine with Grignard reagent of 4-bromotetra- fluoropyridine (Scheme **2-54**) [63].

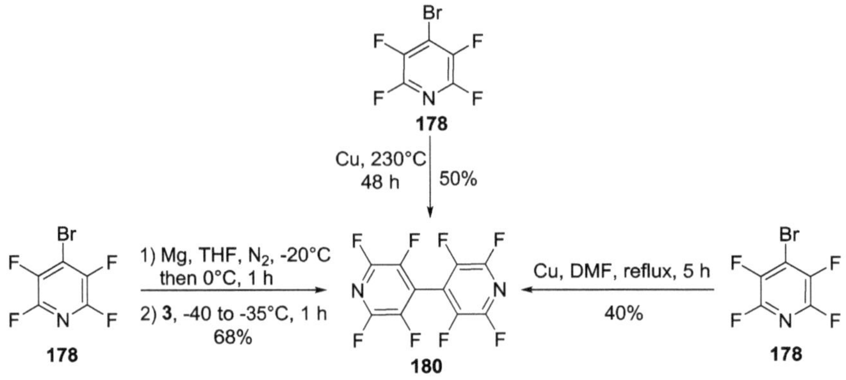

Scheme 2-54. Synthesis of 4,4′-octafluorobipyridine **180**.

Grignard reagent of 4-bromotetrafluoropyridine **178** was used as nucleophile in reaction with carbonyl group and carbondioxide (Scheme **2-55**) [63].

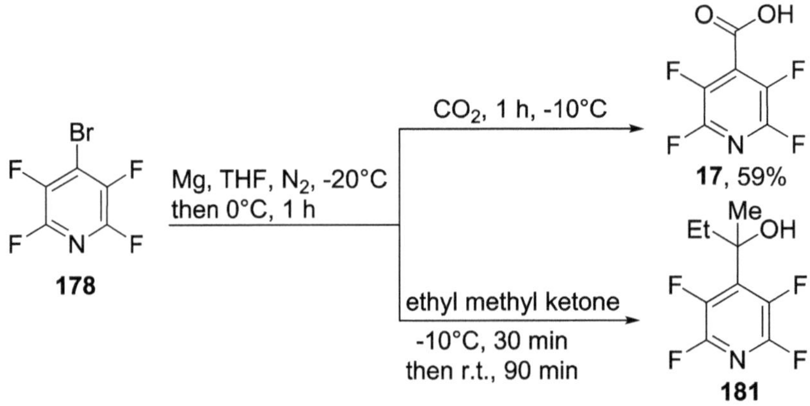

Scheme 2-55. Reactions of grignard reagent of 4-bromotetrafluoropyridine **178**.

4-Bromotetrafluoropyridine **178** reacted with alkyl amines, benzyl amines, alkoxides, ammonia, sodium hydroxide and benzimidazole at the 2-position of pyridine ring, whereas with thiophenol reacted at the 4-position (Scheme **2-56**) [63, 64]. Reaction of aromatic *N*-centered nucleophiles with this compound obtained mixture of products (Scheme **2-57**) [64].

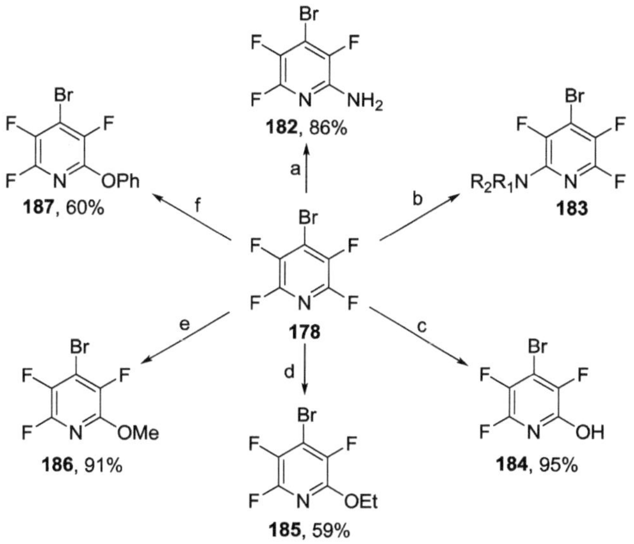

R_1R_2N	yield
MeO(CH$_2$)$_2$NH	76%
cyclopropylNH	56%
MeNH(CH$_2$)$_2$NMe	47%
O(CH$_2$CH$_2$)$_2$N	53%
4-OMe-C$_6$H$_4$CH$_2$NH	74%
2-Br-C$_6$H$_4$CH$_2$NH	61%

a) aq. NH3, 85 °C, 2 h; b) R$_1$R$_2$NH, DIPEA, THF, MW heating; c) KOH, r-BuOH, reflux, 2h; d) EtONa, DIPEA, THF, r.t., 2 h; e) Na/MeOH, 0°C to r.t. 30 min; f) PhONa, DIPEA, THF, 0°C-r.t., 7 h.

Scheme 2-56. Reaction of 4-bromotetrafluoropyridine **178** with with alkyl amines, benzyl amines, alkoxides, ammonia and sodium hydroxide.

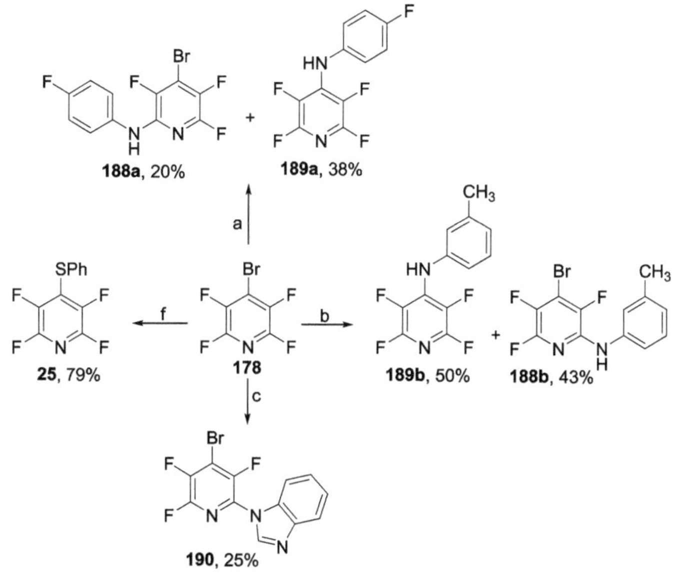

a) 4-F-C$_6$H$_4$NH$_2$, DIPEA, DMSO, MW, 160°C, 3 h; b) 3-CH$_3$-C$_6$H$_4$NH$_2$, DIPEA, DMSO, MW, 160°C, 1 h; c) Benzimidazole, Et$_3$N, CH$_3$CN. r.t., 2 d; f) PhSH, K$_2$CO$_3$, THF, r.t., 12 h.

Scheme 2-57. Reaction of 4-bromotetrafluoropyridine **178** with aromatic amines, benzimidazole and thiophenol.

Both of nitro and fluorine groups of 4-nitrotetrafluoropyridine **179** were replaced in reaction with ammonia (Scheme **2-58**) and sodium methoxide (Scheme **2-59**) [65]. Reduction of nitroamines **191** and **192** by dihydrogen and raney Ni produced corresponding diamines (Scheme **2-58**).

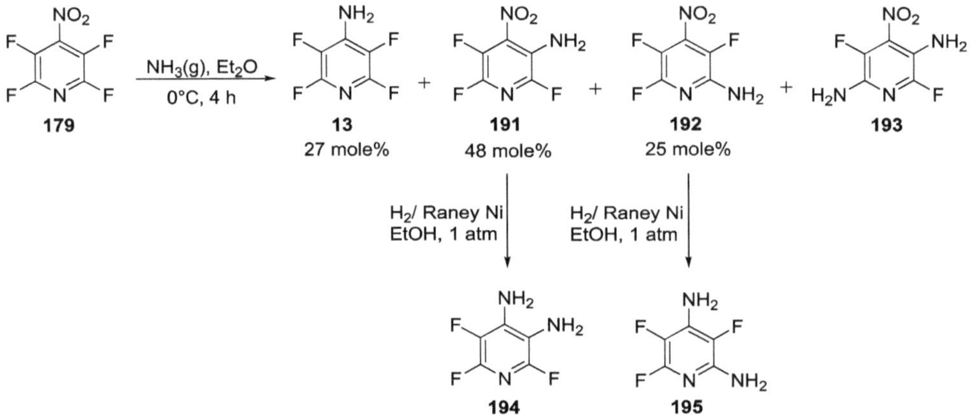

Scheme 2-58. Reaction of 4-nitrotetrafluoropyridine **179** with NH_3 (g) followed by reduction of nitro group.

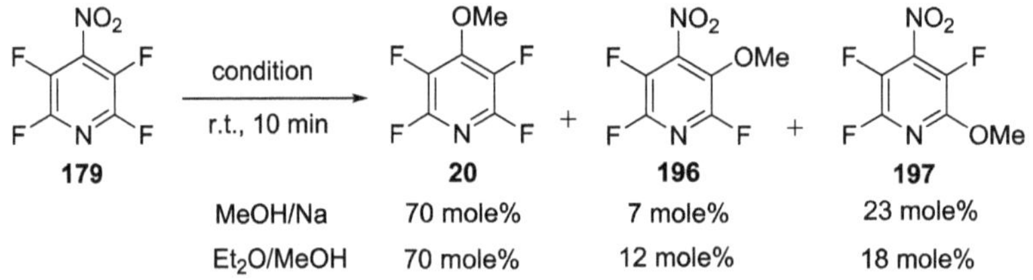

Scheme 2-59. Reaction of 4-nitrotetrafluoropyridine **179** with MeOH.

N-Fluorocarboxamides have been used as selective electrophilic fluorinating agents in preparation of organofluorine compounds [66, 67]. Perfluoro-[*N*-fluoro-*N*-(4-pyridyl)acetamide] **199**, prepared *via* direct fluorination of the sodium salt **198**, used as site-selective electrophilic fluorinating agent of diethyl sodio(phenyl)malonate, 1-morpholinocyclohexene, phenol and anisole (Scheme **2-61**) [68]. The sodium salt **198** was produced from the trifluoroacetylation of 4-aminotetrafluoropyridine **13** or direct treating pentafluoropyridine **3** with the monosodium salt of trifluoroacetamide (scheme 2-**60**).

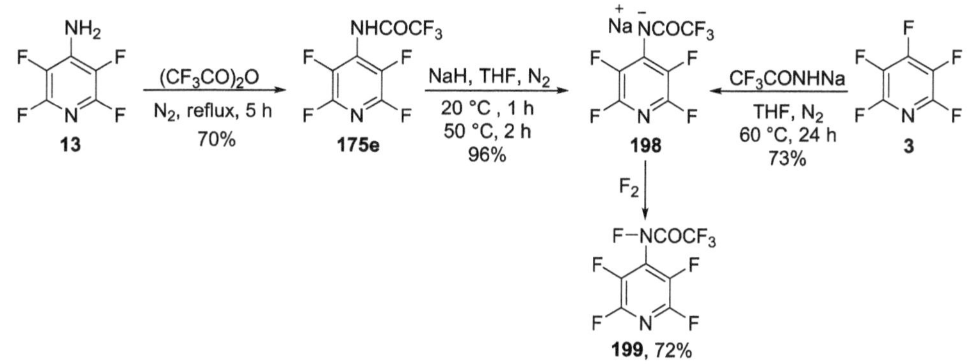

Scheme 2-60. Synthesis of perfluoro-[*N*-fluoro-*N*-(4-pyridyl)acetamide] **199**.

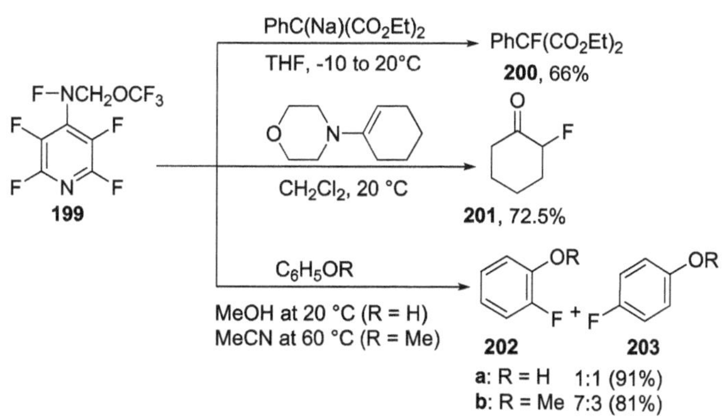

Scheme 2-61. Electrophilic fluorination using perfluoro-[*N*-fluoro-*N*-(4-pyridyl)acetamide] **199**.

Similar to compound **199**, perfluoro-[*N*-(4-pyridyl)methanesulphonamide] **205** have been applied as electrophilic fluorinating agent for formation of fluorinated diethyl sodio(phenyl)malonate, benzene and anisole (Schemes **2-62-2-63**), while it prepared from treatment of pentafluoropyridine **3** with trifluoromethane-sulphonamide followed by F_2 (Scheme **2-62**) [69].

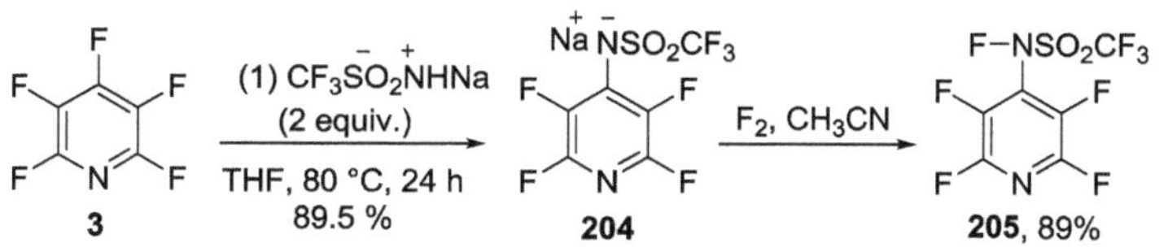

Scheme 2-62. Synthesis perfluoro-[*N*-(4_pyridyl)methanesulphonamide **205**.

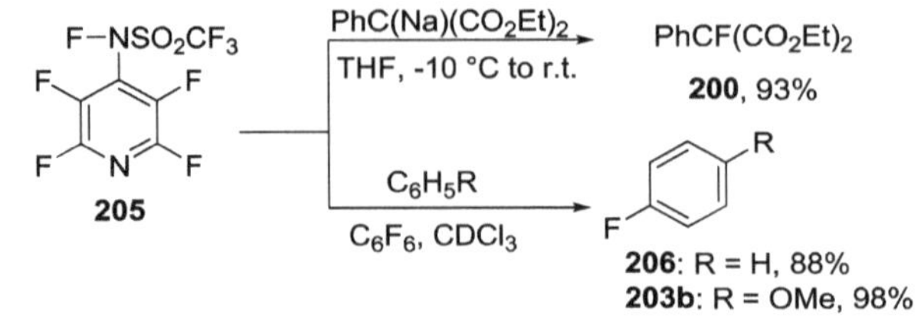

Scheme 2-63. Electrophilic fluorination using perfluoro-[*N*-(4_pyridyl)methanesulphonamide **205**.

Tetrafluoropyridine-4-diazonium fluoride (prepared from reaction of **13** with sodium nitrite in hydrofluoric acid) is an electrophilic species that could be coupled with nucleophilic compounds [70]. Its azo-coupling with mesitylene and anisole gave azo dyes **207a** and **207b** (Scheme **2-64**).

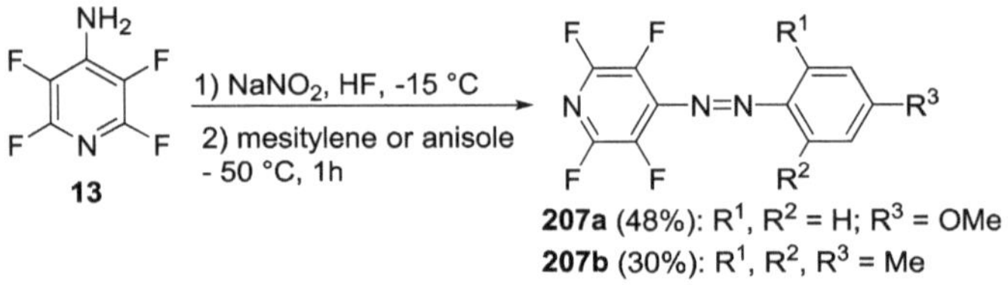

207a (48%): R^1, R^2 = H; R^3 = OMe
207b (30%): R^1, R^2, R^3 = Me

Scheme 2-64. Synthesis of perfluorinated azo dyes **207**.

Pyrolysis of 4-(dichloroamino)tetrafluoropyridine **208** was obtained from the reaction of 4-aminotetrafluoropyridine **13** with *t*-butylhypochlorite, gave octafluoro-4,4'-azopyridine **209** (Scheme **2-65**) [71].

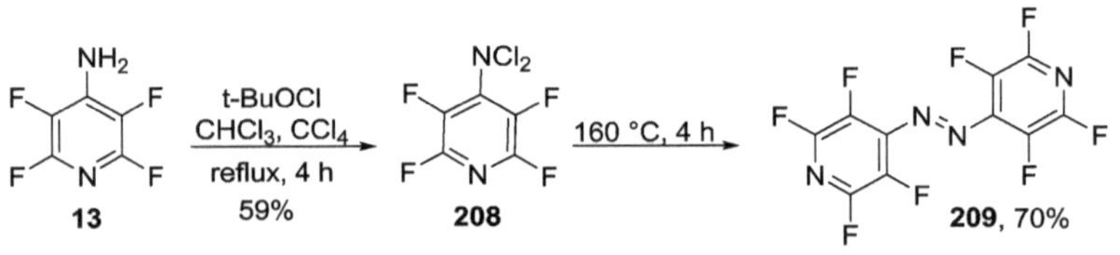

Scheme 2-65. Synthesis of 4-(dichloroamino)tetrafluoropyridine **209**.

4-(dichloroamino)tetrafluoropyridine **208** have been condensed with nitrosoarenes **210a-d** at the presence of benzyltriethylammonium chloride or CuCl and produced perfluorinated azoxy-compounds **211a-d** as main products (Scheme 2-66) [72]. These azoxy-compounds on the reaction with triethyl phosphite gave corresponding tetrafluoro-4-(arylazo)pyridines **207** (Scheme **2-67**), while at the reverse reaction, azo-compound **207b** converted to the corresponding azoxy-compound **211c** on treatment with TFAA and H_2O_2 (Scheme **2-68**).

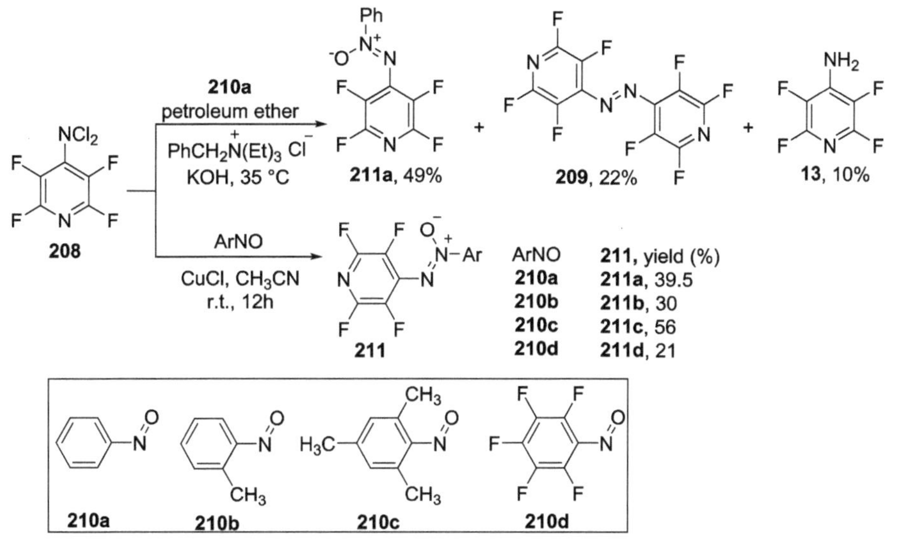

Scheme 2-66. Reaction of 4-(dichloroamino)tetrafluoropyridine **208** with titrosoarenes.

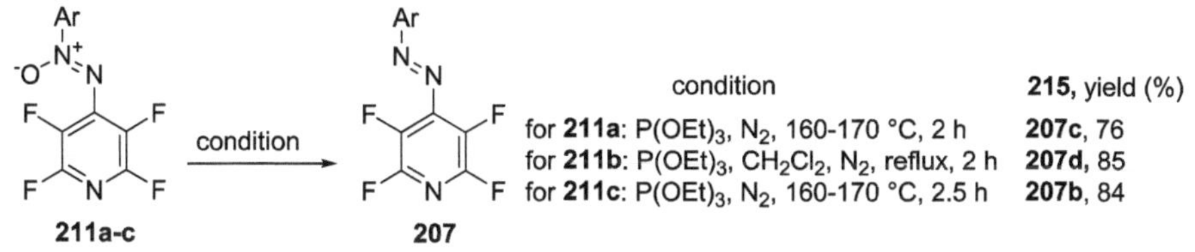

Scheme 2-67. Deoxygenation of tetrafluoro-4-(aryl-ONN-azoxy)pyridines **211a-c**.

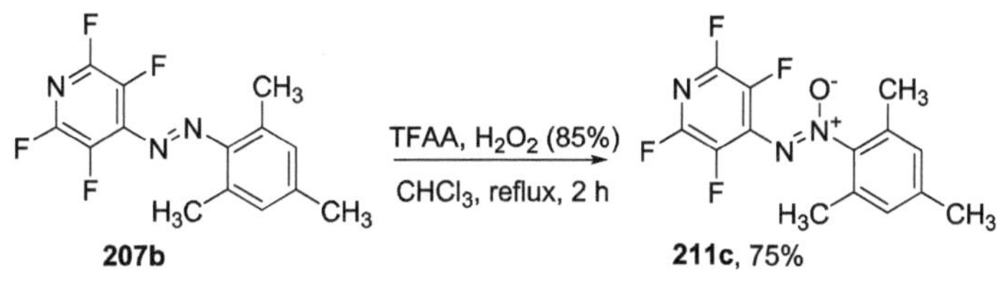

Scheme 2-68. Oxidation of tetrafluoro-4-(2,4,6-trimethylphenylazo)pyridine **207b**.

Pentafluoropyridine **3** reacted with aromatic amines at 4-position and gave tetrafluoro-N-(aryl)pyridine-4-amine derivatives **189** (Scheme **2-69**) and its reaction with cyclohexylamine produced N-cyclohexyl-2,3,5,6-tetrafluoropyri-in-4-amine at high yield (Scheme **2-70**) [62].

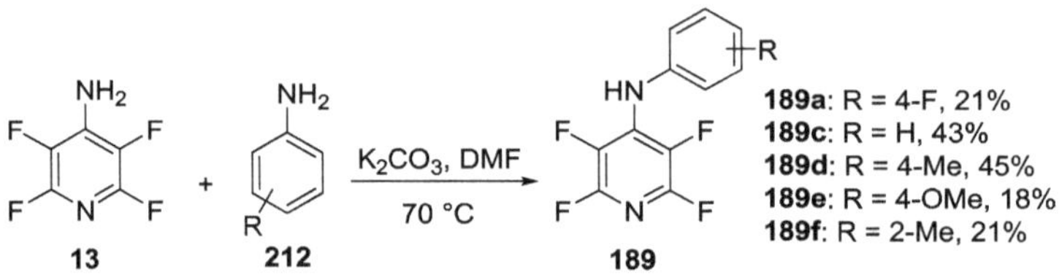

Scheme 2-69. Reaction of pentafluoropyridine **3** with aromatic amines **212**.

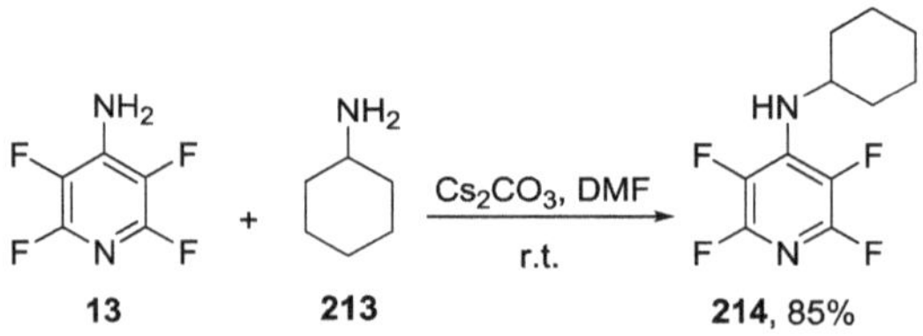

Scheme 2-70. Reaction of pentafluoropyridine **3** with cyclohexylamine **213**.

Pentafluoropyridine **3** is very reactive toward i-Pr$_2$NH at the presence of LDA in THF and gave a mixture of mono-, di- and tri-substituted products (Scheme **2-71**) [30].

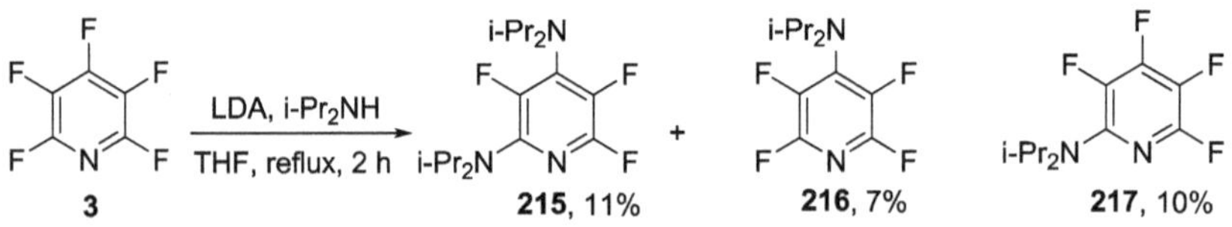

Scheme 2-71. Reaction of pentafluoropyridine **3** with i-Pr$_2$NH.

Continuous flow processes are selective methods for synthesis of a great number of industrial products for the purpose of downtime, increased control, quality control and improved safety. The latest developments in microreactor technology and the application of such devices as continuous flow reactor systems can persuade chemists to use continuous flow procedures as laboratory techniques [73]. Such systems have been designed and applied to carry out nucleophilic reactions on pentafluoropyridine (Schemes **2-72** and **2-73**) [73].

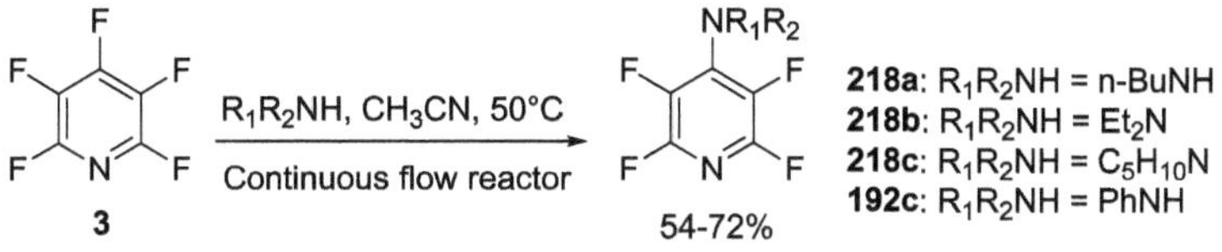

Scheme 2-72. Synthesis of 2-alkoxy-4-aminotrifluoropyridine derivatives **218** and **192c**.

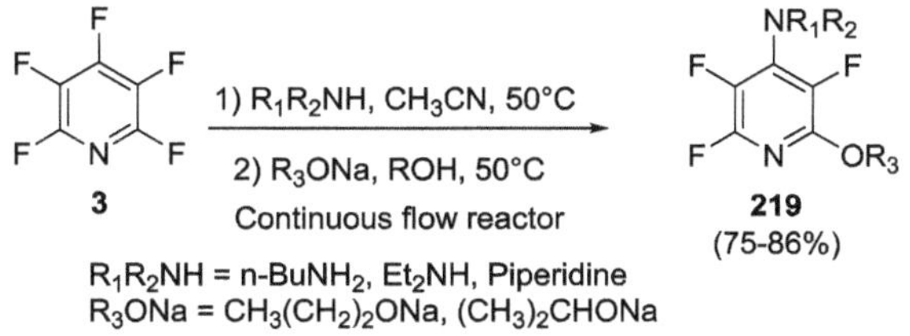

Scheme 2-73. Synthesis of 2-alkoxy-4-dialkylamino trifluoropyridine derivatives **219**.

4-(dimethylamino)pyridine **220** is a useful compound in organic chemistry because of its catalyzing, activating, and stabilizing properties [74 - 76]. It is used for activation of perhalogenated heteroaromatic compounds in order to prepare inaccessible functionalized heteroaromatics [77 - 80]. Reactions of compounds **220** with pentaflouropyridine produced pyridinum salts **221** (Scheme 2-74) as well as pentacationic species **222** used in five equivalents (Scheme 2-75) [81]. Pyridinum salt **221a** reacted successfully with O, S and N nucleophiles and produced multisubstituted pyridine derivatives (Scheme **2-76**) [81].

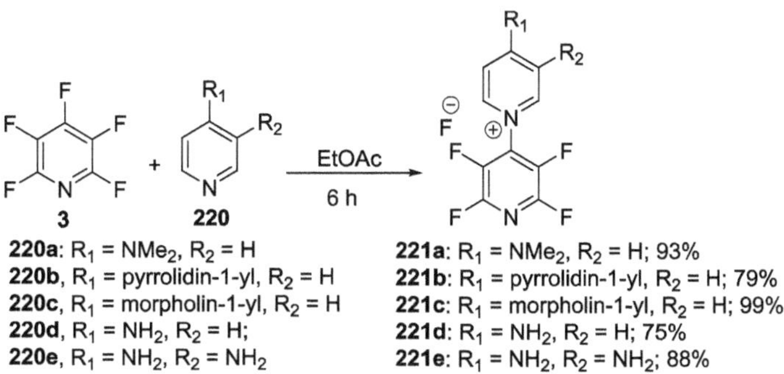

Scheme 2-74. Synthesis of perflouropyridinum salts **221**.

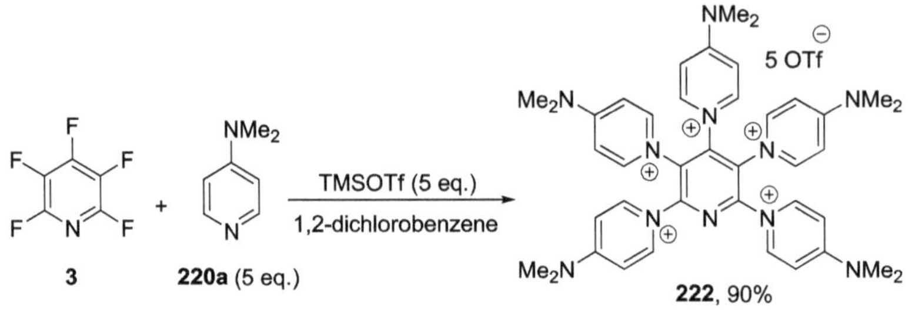

Scheme 2-75. Synthesis of pentacationic species **222**.

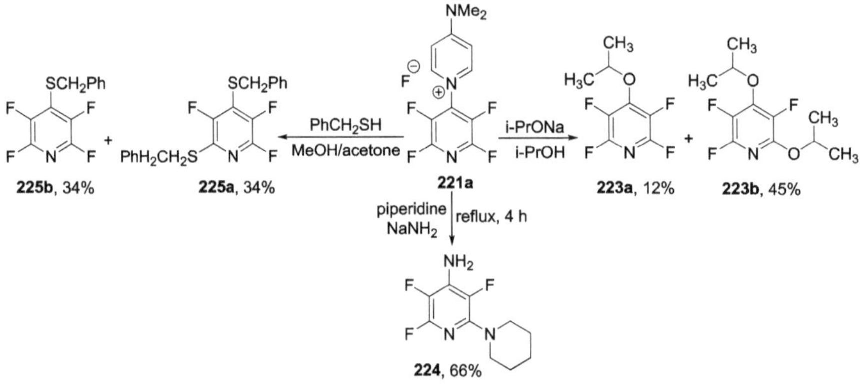

Scheme 2-76. Reaction of various nucleophiles with pyridinum salt **115a**.

Also salt **221a** was prepared from reaction of pentafluoropyridine with 4-(dimethylamino)pyridine in acetonitrile as a solvent (Scheme **2-77**) [82]. Salt **221a** acts as producer reagent of nucleophilic fluorine and produced fluorinated compounds [82].

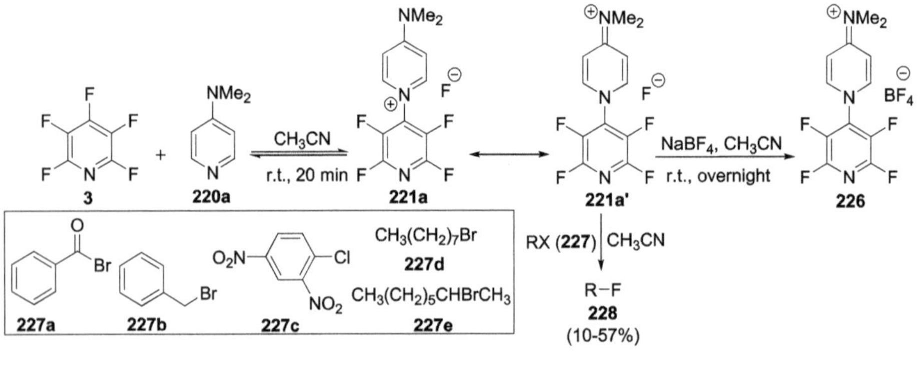

Scheme 2-77. Fluorination of organohalides using **221a′**.

4-azidotetrafluoropyridine **229** was prepared on reaction of pentafluoropyridine with NaN_3 or nitrosation of tetrafluoro-4-hydrazinopyridine **15** (Scheme **2-78**) [83]. This compound carried out simple Staudinger reaction, addition reactions to double and triple bonds and insertion to C-H bond (Scheme **2-79**) [83]. In addition, its reaction with ethylacetoacetate formed triazole compound **240** (Scheme **2-80**) [84].

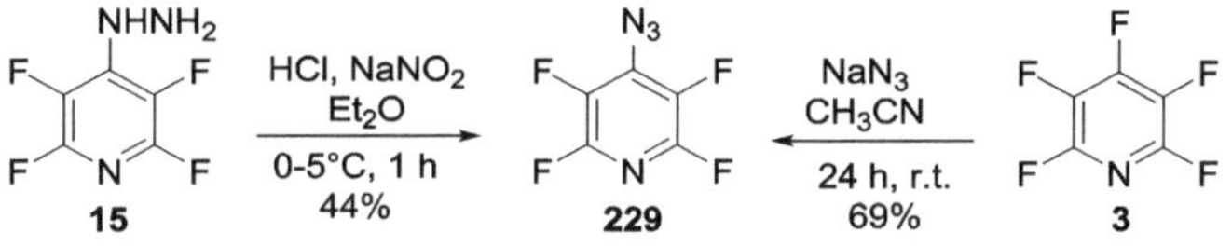

Scheme 2-78. Synthesis of 4-azidotetrafluoropyridine **229**.

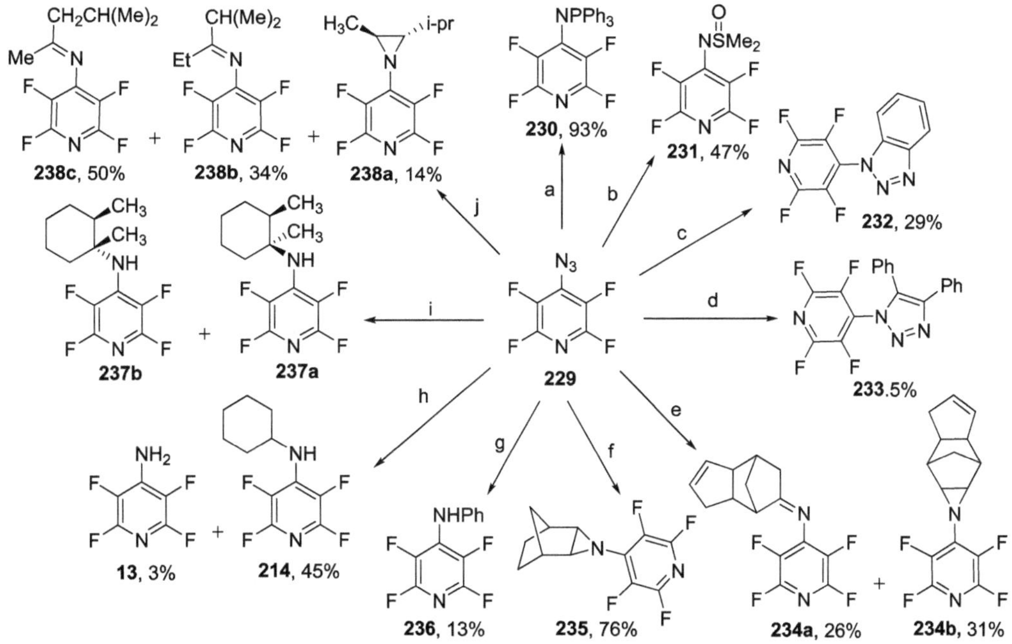

a) PPh_3, Et_2O, reflux, 4 h; b) DMSO, 160°C, <6 h; c) Anthranilic acid, acetone, CH_2Cl_2, n-butyl nitrite; d) diphenylacetyle-ne, CCl_4, reflux, 20 h; e) cyclopentadiene dimer, petroleum ether, r.t., 4 d; f) norbornene, petroleum ether, r.t., 72 h; g) benzene, 175°C, 10 h; h) cyczohexane, 170°C, 5 h; i) cis- or trans-1,2-dimethylcyclohexane, Δ; j) trans-MeCH=CHCHMe, 176°C.

Scheme 2-79. Reactions of 4-azidotetrafluoropyridine **229**.

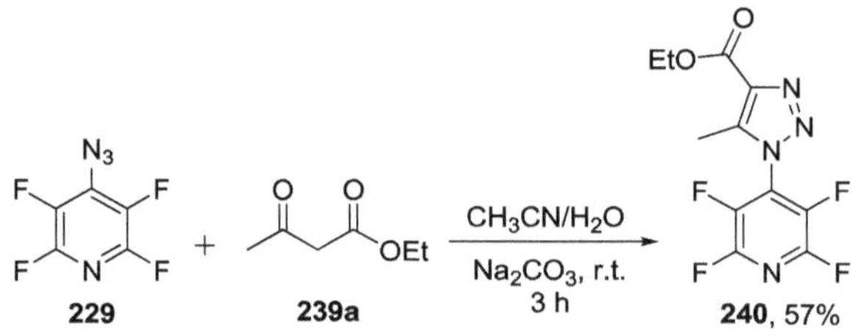

Scheme 2-80. Reactions of 4-azidotetrafluoropyridine **229** with ethylacetoacetate **239a**.

Various azide compounds can react with thiocarboxylic acids to form amide molecules with releasing elemental sulfur and nitrogen gas. Azides including electron-withdrawing groups generally react faster than the corresponding electronrich compounds [85]. 4-azidotetrafluoropyridine **229** has reacted with thioacetic acid at room temperature in high degree of chemoselectivity and gave corresponding amide **178a** (Scheme **2-81**) [85]. The proposed amidation mechanism is shown in Scheme (Scheme **2-82**).

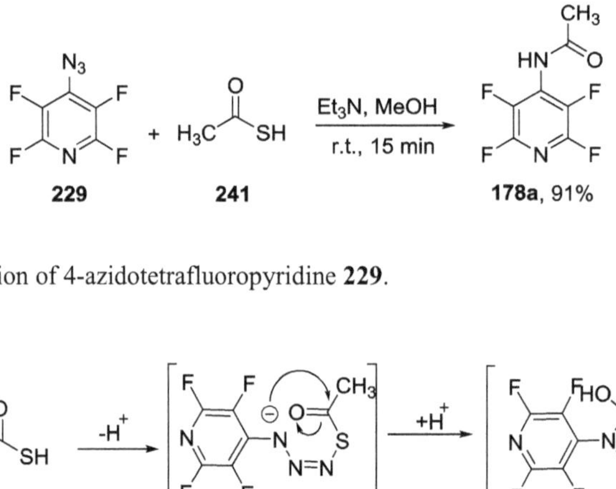

Scheme 2-81. Amidation of 4-azidotetrafluoropyridine **229**.

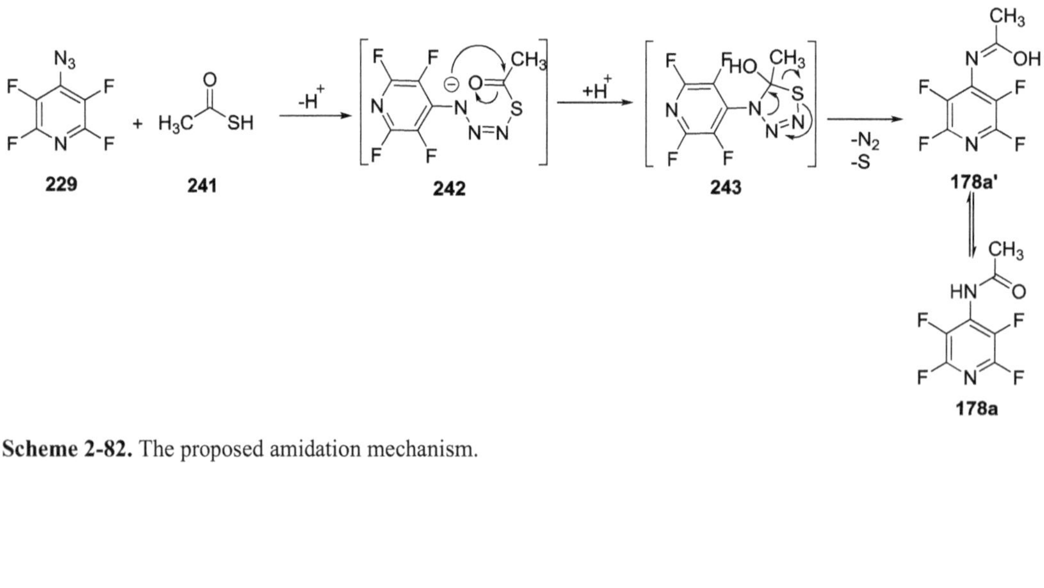

Scheme 2-82. The proposed amidation mechanism.

Tetrafluoro-4-(pentafluorophenylazo)pyridine **207e** can be achieved by reactions involving 4-azidotetrafluoropyridine and pentafluoroaniline that which converted to *N*-(pentafluorophenyl)-*N'*-(tetrafluoro-4-pyridyl) hydrazine **245** on hydrogenation by Pd-C (Scheme **2-83**) [71].

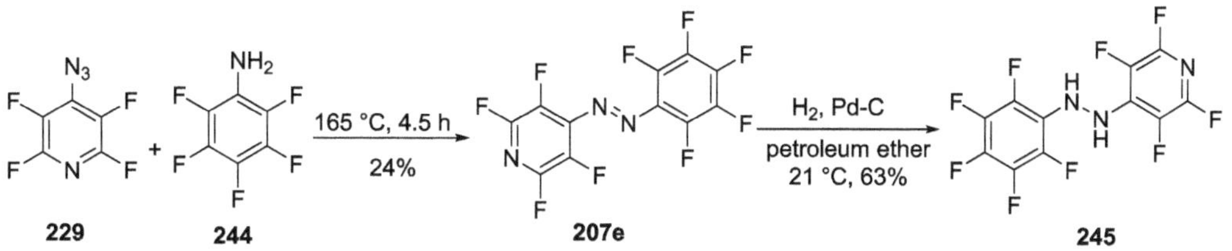

Scheme 2-83. Synthesis of tetrafluoro-4-(pentafluorophenylazo)pyridine **207e** and *N*-(pentafluorophenyl)-*N'*-(tetrafluoro-4-pyridyl)hydrazine **245**.

Reaction of 4-azidotetrafluoropyridine with pentafluoronitrosobenzene gives azoxy-compound **211d** (Scheme **2-84**) [72].

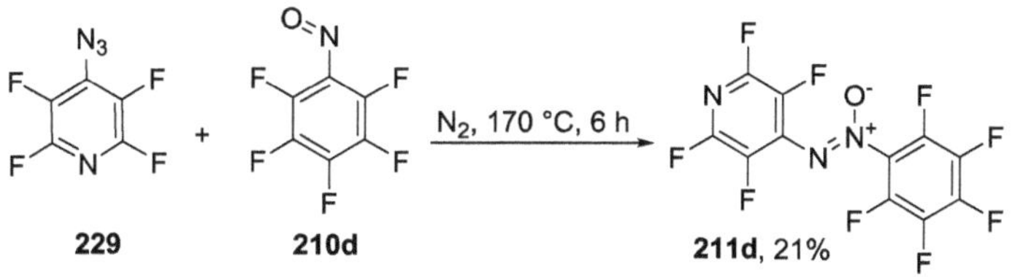

Scheme 2-84. Reaction of 4-azidotetrafluoropyridine **229** with pentafluoronitrosobenzene **210d**.

Squarilium dyes features are good solubility in low polarity solvents, a strong, narrow absorption in the Vis/NIR region, well-documented photoconducting capabilities and remarkable chemical stability [86, 87]. Reaction of hydrazone **247** with pentafluoropyridine and fallowed with squaric acid led to synthesis of pyrrolic squaraine dye **249** (Scheme **2-85**) [88].

The reaction of xanthate **3** with *N*-protected-*N*-allyl-4-aminotetrafluoropyridines **250** and **251** lead to compounds **253** and **245a** respectively, which upon treatment with lauroyl peroxide (DLP) giving mixture of azaindolines **263** and **264a** respectively (Scheme **2-86**) [89]. Similarly, the syntheses of azafluoroindolines **264b-j** were carried out by the reaction of xanthates **252b-j** with perfluoropyridine **251** (Scheme **2-87**).

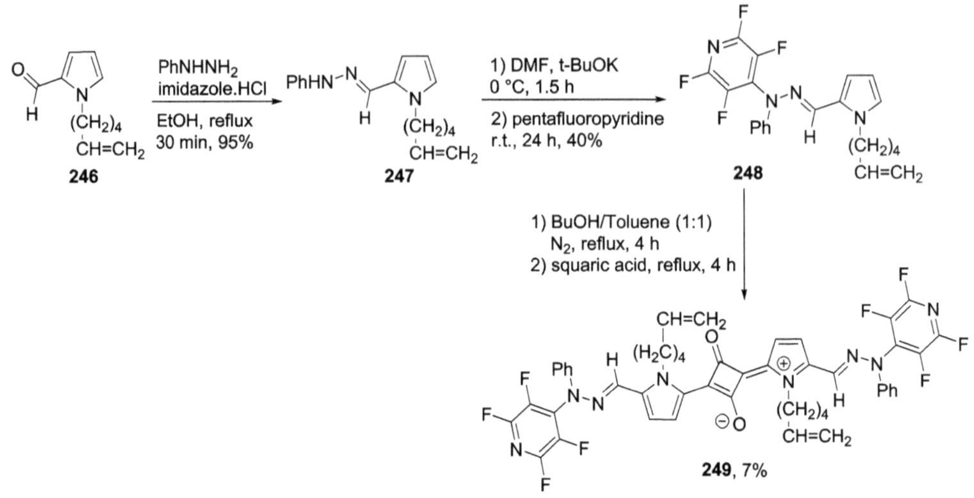

Scheme 2-85. Synthesis of perfluoropyridine-pyrrolic squaraine dye **249**.

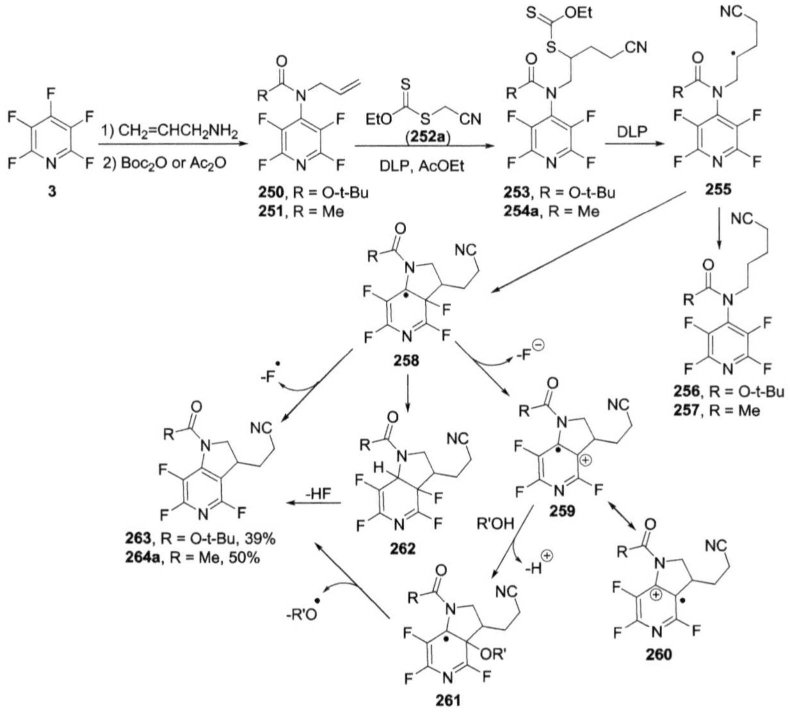

Scheme 2-86. Synthesis of azafluoroindoline by a radical ipso cyclization and fluorine atom elimination.

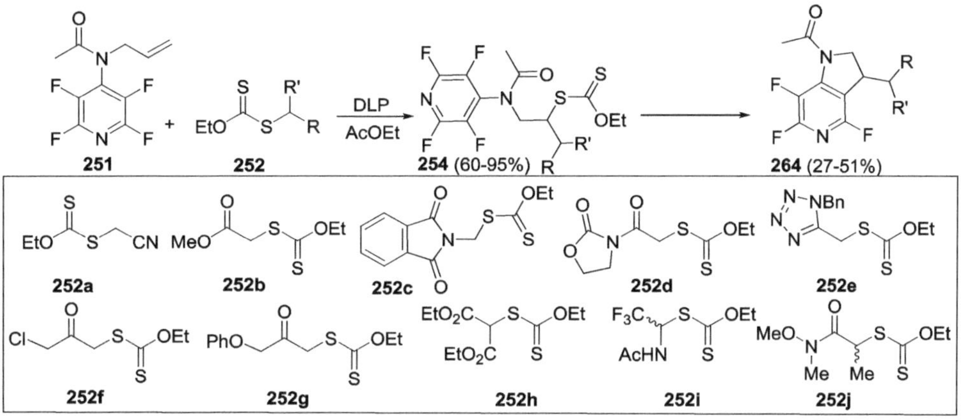

Scheme 2-87. Formation of fluoroazaindolines **264**.

The reaction of 2-*N*-allylamine pyridine with xanthate **252a** results in the formation of compound **266** [89], which converted to difluoroazaindoline **267** *via* a radical ipso cyclization-demethylation (scheme 2-**88**). The proposed mechanism for formation of 267 shown in scheme (2-**89**).

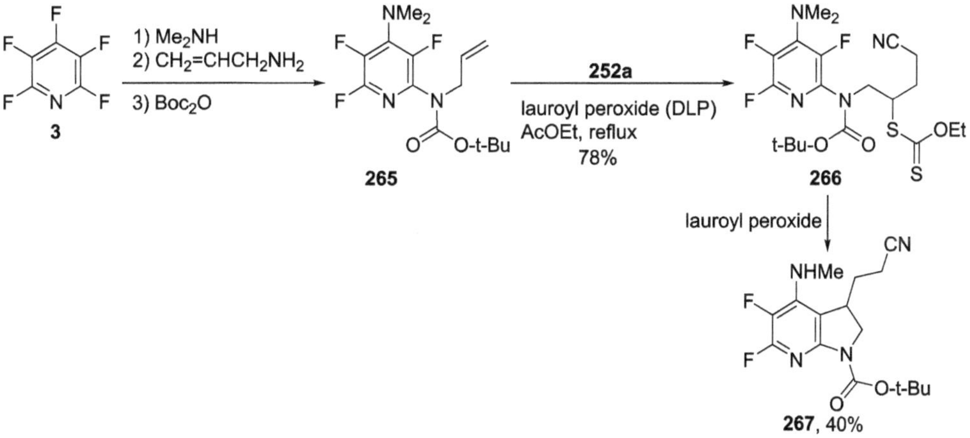

Scheme 2-88. Radical ipso cyclization-demethylation.

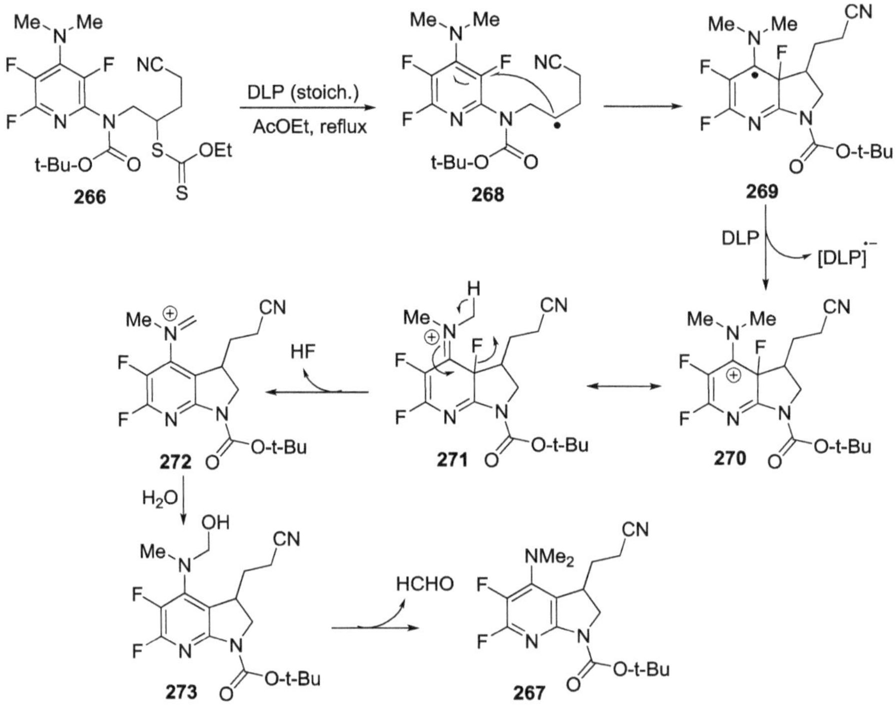

Scheme 2-89. The plausible mechanism for radical ipso cyclization-demethylation.

Azaindoles and related derivatives have attracted considerable interest in organic synthesis and medicinal chemistry [90 - 97]. The classical indole syntheses are not easily led to synthesis of their aza analogues, due to the limited availability of the essential precursors and reactivity problems. Zard and co-workers have reported the preparation of fluoroazaindolines *via* useful radical *ipso*-substitution of a carbon–fluorine bond [98]. 7-Azaindolines **276-278** have been prepared by lauroyl peroxide (DLP) initiated radical addition of xanthate **252k** to carbamate protected 2-*N*-allylamine pyridine **274a** and **274b**, that which easily accessible from pentafluoropyridine (2-**90**). Radical addition of xanthates to acetyl protected 2-*N*-allylamine pyridines leading to formation of 7-azainolines and 7-azaindoles (Table **2-1**). Similarly, corresponding compound **283** leads to 7-azainoline **285** and 7-azaindole **286** (Scheme **2-91**).

Table 2-1. Synthesis of 7-azaindolines 281 and 7-azaindoles 282 by using 4-amino perfluoropyridine derivatives 279.

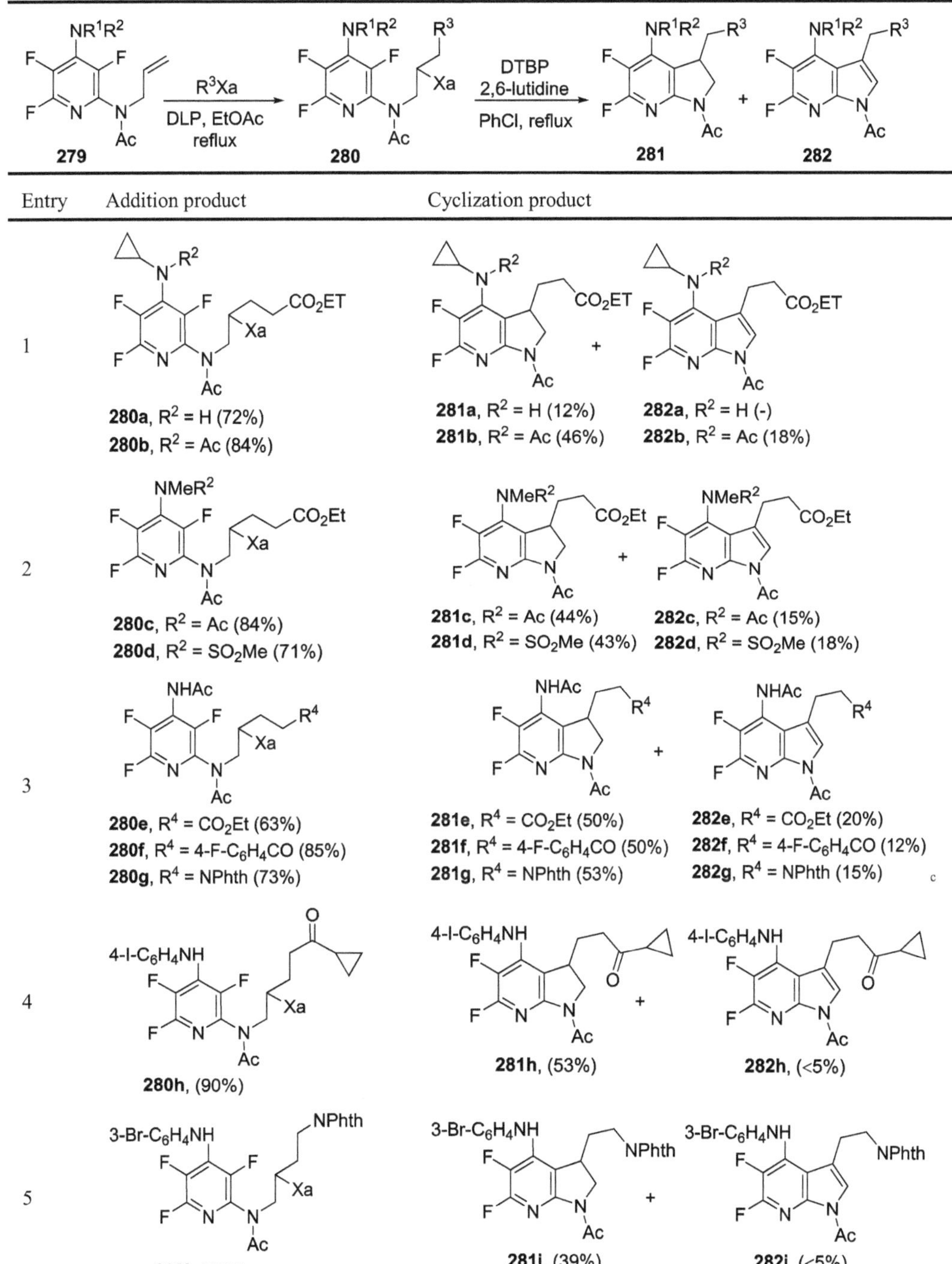

Entry	Addition product	Cyclization product
1	**280a**, R^2 = H (72%) **280b**, R^2 = Ac (84%)	**281a**, R^2 = H (12%) **282a**, R^2 = H (-) **281b**, R^2 = Ac (46%) **282b**, R^2 = Ac (18%)
2	**280c**, R^2 = Ac (84%) **280d**, R^2 = SO$_2$Me (71%)	**281c**, R^2 = Ac (44%) **282c**, R^2 = Ac (15%) **281d**, R^2 = SO$_2$Me (43%) **282d**, R^2 = SO$_2$Me (18%)
3	**280e**, R^4 = CO$_2$Et (63%) **280f**, R^4 = 4-F-C$_6$H$_4$CO (85%) **280g**, R^4 = NPhth (73%)	**281e**, R^4 = CO$_2$Et (50%) **282e**, R^4 = CO$_2$Et (20%) **281f**, R^4 = 4-F-C$_6$H$_4$CO (50%) **282f**, R^4 = 4-F-C$_6$H$_4$CO (12%) **281g**, R^4 = NPhth (53%) **282g**, R^4 = NPhth (15%)
4	**280h**, (90%)	**281h**, (53%) **282h**, (<5%)
5	**280i**, (72%)	**281i**, (39%) **282i**, (<5%)

(Table 2-1) cont.....

6	**280j**, (53%)	**281j**, (38%) +	**282j**, (14%)
7	**280k**, (56%)	**281k**, (38%) +	**282k**, (19%)
8	**280l**, (82%)	**281l**, (61%) +	**282l**, (18%)
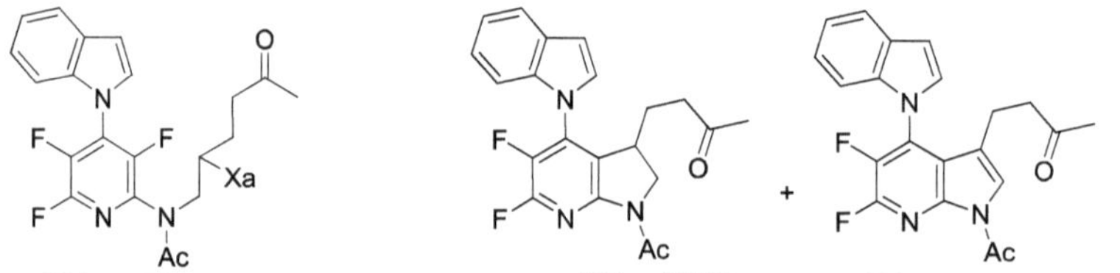	**280m**, (75%)	**281m**, (42%) +	**282m**, (18%)

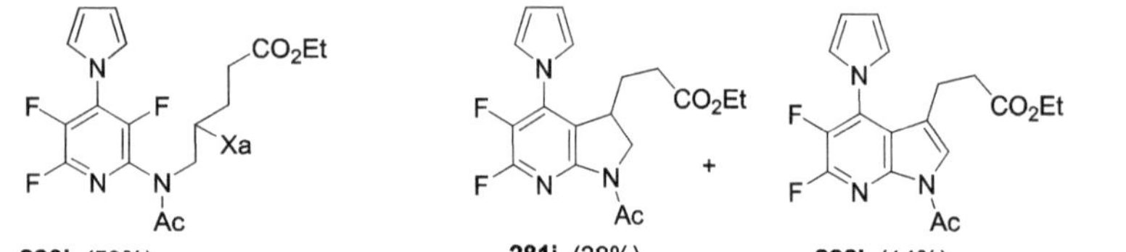

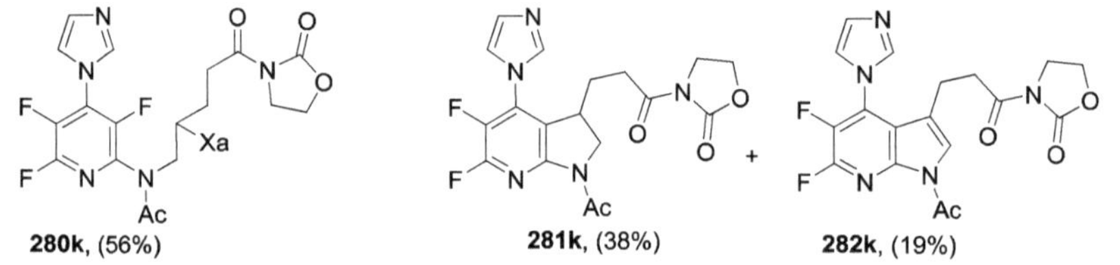

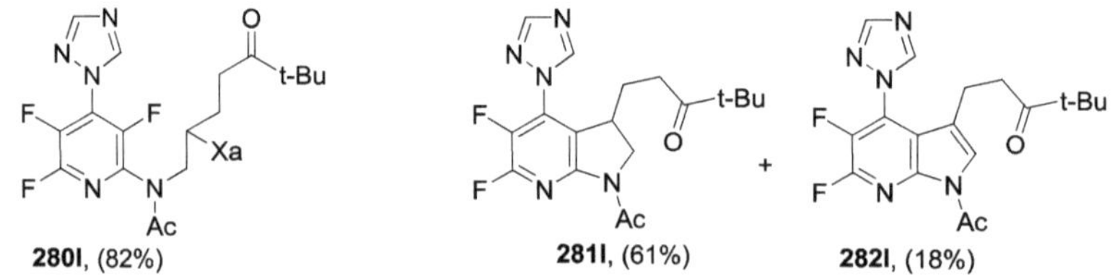

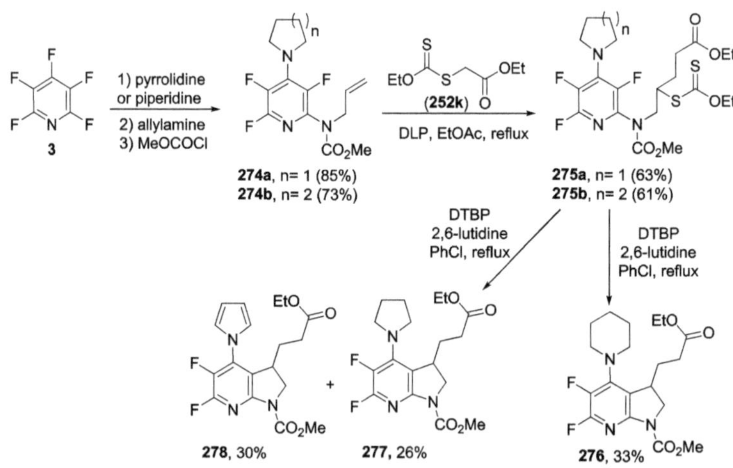

278, 30%   +   **277**, 26%   **276**, 33%

274a, n= 1 (85%)
274b, n= 2 (73%)

275a, n= 1 (63%)
275b, n= 2 (61%)

Scheme 2-90. Synthesis of 7-azaindolines.

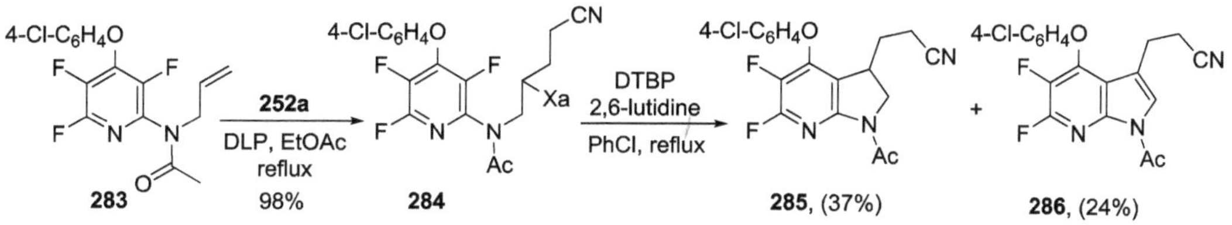

Scheme 2-91. Synthesis of 7-azaindoline **285** and 7-azaindole **286** by 4-aryloxy perfluoropyridine **283**.

Radical addition of compound **252l** to **287** resulted in low yield formation of tetrahydro-azaquinolines **289** (Scheme **2-92**) [98].

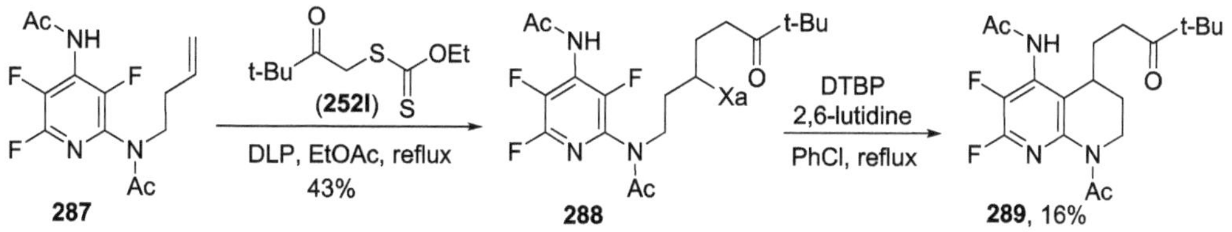

Scheme 2-92. Synthesis of tetrahydro-azaquinoline **289**.

N-perfluoropyridyl-*S*,*S*-diphenylsulfilamines **291** and **292** can be achieved by reactions involving *S*,*S*-diphenylsulfilimine, pentafluoropyridine and 2,3,5,6-tetrafluoropyridine, respectively *via* nucleophilic attack on 4- and 2-postions of pyridine ring (Scheme **2-93**) [99].

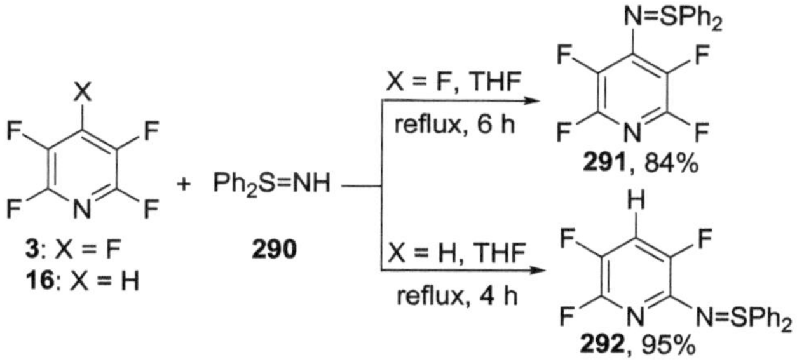

Scheme 2-93. Synthesis of N-perfluoropyridyl-S,S-diphenylsulfilamines **291** and **292**.

4.5. Reaction of Pentafluoropyridine 3 with Halogenating Reagents (Cl, Br, I)

Bromination of pentafluoropyridine and 4-isoperfluoropropyl tetrafluoropyridine **80** has been carried out *via* heating each in excess of HBr and AlBr$_3$ (Schemes **2-94** and **2-95**) [100].

Scheme 2-94. Bromination of pentafluoropyridine **3**.

Scheme 2-95. Bromination of 4-isopropyltetrafluoropyridine **80**.

Reactions of bromofluoropyridine **137** are based on hardness or softness of nucleophiles. The hard nucleophiles attack on the C–F bond and the soft nucleophiles attack on the C–Br bond of compound **137** (Scheme **2-96**) [100].

Scheme 2-96. Reaction of compound **294** with various nucleophiles.

Compounds **137** and **293** undergo metathesis with *n*-BuLi and gives corresponding lithium reagent [100, 101]. These lithium reagents as nucleophiles can be reacted with electrophiles species (Schemes **2-97** and **2-98**).

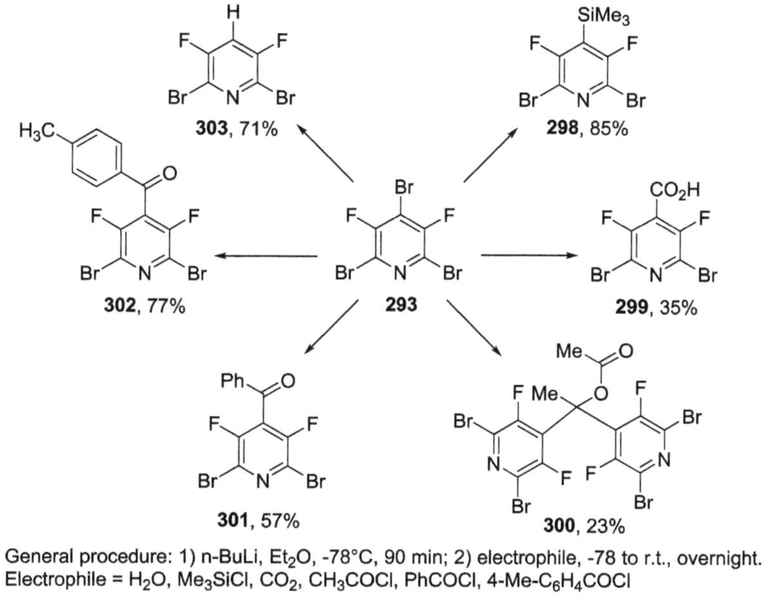
303, 71%
298, 85%
302, 77%
293
299, 35%
301, 57%
300, 23%
General procedure: 1) n-BuLi, Et2O, -78°C, 90 min; 2) electrophile, -78 to r.t., overnight.
Electrophile = H2O, Me3SiCl, CO2, CH3COCl, PhCOCl, 4-Me-C6H4COCl

Scheme 2-97. Preparation and reactions of lithium reagent of 2,4,6-tribromo-3,4-difluoropyridine **293**.

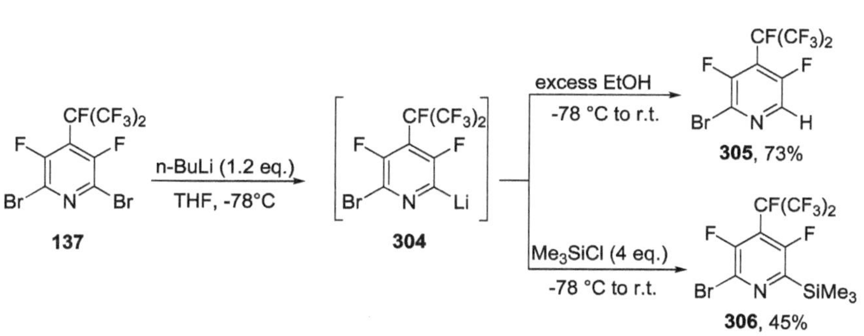
n-BuLi (1.2 eq.)
THF, -78°C
137
304
excess EtOH
-78 °C to r.t.
305, 73%
Me3SiCl (4 eq.)
-78 °C to r.t.
306, 45%

Scheme 2-98. Preparation and reactions of lithium reagent of compound **137**.

Also, compounds **137** and **293** carried out cross-coupling reactions and produce alkylethynyl and aryl fluoropyridines, respectively (Schemes **2-99** and **2-100**) [100].

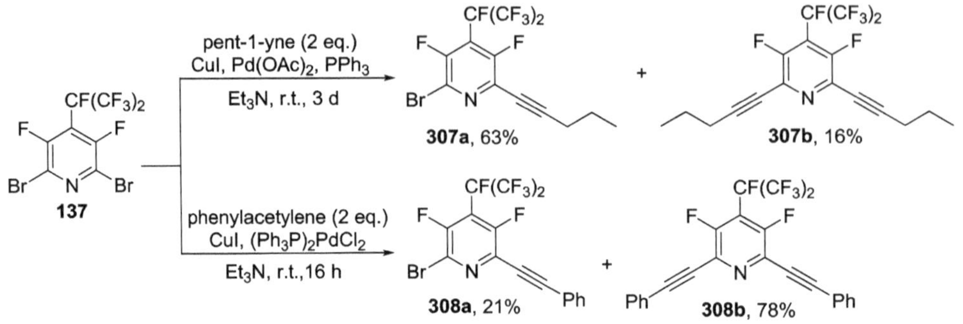

Scheme 2-99. Cross-coupling reactions of **137** with acetylens.

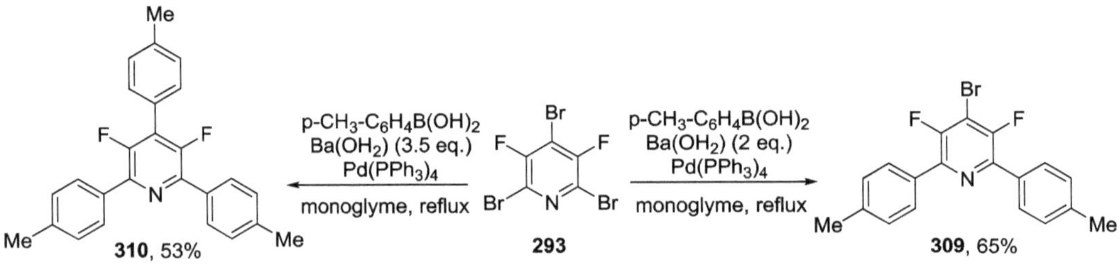

Scheme 2-100. Cross-coupling reactions of **293** with arylbronic acide.

2,3,5,6-tetrafluoro-4-iodopyridine **311** has obtained from the reaction of pentafluoropyridine with sodium iodide or oxidation of 2.3.5.6-tetrafluoro-4-hydrazinopyridine **15** (Scheme **2-101**) [102]. Compound **311** readily converted into 2,3,5,6-tetrafluoropyridylrnagnesium iodide or 2,3,5,6-tetrafluoropyridyllithium, which reacted with electrophilic types and gives various substituted perfluoropyridines (Scheme **2-102**). In addition, it has been afforded perfluoro-4.4'-bipyridyl by the Ullmann technique.

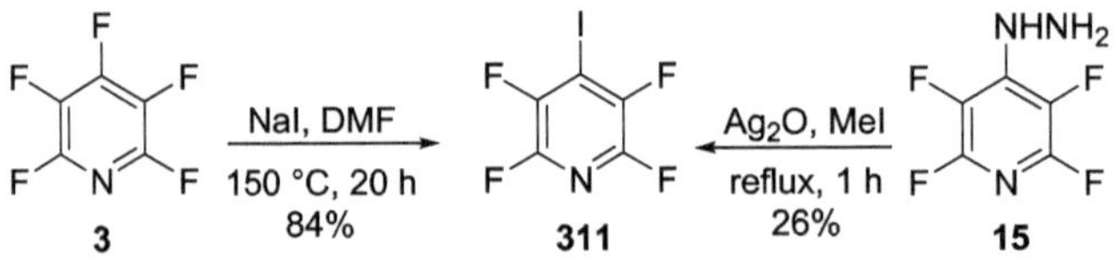

Scheme 2-101. Synthesis of tetrafluoro-4-iodopyridine **311**.

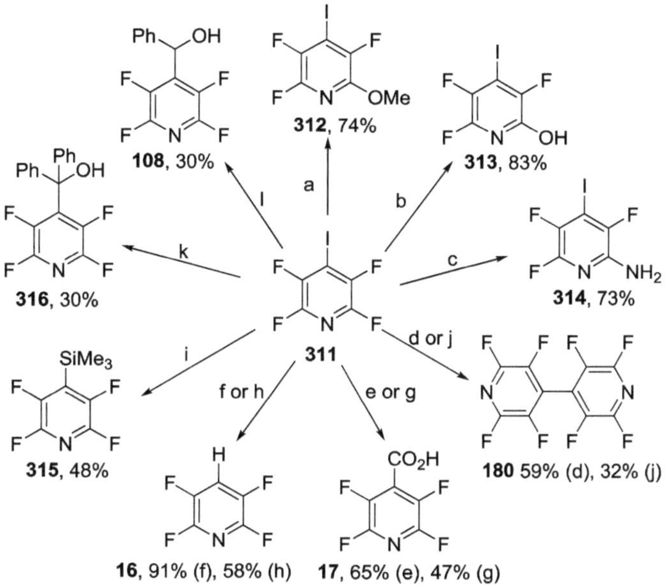

Scheme 2-102. Various reactions of tetrafluoro-4-iodopyridine **311**.

a) NaOMe, MeOH, 20 °C, 1h; b) KOH, t-BuOH, reflux, 2 h; c) aq. NH$_3$, 80-90 °C, 27 h; d) Cu, 200 °C, 27 h; e) n-BuLi, -35 °C, Et$_2$O/benzene, 4 h; then CO$_2$, -10 °C; f) NaI, DMF, 150 °C, 40 h; g) Mg, THF, r.t., 30 min; then -15 °C, 2 h; then CO$_2$, 2 h; h) Mg, THF, r.t., -15 °C, 3.5 h and -5 °C, 1.5 h; then H$_2$SO$_4$; i) Mg, THF, -15 °C, 6 h; then Me$_3$SiCl, -15 °C, 2 h and r.t., 1 h; j) Mg, THF; then pentafluoropyridine, -40 °C, 3 h; k) Mg, THF; then Ph$_2$CO, -20 °C, 3h; l) Mg, THF; then PhCHO, -15 to -15 °C.

Scheme 2-102. Various reactions of tetrafluoro-4-iodopyridine **311**.

Pentafluoropyridine **3** have been chlorinated selectively at the 4-position by benzyltributylammonium chloride in the presence of TMSCl to afford **318** in quantitative yield by ^{19}F NMR (Scheme **2-103**) [103]. 4-chlorotetrafluoropyridine **318** has the potential for coupling reactions that would be difficult or impossible with the fluoroarene starting material (Scheme **2-104**) [103]. In contrast to pentafluoropyridine that carried out substitution reaction with lithiates, **318** underwent halogen–lithium exchange, and gave smooth addition to benzaldehyde (Scheme **2-104**).

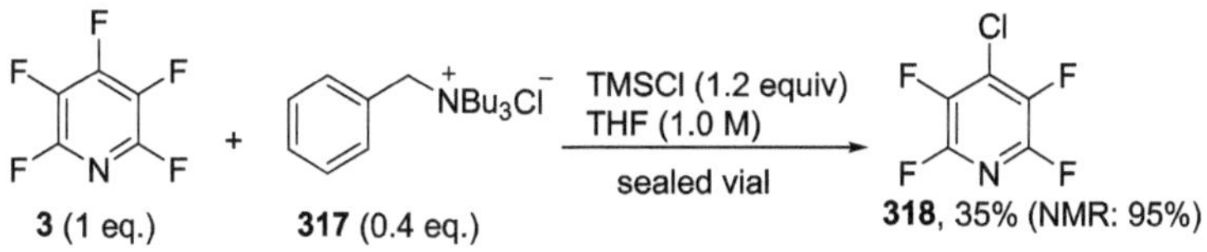

Scheme 2-103. The catalytic chlorination of pentafluoropyridine **3**.

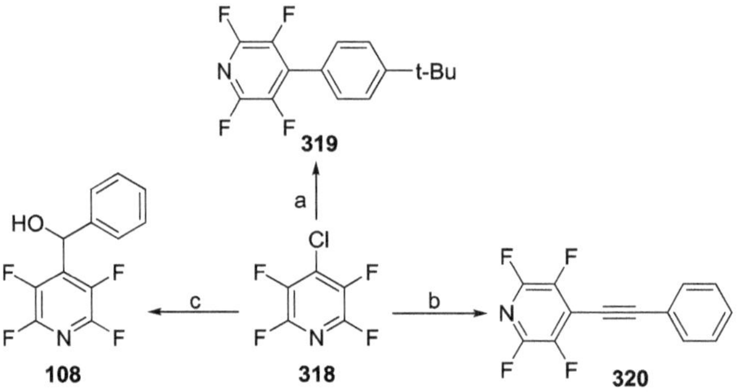

a) 4-t-Bu-C$_6$H$_4$B(OH)$_2$ 1.2 equiv, Pd(OAc) 5 mol%, PPh$_3$ 10 mol%, K$_2$CO$_3$ 207 equiv, DME 0.75 M, sealed vial, 80 °C, Ar, overnight, 70%; b) phenylacetylene 1.2 equiv, Pd(pph)$_2$Cl$_2$ 2 mol%, Cs$_2$CO$_3$ 1 equiv, t-Bu$_3$P 4 mol%, DBU 10 mol%, DMF 0.3 M, MW reactor, 150 °C, 10 min, 80%; c) BuLi 1.2 equiv, THF 0.5 M, -78 °C and then PhCHO 1.2 equiv, 62%

Scheme 2-104. Synthetic utility of 4-chlorotetrafluoropyridine **318**.

4.6. Reduction of Perfluorinated Pyridines

Reduction of pentafluoropyridine with LiAlH$_4$ or diisobutylaluminium hydride (DIBAL) gives rise to compounds **16**, **321** and **322** [104]. Substitution of hydrogen has been mainly occurred at the 4-position of pyridine ring using LiAlH$_4$ in the presence of crown ether or DIBAL (Scheme **2-105**). 3,5-dichlorotrifluoropyridine **85** has efficiently converted to 2,3,5,6-tetrafluoropyridine on reaction with DIBAL (Scheme **2-106**).

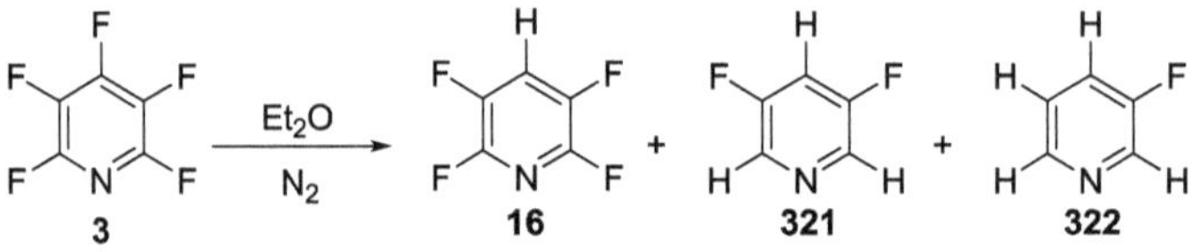

	16	321	322
a:	40%	30%	20%
b:	70%	30%	
c:	77%		

a) LiAlH$_4$, Et$_2$O, N$_2$, 0 °C, then r.t., 28 h; b) LiAlH$_4$, N$_2$, Et$_2$O, 12-crown-4 polyether, 0 °C, then r.t., 19 h; c) DIBAL, diglyme, 100 °C, 24 h

Scheme 2-105. Reduction of pentafluoropyridine **3** under different conditions.

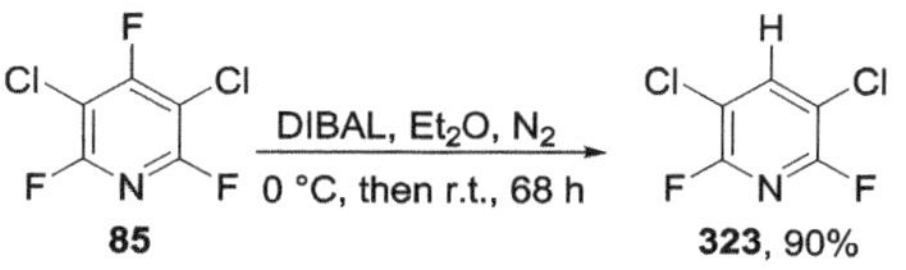

Scheme 2-106. Reduction of 3,5-dichlorotrifluoropyridine **85**.

The catalytic homogeneous hydrodefluorination (HDF) reactions of pentafluoropyridine have proceeded regioselectively at the *para* C-F bond of pyridine ring using a nickel catalyst and triethyl phosphine and results in formation of 2,4,5,6-tetrafluoropyridine **16** (Scheme **2-107**) [105].

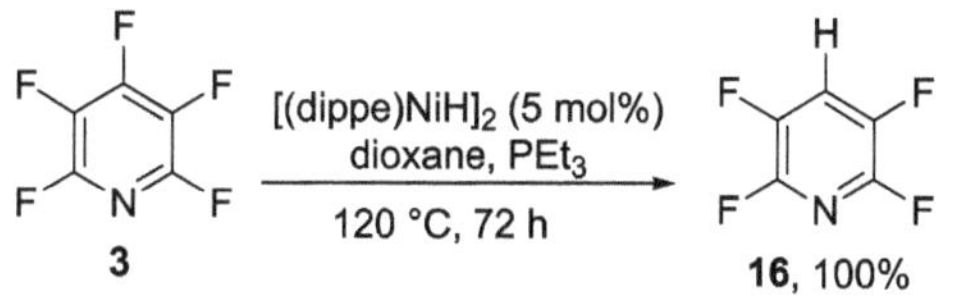

Scheme 2-107. Hydrodefluorination of pentafluoropyridine **3**.

3-chlorotetrafluoropyridine **5** underwent reduction at C-Cl bond using 0.5% palladium on alumina produced 2,3,4,6-tetrafluoropyridine **324** (Scheme **2-108**) [106].

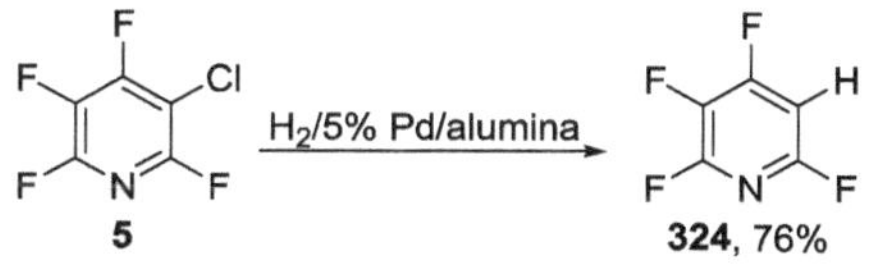

Scheme 2-108. Reduction of 3-chlorotetrafluoropyridine **324** with Pd/alumina.

The removal of fluorine from polyfluoropyridines **3** and **5** proceeded selectively at 4-F position of ring by Zn and $NaBH_4$, respectively, (Schemes **2-109** and **2-110**) [107]. Compounds **5** and **85** have been underwent removal of chlorine by Pd/C in the presence of ammonium formate as the hydrogen source (Schemes 2 - 110 and 2 - 111) [107].

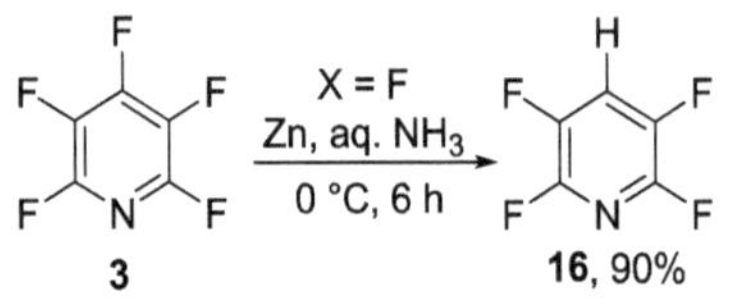

Scheme 2-109. Reduction of pentafluoropyridine **3** with Zn/NH$_3$.

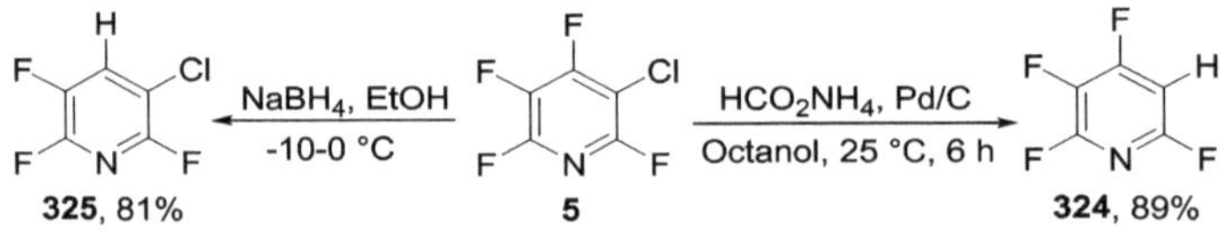

Scheme 2-110. Reduction of 3-chloro-2,4,5,6-tetrafluoropyridine **325** using Pd/C and NaBH$_4$.

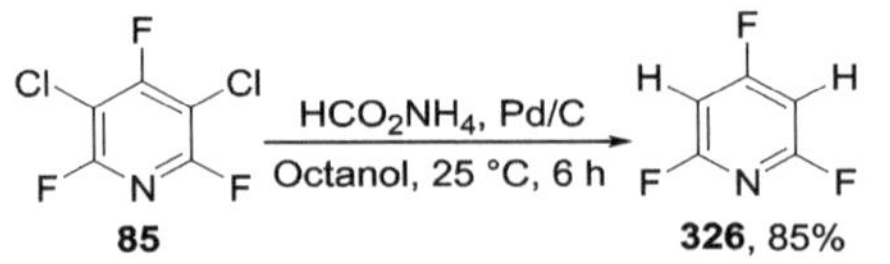

Scheme 2-111. Reduction of 3,5-dichloro-2,4,6-trifluoropyridine **85**.

Compounds **323** and **325** on treatment with hydrazine monohydrate gives 2-hydrazino derivatives (Schemes 2 - 112 and 2 - 113), while compound **324** results in the formation of 4-hydrazinotrifluoropyridine **329** (Scheme 2 - 114) [107].

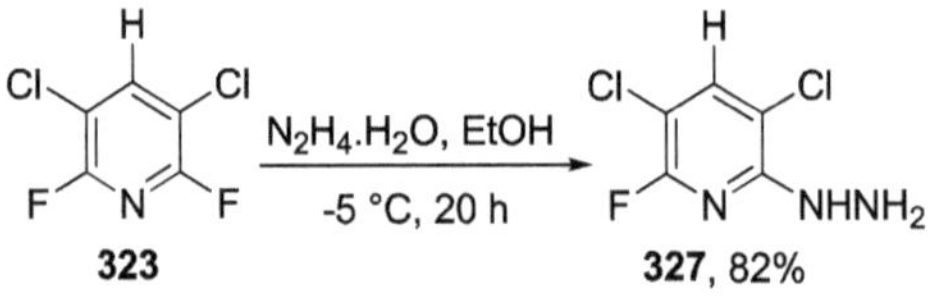

Scheme 2-112. Reaction of compound **323** with hydrazine monohydrate.

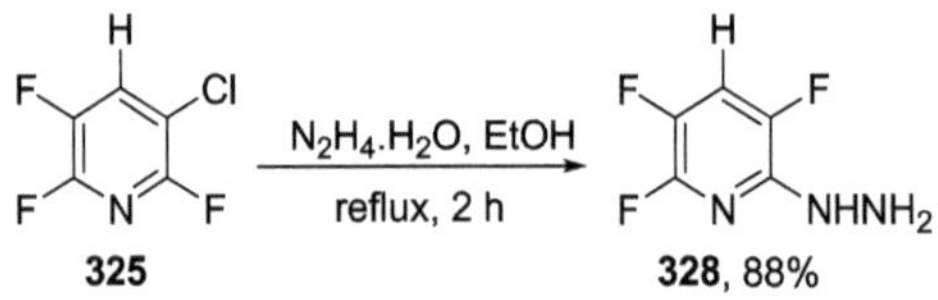

Scheme 2-113. Reaction of compound **325** with hydrazine monohydrate.

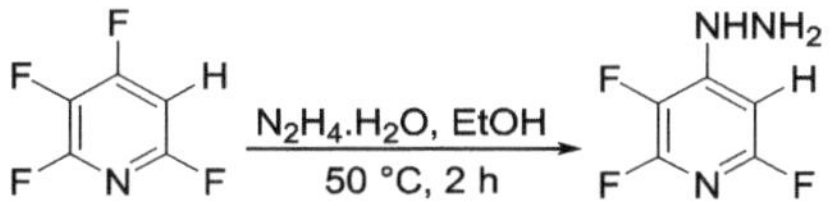

Scheme 2-114. Reaction of compound **324** with hydrazine monohydrate.

5. REACTION OF PERFLUOROPYRIDINES WITH VARIOUS MULTIDENTATE NUCLEOPHILES

5.1. Synthesis of Perfluorinated Heterocyles

Reaction of perfluorinated compounds with various nucleophiles produced range of products depending on the hardness or softness of nucleophile. Generally, the soft nucleophiles prefer the softer C-F bonds and the hard nucleophiles prefer the harder nucleophiles. Chambers *et al.* have been suggested the explanation of the 'hardness' and 'softness' of nucleophiles for determination of the attack position in polyfluorinated pyridines [101, 104]. Base on hard–hard interaction principle, the reaction of pentafluoropyridine with enolates has been selectively occured at the 4-position of pyridine ring by the oxygen site of enolate (Scheme 2 - 115) [108].

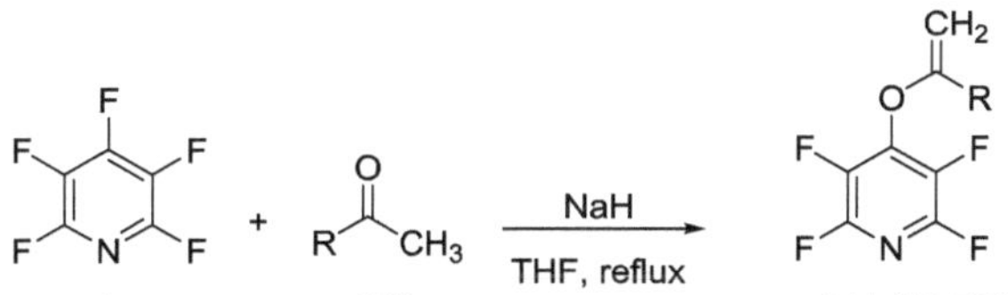

R = aryl and heteroaryl

Scheme 2-115. Reaction of various enolates with pentafluoropyridine **3**.

Anion derived from ethylacetoacetate reacts with pentafluoropyridine from C site and produced non-cyclic product **342** (Scheme 2 - 116) [109].

3 **239a** **342**, 8%

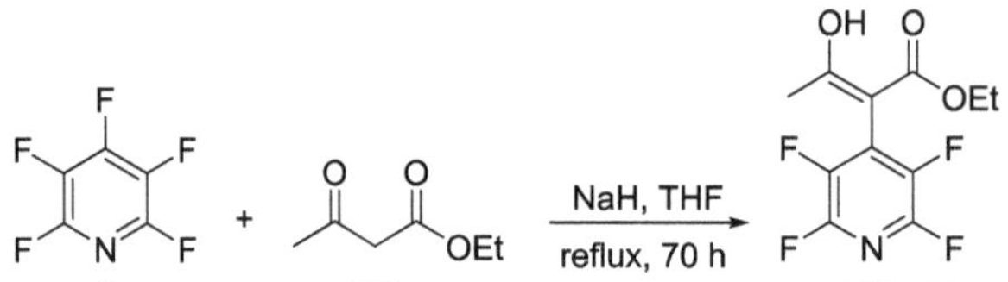

Scheme 2-116. Reaction of pentafluoropyridine **3** with ethylacetoacetate **239a**.

The oxazolone enolate is capable to participation in nucleophilic aromatic substitution and be utilized for synthesis of non-natural fluorinated amino acid derivatives [110]. Reaction of oxazolone enolates with pentafluoropyridine occurs preferentially by nucleophilic attack at the 4-position of pyridine ring (Scheme 2 - 117).

3 (1.025 eq.) **343** (1.0 eq.) **344**

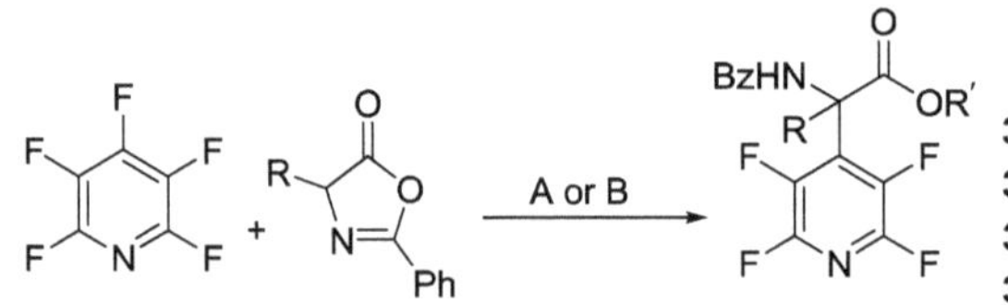

344a: A, R = H, R' = Et, 79%
344b: B, R = CH_3, R' = Me, 80%
344c: B, R = $(CH_3)_2CHCH_2$, R' = Me, 74%
344d: B, R = $PhCH_2$, R' = Me, 71%
344e: B, R = $CH_3SCH_2CH_2$, R' = Me, 79%

A: 1) TMG (2.05 equiv.), CH_3CN, -20 °C, 0.5 h; 2) TFA, EtOH, 1 h.
B: 1) DIPEA (210 equiv.), CH_3CN, 0.5 h; 2) TFA, MeOH.

Scheme 2-117. Synthesis of *N*-benzoyl perfluoroaryl-amino esters **344**.

Substitution of 4-chlorotetrafluoropyridine **318** with enolate anion derived from **343a** occurs primarily at the C-Cl bond rather than C-F bond (Scheme 2 - 118) [110].

318 (1.2 eq.) **343a** (1 eq.) **344a** (ratio 3:1) **345**

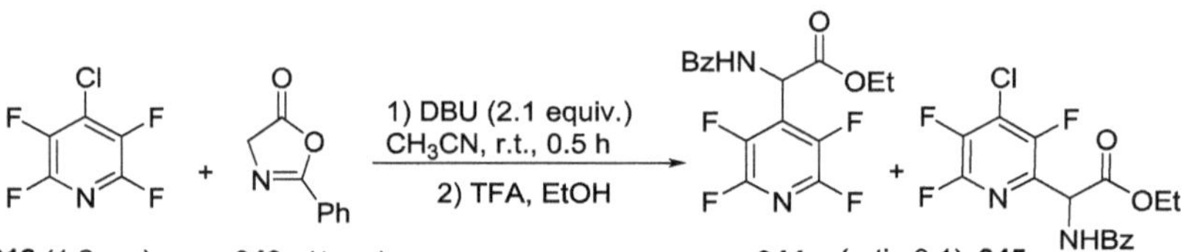

Scheme 2-118. Reaction of oxazolone **2a** with 4-chlorotetrafluoropyridine **318**.

Reaction of oxazolone **343a** with 3-chlorotetrafluoropyridine **5** was shown a preference for substitution of the 4-fluoro over 3-chloro as leaving group (Scheme

2 - 119) [110].

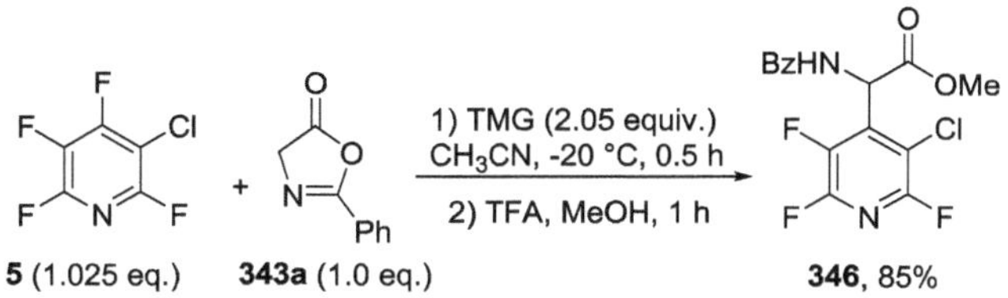

Scheme 2-119. Synthesis of *N*-benzoyl perfluoroaryl-amino ester **346**.

The amino acid derivatives **348a** and **348b** are formed by the reaction of pentafluoropyridine with oxaxolone **343a** in the acidic condition, which were further thermal decarboxylation to give aminium chlorides **349a** and **349b** in acetone after 1 h (Scheme 2-**120**) [110].

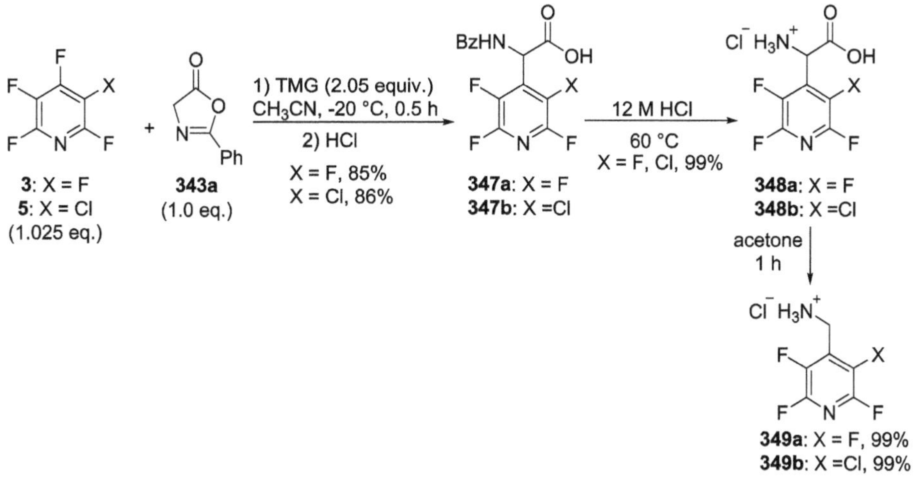

Scheme 2-120. Synthesis of (perfluoropyridin-4-yl)methanaminium chloride **349**.

In the presence of 1,1,3,3-tetramethylguanidine (TMG) as the base, the ring opening to *N*-acylated guanidines has been occurred after perfluoroarylation, which upon heating in HCl underwent debenzoylation and cyclization to products **350a-c** (Scheme 2-**121**) [110].

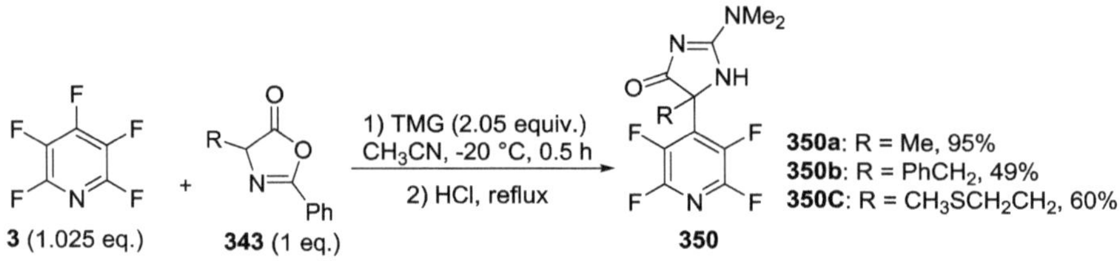

Scheme 2-121. Synthesis of 2-aminohydantoins **350**.

Unsubstituted and substituted Meldrum's Acids (MAs) **351** have been directly reacted with pentafluoropyridine and 3-chloro-2,4,5,6-tetrafluoropyridine **5** from C site in the presence of diisopropylethylamine (DIPEA) and produced ammonium enolate salts **352** and **353** (Schemes 2 - 122 and 2 - 123) [111].

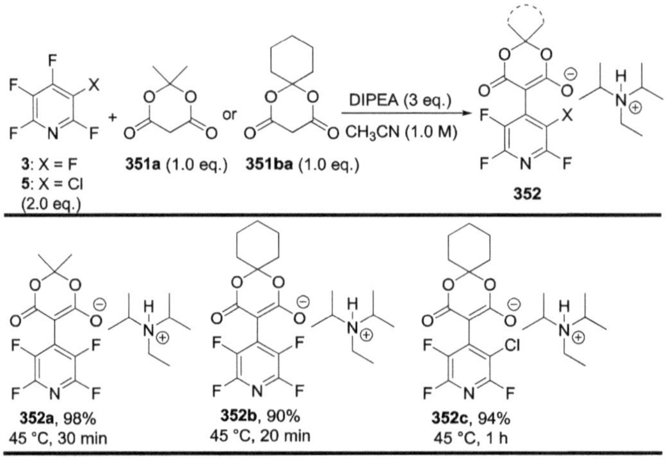

Scheme 2-122. Reaction of unsubstituted MA with perfluoropyridines **3** and **5**.

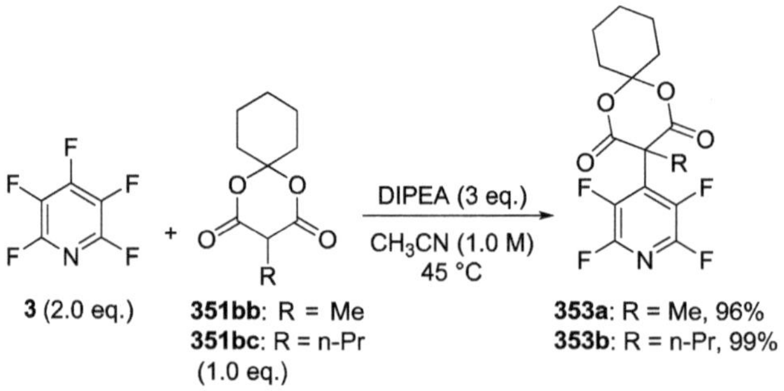

Scheme 2-123. Reaction of substituted MAs with pentafluoropyridine **3**.

The Meldrum's Acid adducts are stable under basic conditions and under acidic conditions underwent hydrolysis and nucleophilic addition. Under acidic conditions, nucleophilic attack of the carbonyl group of ammonium enolate salt **352ba** leads to the ring opening along with decarboxylation (Scheme 2-**124**) [111]. In addition, this salt under acidic condition reacts with amines giving corresponding acetamides (Scheme 2-**125**) [62].

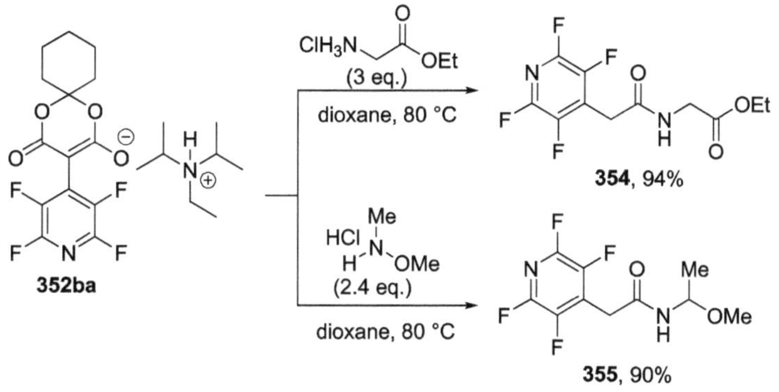

Scheme 2-124. Reactions of **352ba** under acidic conditions.

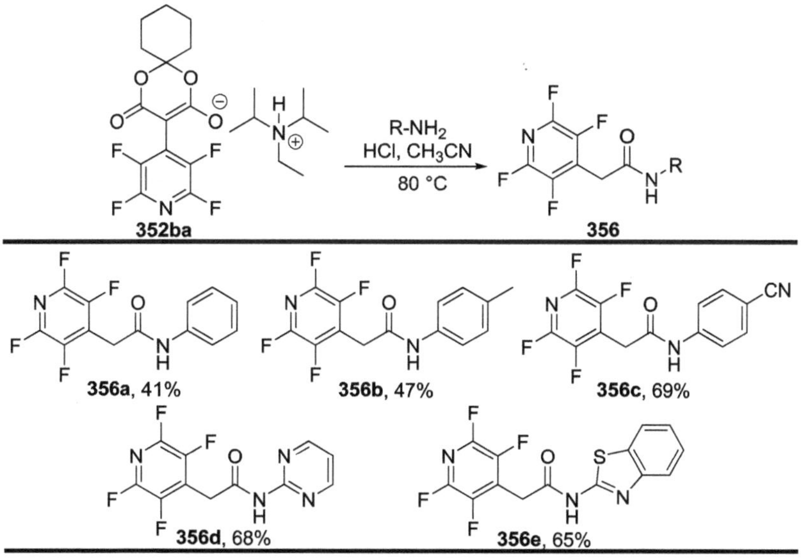

Scheme 2-125. Reaction of **352ba** with amines under acidic conditions.

Amidoximes have three nucleophilic centers (two *N* and one O), and it is clear that the oxygen atom in the amidoxime is a better nucleophile than the nitrogen atoms because of the alpha effect and less hinderers around the oxygen atom. It has been shown that oxygen atom of amidoximes participated in reaction with pentafluoropyridine, although reaction carried out with other sites, depending on reaction conditions [112]. Substituted imidamide systems **358** have been synthesized in a concentrated acetonitrile solution of pentafuoropyridine and amidoximes in a 1:1 molar ratio at reflux condition for 6 h (Scheme 2 - 126), also bis-perfuoropyridylimidamide systems **358** are synthesized using 2:1 molar ratio of pentafluoropyridine **3** and amidoximes **357**, respectively (Scheme 2 - 127).

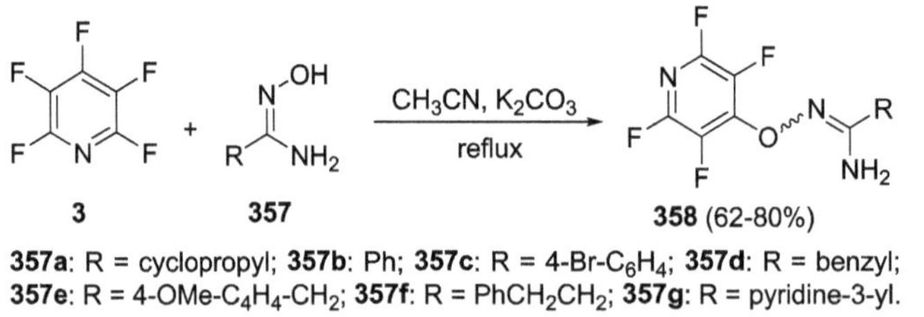

CH3CN, K2CO3
reflux
3
357
358 (62-80%)
357a: R = cyclopropyl; 357b: Ph; 357c: R = 4-Br-C6H4; 357d: R = benzyl;
357e: R = 4-OMe-C4H4-CH2; 357f: R = PhCH2CH2; 357g: R = pyridine-3-yl.

Scheme 2-126. Synthesis of perfluoropyeidineimidamide systems **358** from pentafluoropyridine **3**.

CH3CN, K2CO3
reflux
3 (2 eq.)
357h (1 eq.), R = cyclohexyl
357c (1 eq.), R = 4-Br-C6H4
359, R = cyclohexyl, 70%
360, R = 4-Br-C6H4, 35%

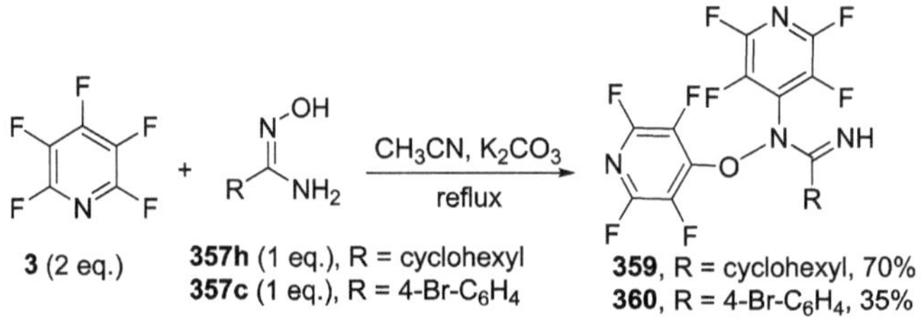

Scheme 2-127. Synthesis of bis-perfuoropyridylimidamide systems **359** and **360** from pentafluoropyridine **3**.

Anion derived from *N*-arylformamides as bidentate nucleophiles reacts with pentafluoropyridine **3** by both oxygen and nitrogen site, depending on the nature of the aromatic ring substituent; with electron releasing group, nucleophilic attack was accomplished by oxygen atom and with an electron withdrawing group, the reaction of *N*-arylformamide anions with pentafluoropyridine **3** proceeded *via* nitrogen site (Scheme 2 - 128) [113]. A rationalization of these observations is shown in Scheme 2 - 129. It is believed that the first step in these reactions is the expected nucleophilic attack by nitrogen of formamides to give the initially formed intermediate **365**, which under reaction conditions converted rapidly to main product **189** and formyl fluoride **366. 366** decomposes to carbon monoxide (CO) and hydrogen fluoride (HF) in reaction condition [114, 115].

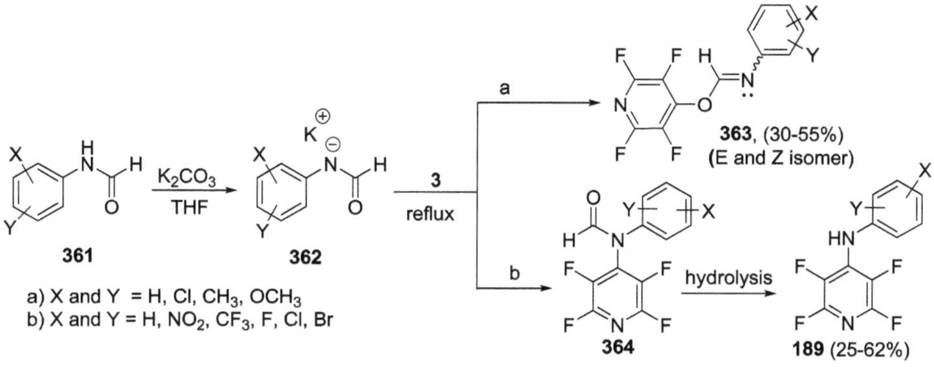

Scheme 2-128. Reaction of formamides **361** with pentafluoropyridine **3**..

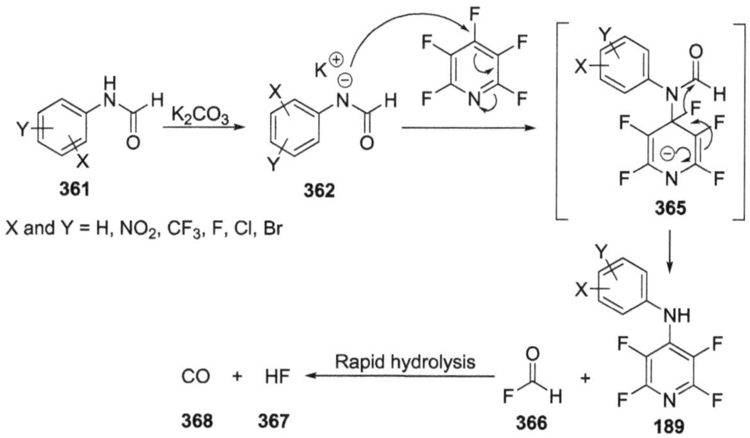

Scheme 2-129. The proposed explanation for observed **189**.

The reaction of pentafluoropyridine **3** with *N*-phenylbenzamidine **368a** gives *N'*-(perfluoropyridin-4-yl)-*N*-phenylbenzimidamide **369** and 2,3,5,6-tetrafluoro-*N*-phenylpyridin-4-amine **189c** by a competing elimination reaction (Scheme 2 - 130) [116]. The proposed mechanism for formation of **189c** is shown in scheme 2 - 131. Attack is occurred by the more nucleophilic secondary nitrogen of *N*-phenyl benzamidine at the 4-position of the pyridine ring to give intermediate **370**, which under the reaction conditions is converted to the main product **189c**.

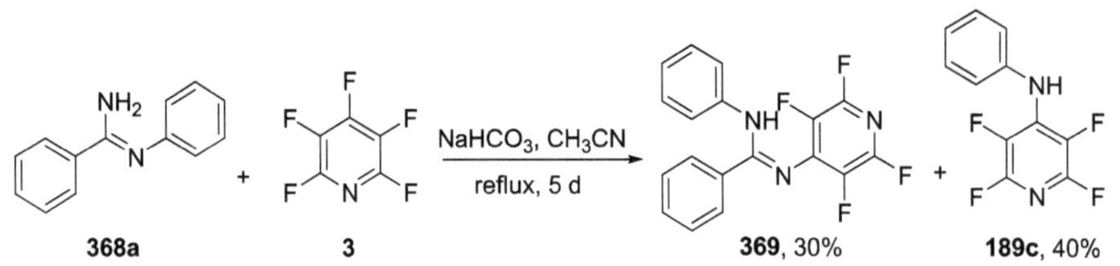

Scheme 2-130. Reaction of *N*-phenylbenzamidine **368a** with pentafluoropyridine **3**.

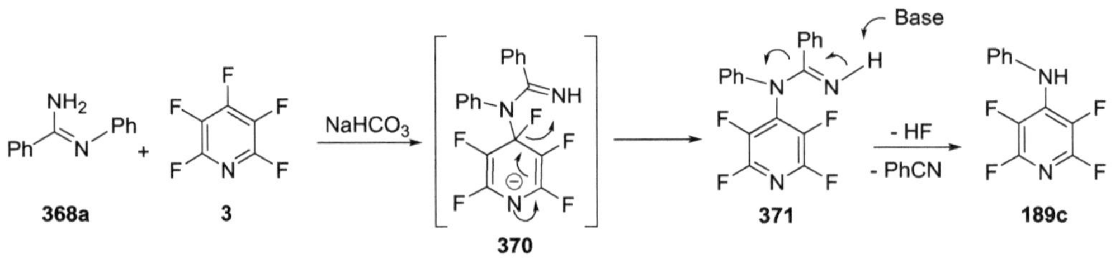

Scheme 2-131. The proposed explanation for the formation of **189c**.

1,1′-binaphthyl-2,2′-diol (BINOL) **372** and its derivatives are high usage chiral reagents [117 - 119]. Their hydroxyl groups can be act as nucleophile in aromatic nucleophilic substitution. Reaction of BINOL with pentafluoropyridine **3** in the presence of potassium carbonate leads to product **373** in high yield, while product **374** formed in mole ratio 2:1 (pentafluoropyridine to BINOL) (Scheme 2 - 132). Compound **374** is easily functionalized by reaction with various nucleophiles (Scheme 2 - 133) [120].

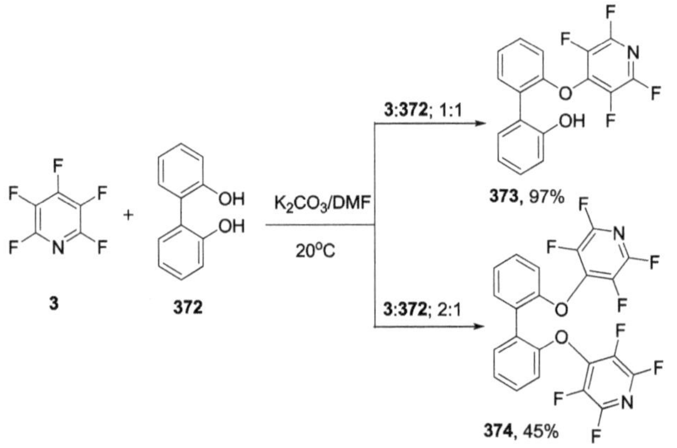

Scheme 2-132. Reaction of BINOL **372** with pentafluoropyridine **3**.

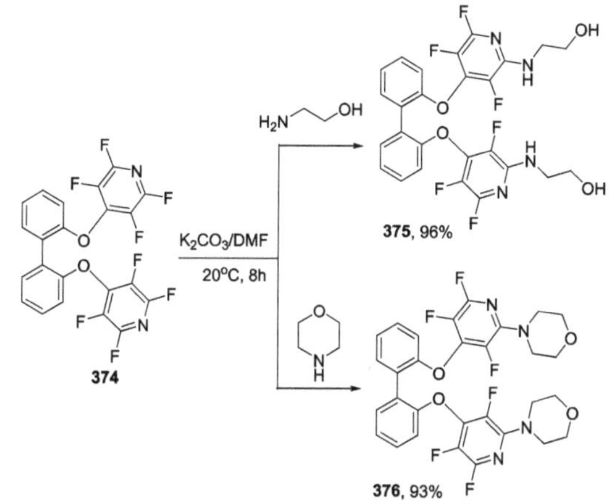

Scheme 2-133. Reaction of diether **374** with ethanolamine and morpholine.

Reaction of pentafluoropyridine with bidentate nucleophiles in water as a green solvent results in the formation of bis-perfluoropyridine derivatives in high yield (Scheme 2 - 134) [121].

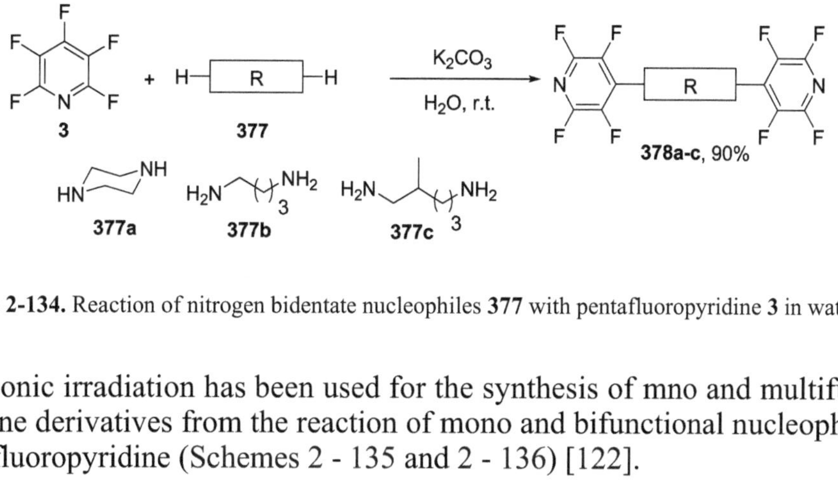

Scheme 2-134. Reaction of nitrogen bidentate nucleophiles **377** with pentafluoropyridine **3** in water.

Ultrasonic irradiation has been used for the synthesis of mno and multifunctional pyridine derivatives from the reaction of mono and bifunctional nucleophiles with pentafluoropyridine (Schemes 2 - 135 and 2 - 136) [122].

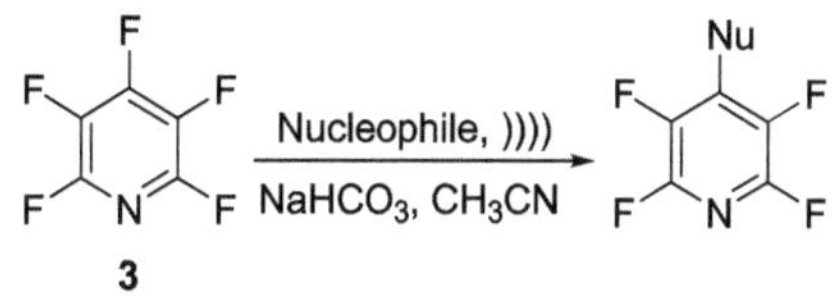

11: Nu = NMe_2; 94%
24: Nu = SO_2Ph; 93%
218b: Nu = NEt_2; 93%
218c: Nu = NC_5H_{10}; 92%
189c: Nu = NHPh; 72%
379a: Nu = NHMe; 92%
379b: Nu = $NH(CH_2)_4NEt_2$; 94%
379c: Nu = NC_4H_8O; 90%
379d: Nu = NHC_6H_4-4-NH_2; 72%
379e: Nu = NHC_6H_4-3-NH_2; 70%

Scheme 2-135. Synthesis of 4-substitued tetrafluoropyridines under ultrasonic irradiation.

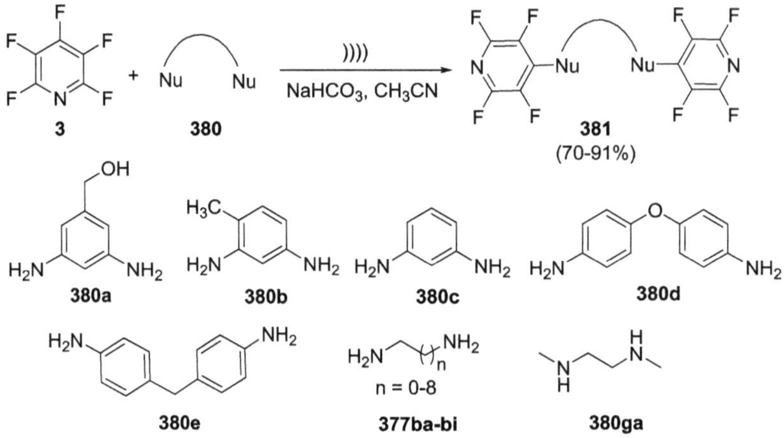

Scheme 2-136. Synthesis of bis-perfluoropyridines **381** under ultrasonic irradiation.

Pyridin-2-ol and pyridin-4-ol compounds have two nucleophilic sites (*N* and *O*) that both sites can be participate as nucleophile in substitution reaction. Their reaction with pentafluoropyridine proceed at both nitrogen and oxygen site depending on the structure of pyridinol (Scheme 2 - 137) [123]. Pyridin-2-ol participated in reaction as ambident nucleophile, while pyridin-4-ol reacted essentially as nitrogen nucleophile. Furthermore, pyririn-3-ol reacted with pentafluoropyridine from oxygen site.

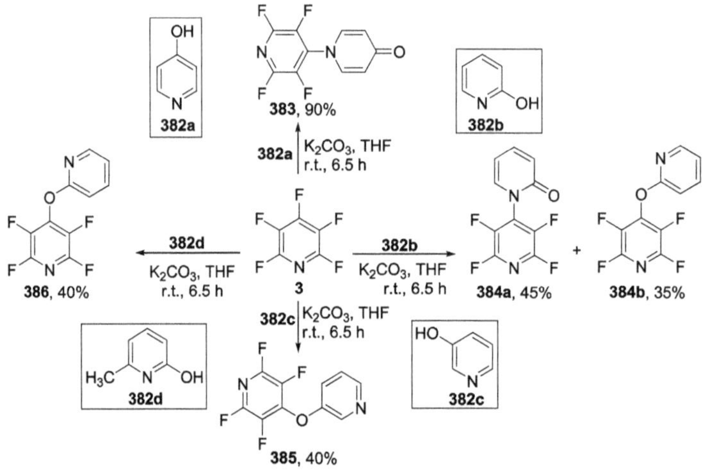

Scheme 2-137. Reactions of pyridinols **382a–d** with pentafluoropyridine **3**.

4,6-diaminopyrimidine-2(1H)-thione **387** reacts chemoselectively with pentafluoropyridine **3** from *S* site and produced 2-[(2,3,5,6-tetrafluoropyridi- -4-yl)-sulfanyl]pyrimidine-4,6-diamine **388**, while its reaction with 2,3,5,6-

tetrafluoro-4-(phenylsulfonyl)pyridine **24** proceeded *via* replacement of $PhSO_2$ group by the *S*-nucleophilic site of **387** (Scheme 2 - 138) [124].

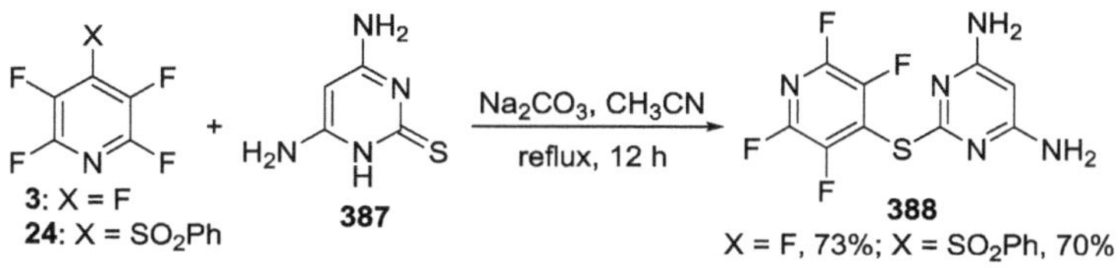

Scheme 2-138. Reaction of 4,6-diaminopyrimidine-2(1H)-thione **387** with pentafluoropyridine **3** and tetrafluoro-4-(phenylsulfonyl)pyridine **24**.

Reaction of pentafluoropyridine **3** and 3-chloro-2,4,5,6-tetrafluoropyridine **5** with guanidine in the presence of NaH gave noncyclized products **390a** and **390b** (Scheme 2 - 139) [125]. Attempts to converting these compounds to cyclized products led to polymeric material.

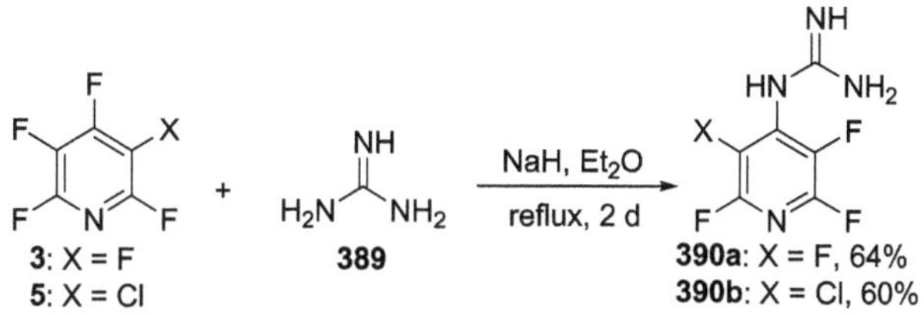

Scheme 2-139. Reaction of perfluoropyridines **3** and **5** with guanidine **389**.

Reaction of pentafluoropyridine **3** and 3-chloro-2,4,5,6-tetrafluoropyridine **5** with urea and thiourea gave products **392a**, **392b** and **28,394**, respectively (Schemes 2 - 140 and 2 - 141) [125]. A rationalisation for formation of these compounds is shown in Schemes 2 - 142 and 2 - 143.

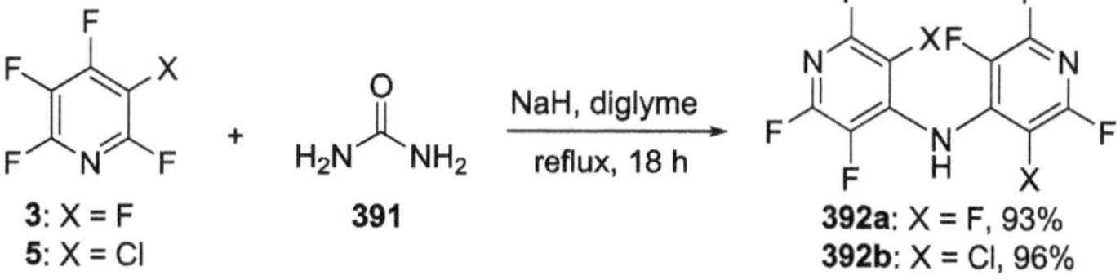

Scheme 2-140. Reaction of perfluoropyridines **3** and **5** with urea **391**.

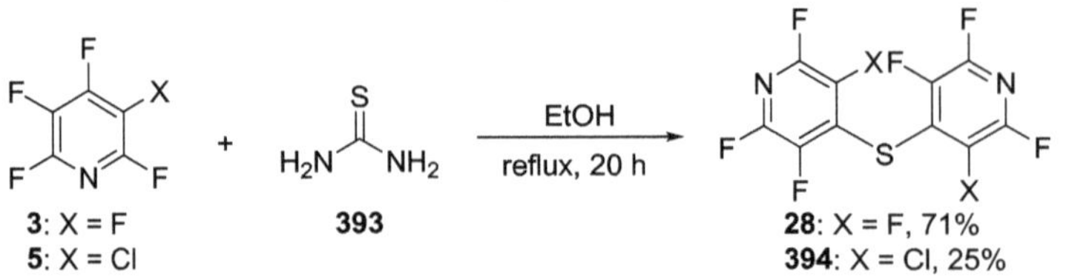

Scheme 2-141. Reaction of perfluoropyridines **3** and **5** with thiourea **393**.

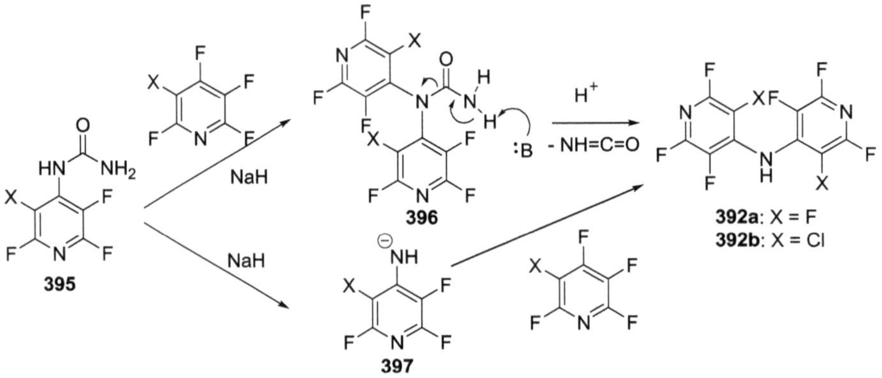

Scheme 2-142. The postulated mechanism for formation **392a** and **392b**.

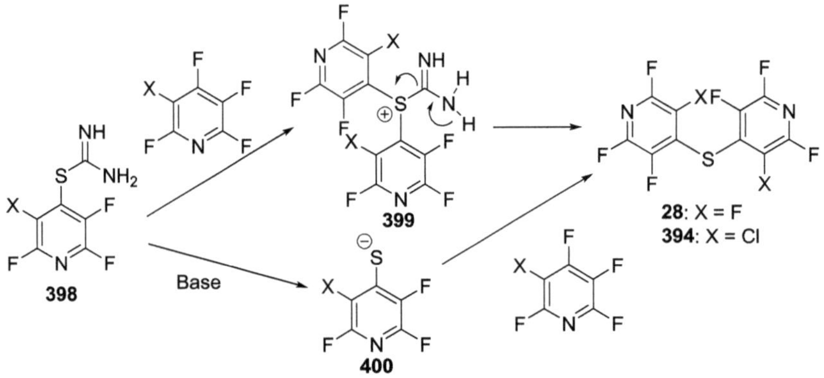

Scheme 2-143. The postulated mechanism for formation **28** and **394**.

Star-shaped multivalent pyridine systems **402** are considerable molecules because of their self-assembly behavior at the graphite surface [126]. The star-shaped compound **402** with perfluoropyridine end group synthesized by using a simple nucleophilic aromatic substitution with pentafluoropyridine (Scheme 2 - 144) [126].

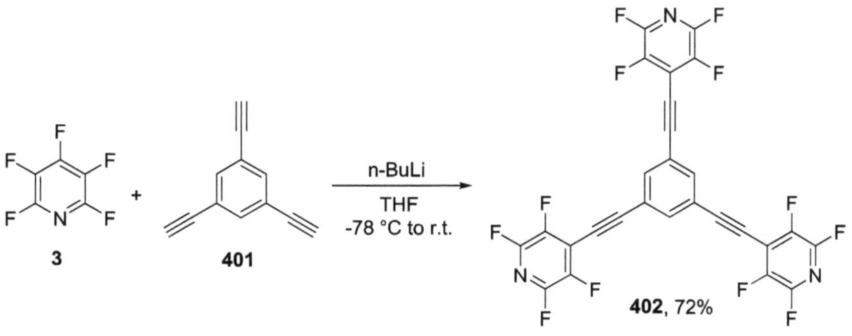

Scheme 2-144. Synthesis of star-shaped compound **402**.

Benzodichalcogenophene (BDC) units are efficient building blocks for polymeric and small molecule semiconductors [127 - 130]. Compounds **403** easily functionalized at its termini with pentafluoropyridine *via* S_{NAr} reactions (Scheme 2 - 145) [131].

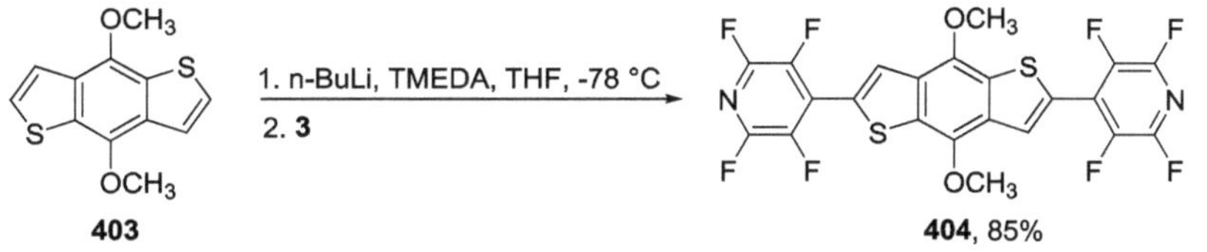

Scheme 2-145. Reaction of pentafluororpyridine **3** with BDC.

Pentafluoropyridine has been successfully applied to access a range of modified peptides [132]. This compound has been readily arylated nucleophilic side chains including cysteine, tyrosine, and lysine in the presence of DIPEA (Scheme 2 - 146). With employing an inorganic base, Cs_2CO_3, is observed a significant increase in peptide "tagged" compared with the use of DIPEA.

Incorporation of tetrafluoropyridine amino acids into dipeptide and tripeptide havs been successfully done [133]. The OH group of Boc-Ser-OMe **408a** as nucleophile has been attacked to pentafluoropyridine and afforded **409a**. The Boc and methyl ester protecting groups have removed selectively on treating with TFA, and the resulting TFA salt immediately coupled to Boc-Ala-OH *via* PyBOP-mediated amide bond formation and give the di-peptide **410a** (Scheme 2 -

147). Similar to synthesis of **409**, compound **409b** was obtained from the reaction of Boc-Ser-OBn **408b** with pentafluoropyridine, which has been converted to tripeptide **411** during several steps (Scheme 2 - 148).

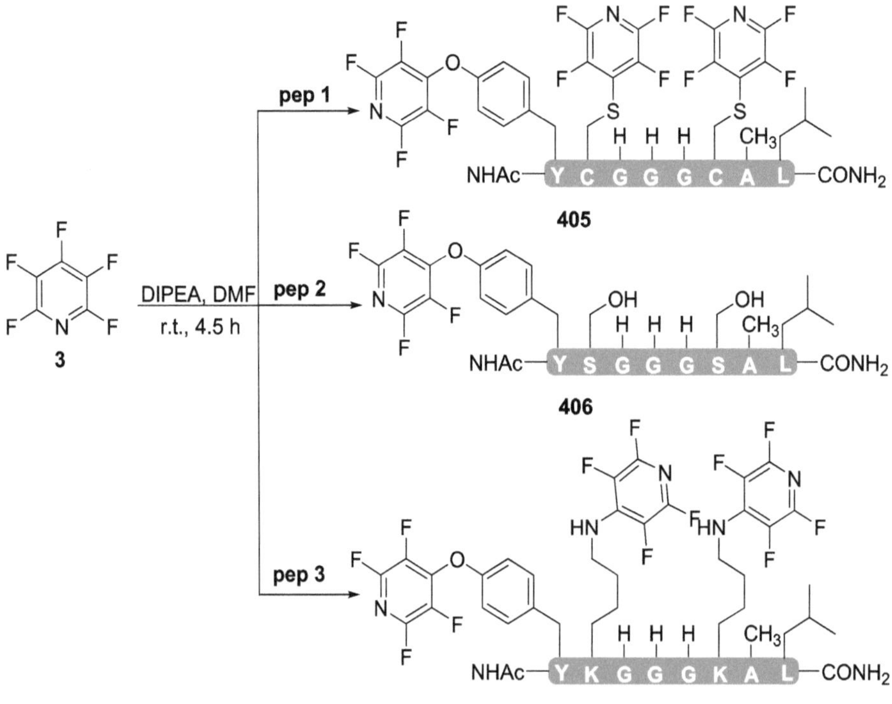

AcNH-[YXGGGXAL]-CONH$_2$: pep 1, X = Cysteine; pep 2, X = Serine; pep 3, X = Lysine.

Scheme 2-146. Main products for the S$_N$Ar reactions of pentafluoropyridine **3** with thiol, hydroxyl and amine based peptides **1-3**.

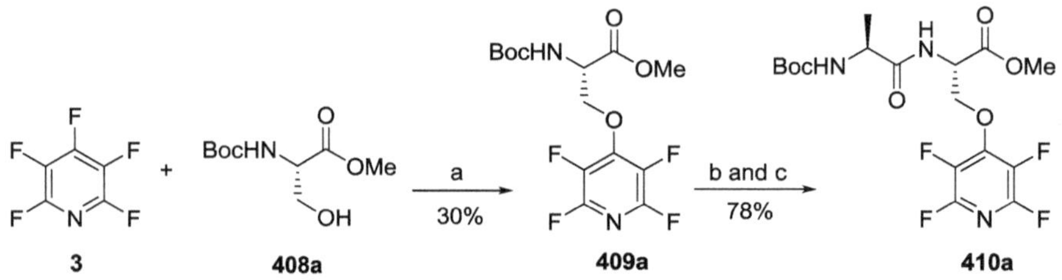

a) K$_2$CO$_3$, CH$_3$CN, r.t., 20 h; b) TFA, CH$_2$Cl$_2$, r.r., 4h; c) Boc-Ala-OH, PyBop, NMM, CH$_2$Cl$_2$, rt, 18 h.

Scheme 2-147. Synthesis of dipeptide **410a**.

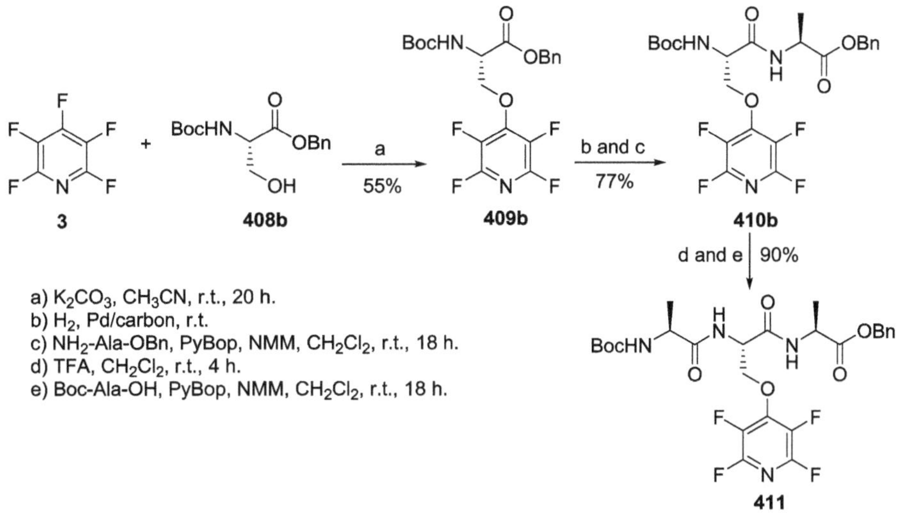

3
408b
409b
410b
411
a
55%
b and c
77%
d and e 90%
a) K_2CO_3, CH_3CN, r.t., 20 h.
b) H_2, Pd/carbon, r.t.
c) NH_2-Ala-OBn, PyBop, NMM, CH_2Cl_2, r.t., 18 h.
d) TFA, CH_2Cl_2, r.t., 4 h.
e) Boc-Ala-OH, PyBop, NMM, CH_2Cl_2, r.t., 18 h.

Scheme 2-148. Synthesis of tripeptide **411**.

Perfluorinated dehydrobutyrine-containing amino acids have been synthesized from the reaction of pentafluoropyridine with threonine [134]. The reaction of pentafluoropyridine **3** with mono-protected L-threonine methyl ester **412** gives exclusively the single elimination product *Z*-isomer of perfluorinated dehydrobutyrine methyl ester **413** and salt **414** (Scheme 2 - 149). With using *N,N*-diisopropylethylamine (DIPEA) instead of K_2CO_3, *N*-substituted tetrafluoropyridine-L-threonine methyl ester **415** and dehydrobutyrine **413** have been formed (Scheme 2 - 149). It has been suggested that the elimination pathway proceeded *via* an E1cb-type mechanism (Scheme 2 - 150). Under the same condition, three compounds have been isolated from reaction of reaction of L-allo-threonine methyl ester **417** with pentafluoropyridine (Scheme 2 - 151).

3
412
413
414
415, 28%
K_2CO_3
65%
CH_3CN
r.t., 24 h
DIPEA
413 + 414

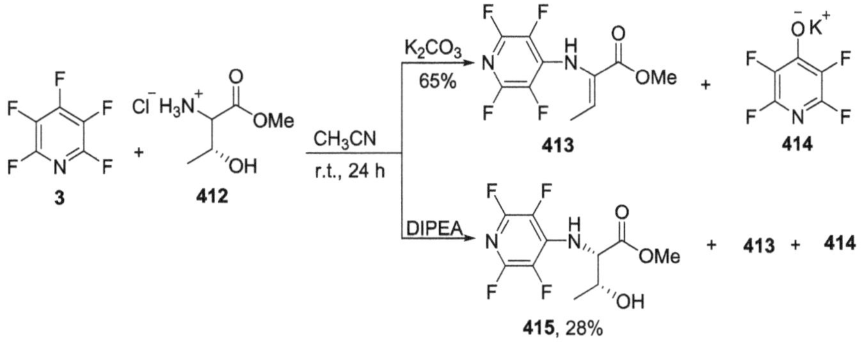

Scheme 2-149. Reaction of pentafluoropyridine **3** with L-threonine methyl ester **412**.

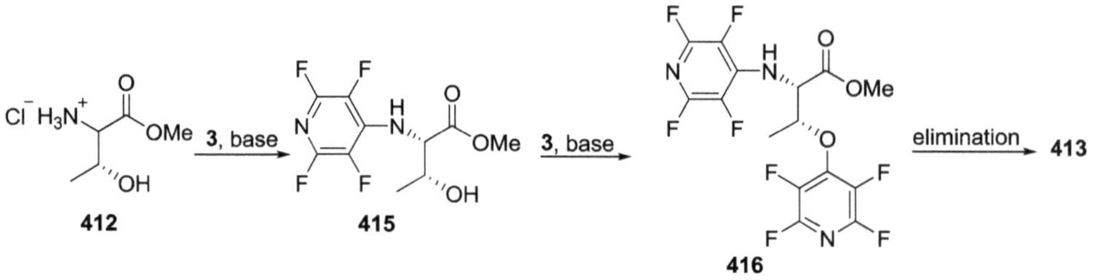

Scheme 2-150. The proposed pathway for formation of compound **413**.

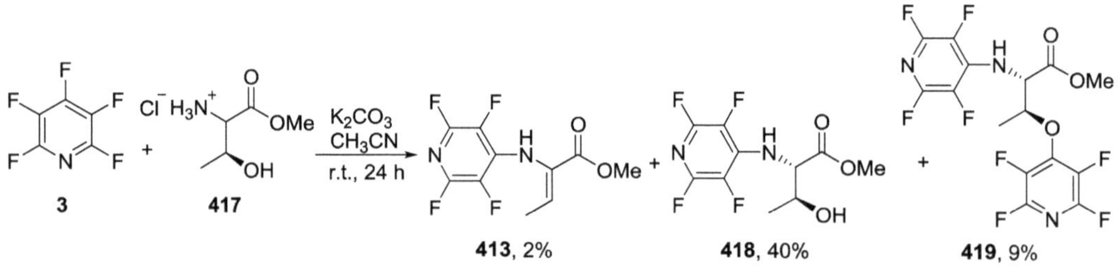

Scheme 2-151. Reaction of L-allo-threonine methyl ester **417** with pentafluoropyridine **3**.

Development of new methods are important for modification of nucleosides, nucleotides, heterocyclic bases and oligonucleotides [135 - 137]. It is believed that an efficient method for modification of arens is their reaction with multiagent molecules. Arens have several nucleophilic atom or group that can participate in nucleophilic reactions. Hydroxyl groups of thymidine **420**, adenosine **424** and uridine **426** have been reacted with pentafluoropyridine and produced corresponding nucleoside ethers (Schemes 2 - 152 to 2-154) [138].

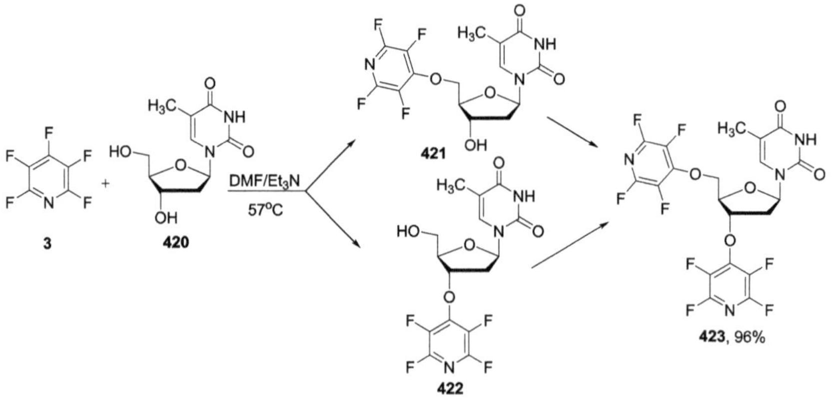

Scheme 2-152. Reaction of **420** with pentafluoropyridine **3**.

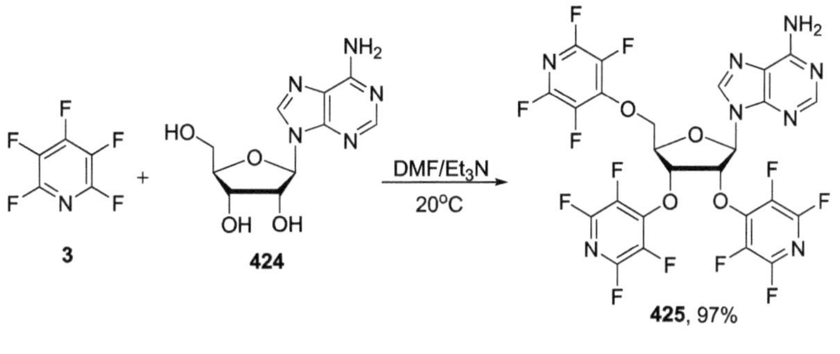

Scheme 2-153. Reaction of **424** with pentafluoropyridine **3**.

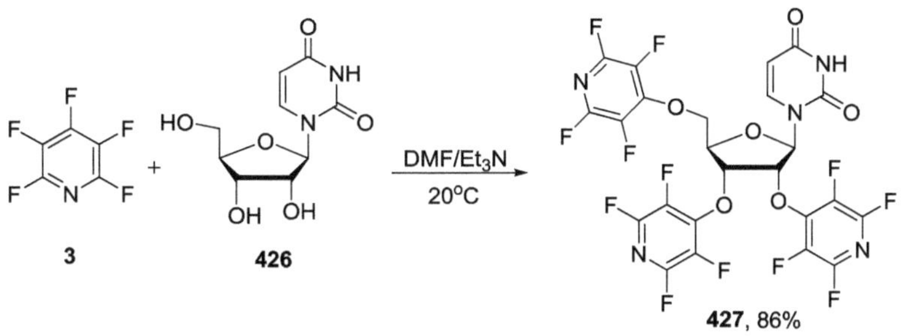

Scheme 2-154. Reaction of **426** with pentafluoropyridine **3**.

Perfluoroarenes are used as reagents for protection of active functional groups. Pentafluoropyridine in the reaction with oestradiol **428** generated perfluoropyridyl ethers **429** and **430** (Schemes 2 - 155 and 2 - 156) [139].

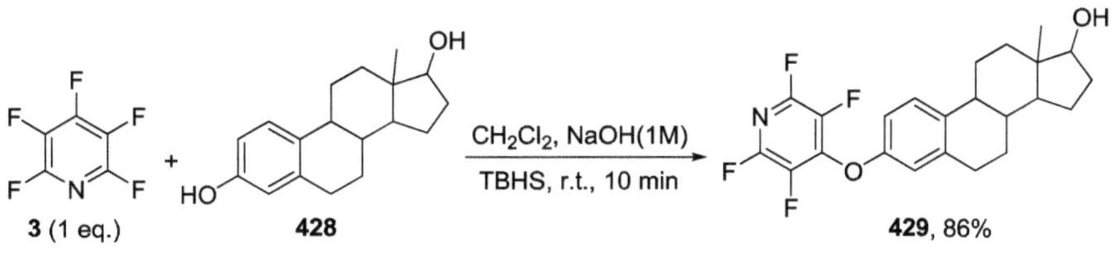

Scheme 2-155. Synthesis of perfluoropyridyl ether **429**.

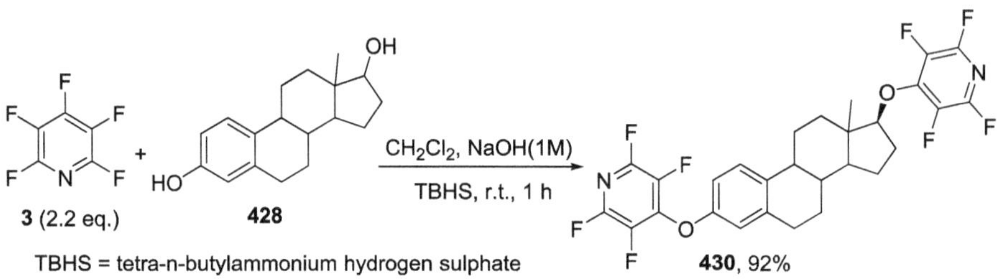

Scheme 2-156. Synthesis of bis(perfluoropyridyl) ether **430**.

2-aminopyridine and 4-aminopyridine selectivity react with pentafluoropyridine and give bis-perfluoropyridyl systems **432** ana **434** (Schemes 2 - 157 and 2 - 158) [140]. The regioselectivity in this process are based on high nucleoplilicity of the secondary or primary amino groups and the activating influence of pyridine ring nitrogen that significantly activates the *ortho* and *para* sites to itself.

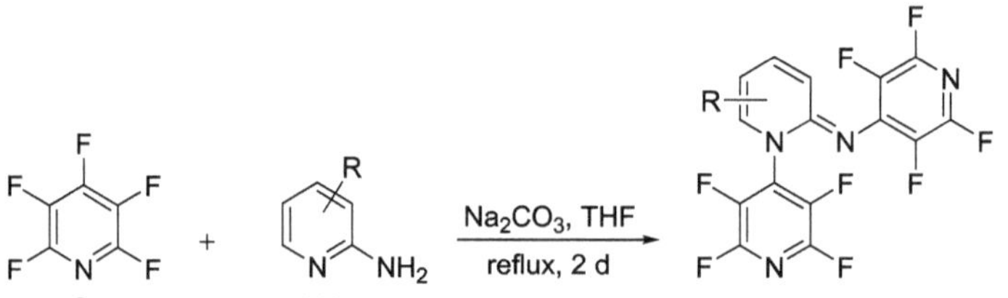

Scheme 2-157. Reaction of pentafluoropyridine **3** with 2-aminopyridine derivatives **431**.

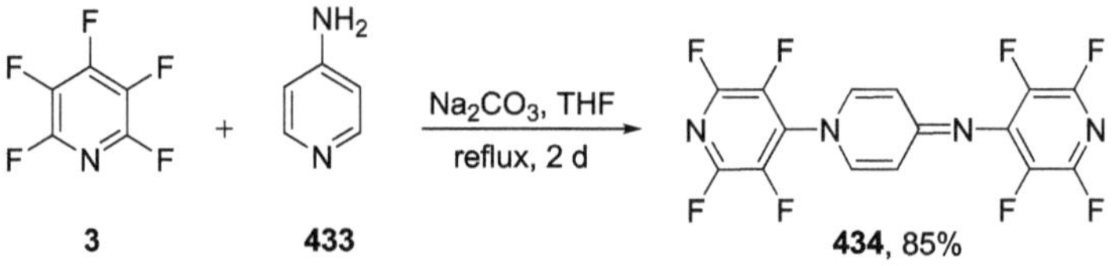

Scheme 2-158. Reaction of pentafluoropyridine **3** with 4-aminopyridine **433**.

5.2. Synthesis of Fluorinated Ring-fused Heterocyles

Perfluoropyridines are useful precursors for preparation of ring-fused heterocyles on their reactions with multidentate nucleophiles [141]. Substitution occur at the

4-position of pyridine ring and following by attack at the adjacent 3-position as shown in scheme 2 - 159. Ring-fused can be react with various nucleophiles and produce a wide variety of analogues fused ring systems. In addition, with blocking of 4-position of pentafluoropyridine and following and then reaction with bidentate nucleophiles can be produce ring-fused systems *via* substitution at 2-position of pyridine and following by ring closure at 3-position of pyridine ring (Scheme 2 - 160) [142]. Ring-fused is active toward nucleophilic attack and produce multisubstituted bicyclic *N*-heterocycles.

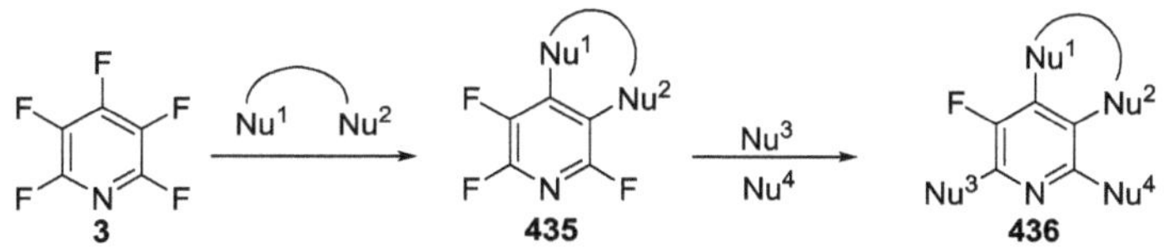

Scheme 2-159. Possible synthetic route for synthesis of fluorinated ring-fused systems and polyfunctional analogues.

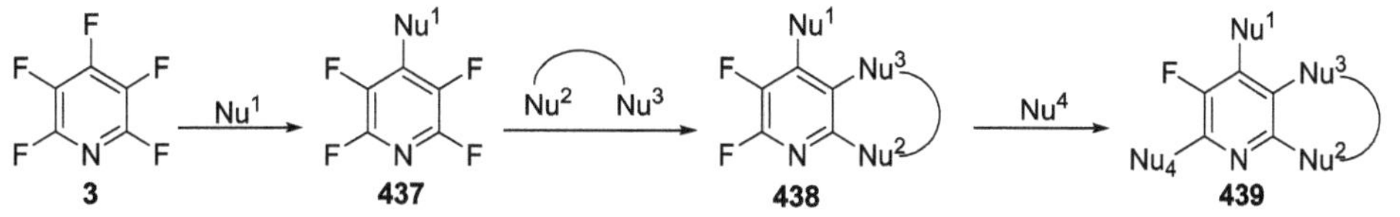

Scheme 2-160. Strategy for synthesis of polyfunctional ring-fused systeme.

Pyridooxadiazine systems **440, 441** have been produced in diluted acetonitrile solution of pentafuoropyridine and amidoximes in 1:1 molar ratio under reflux condition for 24 h (Scheme 2 - 161) [112].

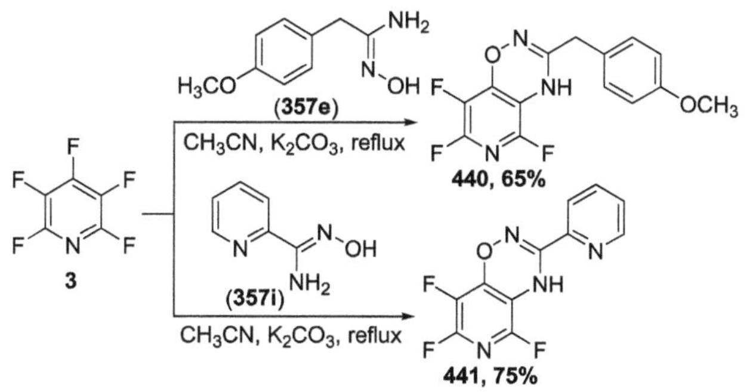

Scheme 2-161. Synthesis of pyridooxadiazine systems **440** and **441** from pentafluoropyridine **3**.

Tricyclic dipyridoimidazoles **442-445** synthesized simply in on step from the reaction of perfluoropyridines **3** and **5** with 2-aminopyridine derivatives (Scheme 2 - 162) [143]. Reaction of 4-cyano- and 4-phenylsulphonyltetrafluoropyridine with aminopyridine **431b** formed mixture of products (Schemes 2 - 163 and 2 - 164) [143].

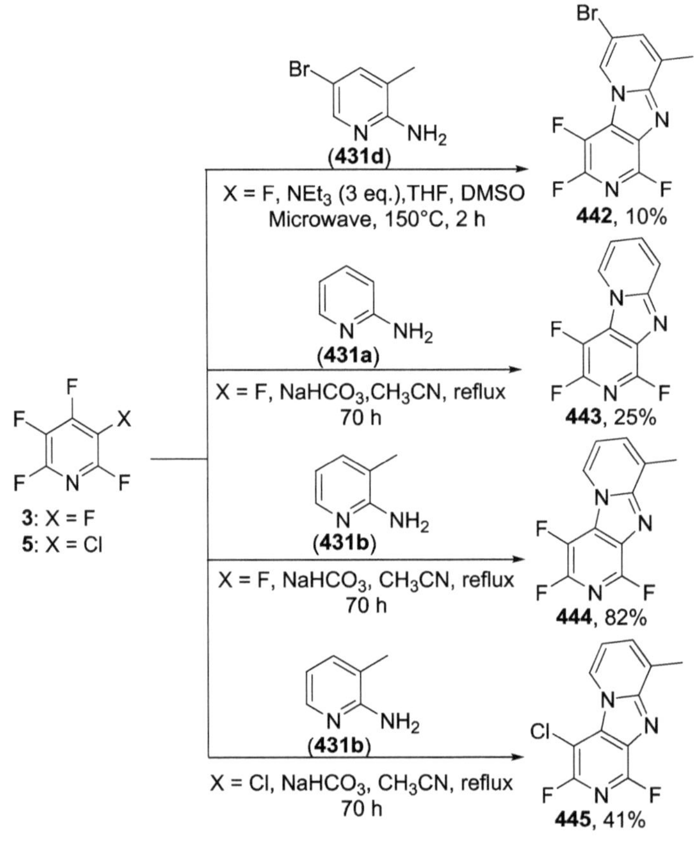

Scheme 2-162. Reaction of pentafluoropyridine **3** and 3-chlorotetrafluoropyridine **5** with 2-aminopyridines.

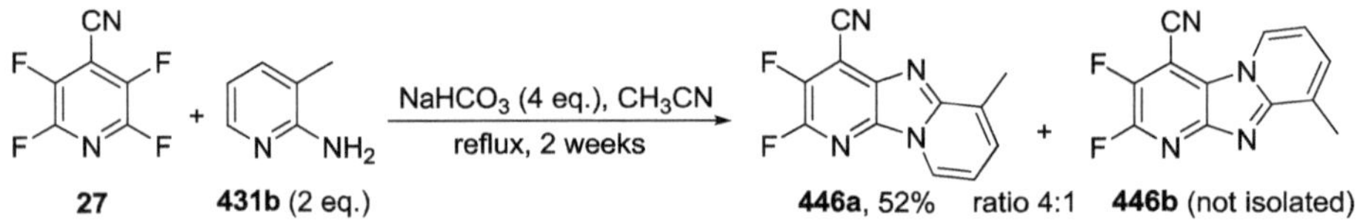

Scheme 2-163. Reaction of 4-cyanotetrafluoropyridine **27** with aminopyridine **431b**.

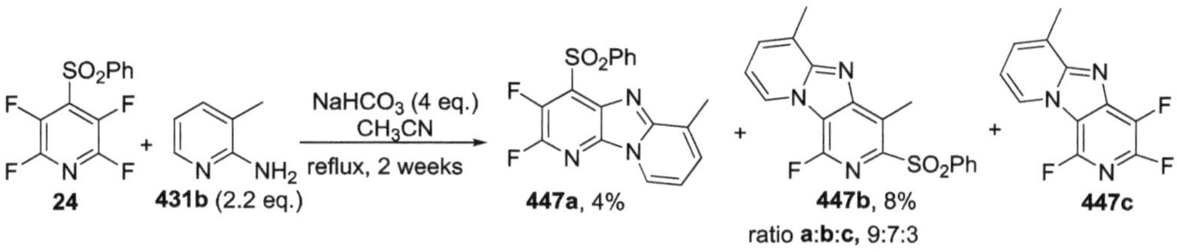
SO2Ph
NaHCO3 (4 eq.)
CH3CN
reflux, 2 weeks
24
431b (2.2 eq.)
447a, 4%
447b, 8%
447c
ratio a:b:c, 9:7:3

Scheme 2-164. Reaction of 4-phenylsulphonyltetrafluoropyridine **24** with aminopyridine **431b**.

Ring-fused systems **444** and **445** reacted selectively at F-2 with nucleophiles [143]. However, LiSPh in reaction with **444** replaced at both F-2 and F-3 (Scheme 2 - 165). Compound **445** in reaction with *n*-BuLi underwent of Li-Cl exchange and participated in reaction with electrophiles (Scheme 2 - 165).

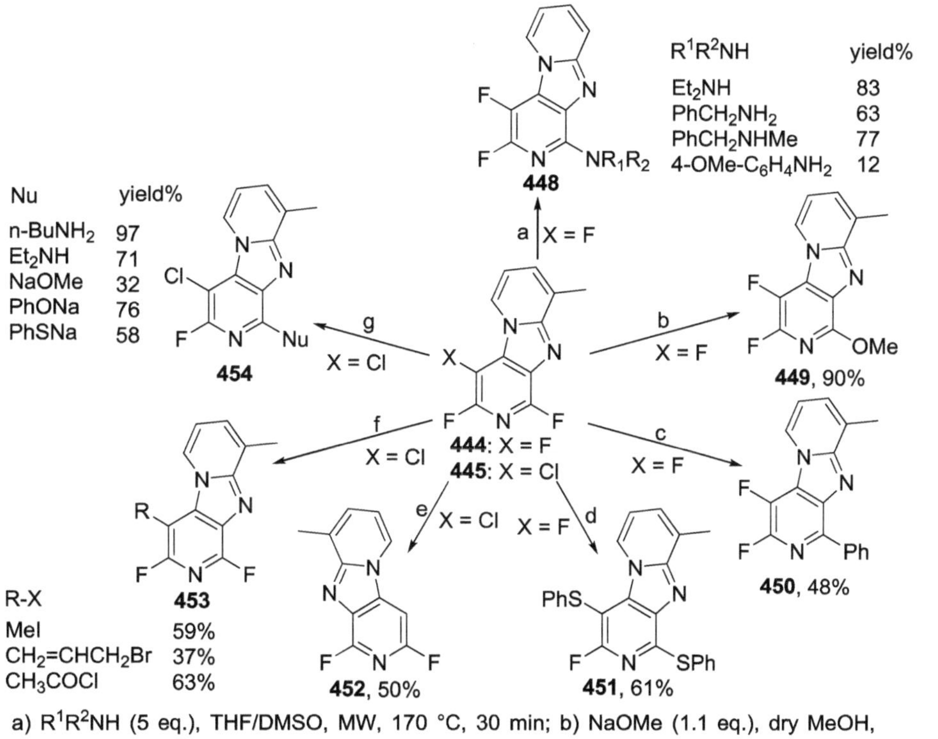
R1R2NH yield%
Et2NH 83
PhCH2NH2 63
PhCH2NHMe 77
4-OMe-C6H4NH2 12
448
Nu yield%
n-BuNH2 97
Et2NH 71
NaOMe 32
PhONa 76
PhSNa 58
454
449, 90%
444: X = F
445: X = Cl
450, 48%
R-X
453
MeI 59%
CH2=CHCH2Br 37%
CH3COCl 63%
452, 50%
451, 61%

a) R^1R^2NH (5 eq.), THF/DMSO, MW, 170 °C, 30 min; b) NaOMe (1.1 eq.), dry MeOH, Et_3N, MW, 140 °C, 30 min; c) PhMgBr (2 eq.), THF, reflux, 93 h; d) LiSPh (2 eq.), THF, reflux, 17 h; e) HCO_2NH_4, Pd, THF, reflux, 48h; f) n-BuLi, THF, -78 °C, 1 h then RX, r.t.; g) Nu, THF/DMSO, MW, 170 °C, 30 min.

Scheme 2-165. Reactions of imidazopyridines **444** and **445**.

Reaction of 4-phenylsulphonyltetrafluoropyridine **24** with 2,6-diaminopyridine **431e** operated less selective than the reactions described above and gave two major products (Scheme 2 - 166) [144].

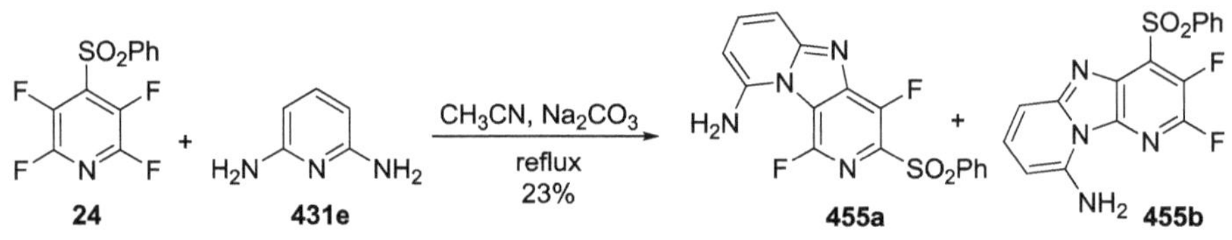

Scheme 2-166. Reaction of 4-phenylsulphonyltetrafluoropyridine **24** with 2,6-diaminopyridine **431e**.

In contrast with pentafluoropyridine **3**, 4-cyanotetrafluoropyridine **27** gives cyclic products on reaction with ethylacetoacetate **239a** and ethyl 3-oxo-3-phenylpropanoate **239b** (Scheme 2 - 167) [109]. Ring-fused system **456** reacted selectively with diethylamine at the *ortho* position of pyridine ring (Scheme 2 - 168).

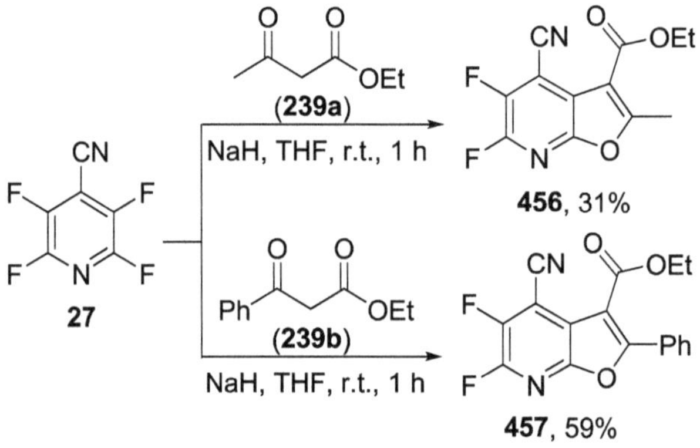

Scheme 2-167. Reaction of 4-cyanotetrafluoropyridine **27** with ethylacetoacetate **239a** and ethyl 3-oxo-3-phenylpropanoate **239b**.

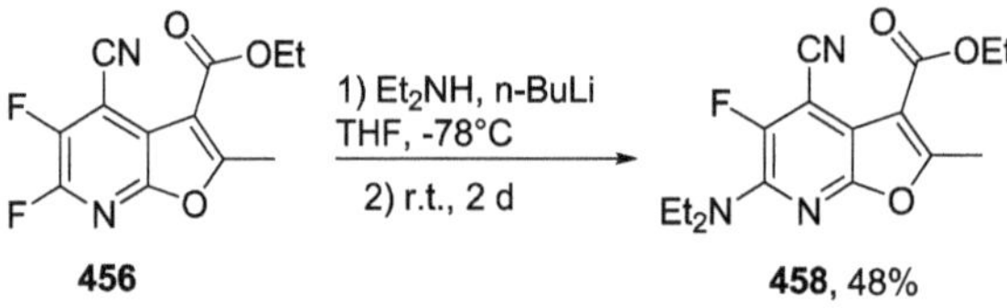

Scheme 2-168. Reaction of diethylamine with **456**.

4-phenylsulfonyltetrafluoropyridine **24** reacts with enolate derived from methyl-4-pyridylketone **340a** from the carbon site and produced corresponding ring-fused system **459a** as major product (Scheme **2 - 169**) [108]. Attacking of C–F bond at 2-position by the carbon site of enolate explained based on chelating system formed between ring nitrogen and salt (Scheme **2 - 170**).

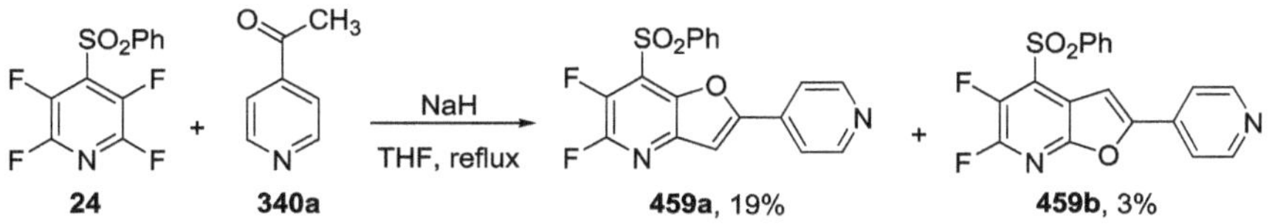

Scheme 2-169. Reaction of methyl-4-pyridylketone **340a** with 4-phenylsulfonyltetrafluoropyridine **24**.

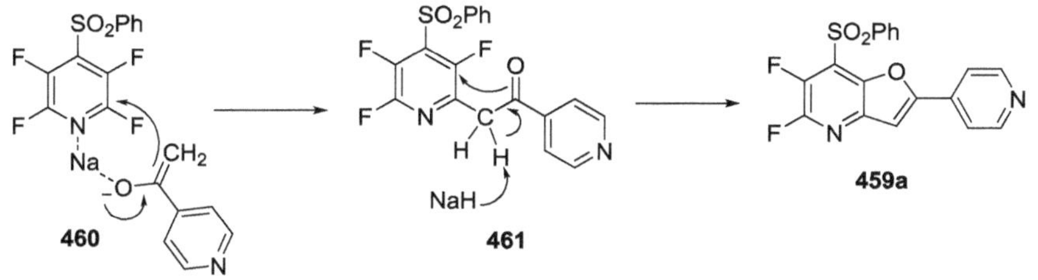

Scheme 2-170. Proposed mechanism for formation of compound **459a**.

Tetrahydropyridido[3,4-*b*]pyrazine **462a-b** is synthesized simply by the reaction of pentafluoropyridine **3** with secondary diamines at reflux conditions [141] or ultrasonic irradiation conditions (Scheme **2 - 171**) [122]. Whereas reaction with ethylenediamine give non-cyclic product **463** (Scheme **2 - 172**) [141]. These results explained by the further nucleophilicity of secondary amine compared to primary amines.

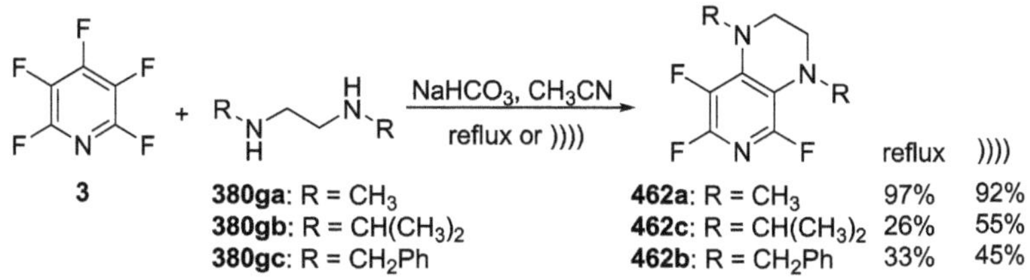

Scheme 2-171. Reaction of pentafluoropyridine **3** with secondary diamines.

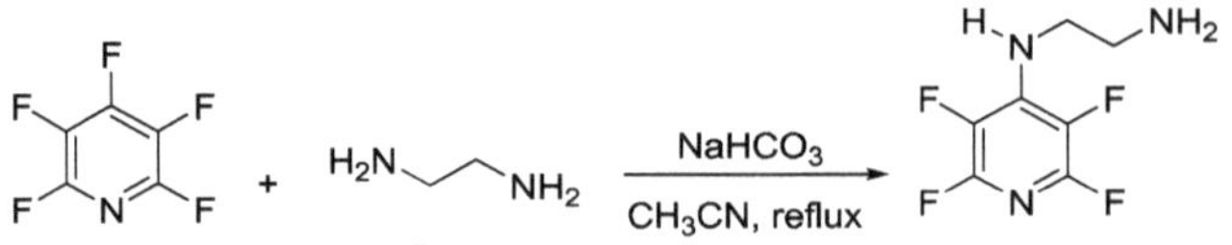

Scheme 2-172. Reaction of pentafluoropyridine **3** with secondary ethylenediamine.

Various nucleophiles react with **462a** at both 2- and 6-positions of pyridine (Table **2-2**) [141]. 6-position of pyridine is more reactive than 2-position due to activating effect of *meta* and *ortho* fluorine atoms and ring nitrogen (Fig. **2-3**). Compound **464a** reacts with nucleophiles at the 2-position of pyridine ring (Table **2-3**) [141].

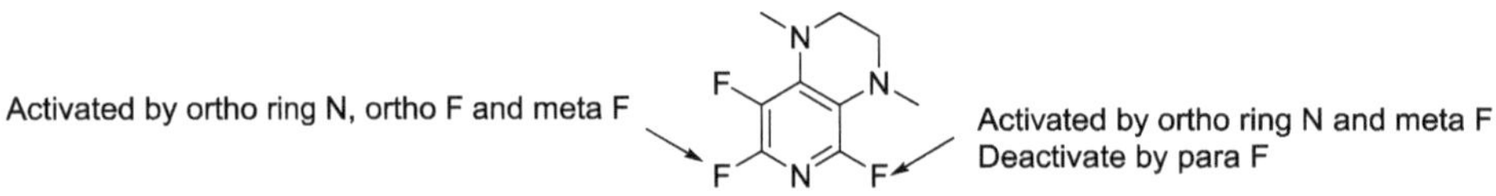

Fig. (2-3). Activating influences on **462a** for nucleophilic aromatic substitution reactions.

Table 2-2. Nucleophilic substitution reactions of 462a with various nucleophiles.

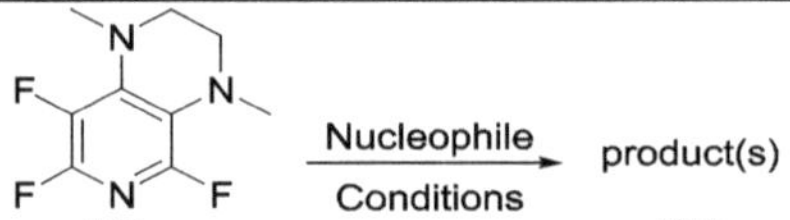

Nucleophile/conditions	Product(s)
MeONa/MeOH, reflux, 2 d	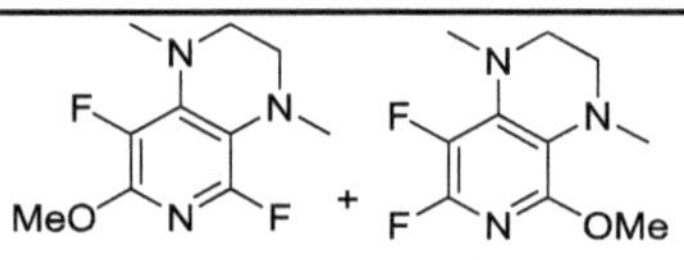 **464a** + **464b** 76%, 10:1

(Table 2-2) cont.....

EtONa/EtOH, reflux, 2 d	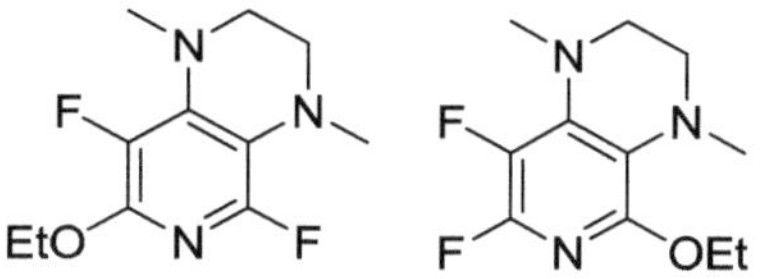 **464c** **464d** 80%, 8:1
t-BuOK/THF, 90˚C	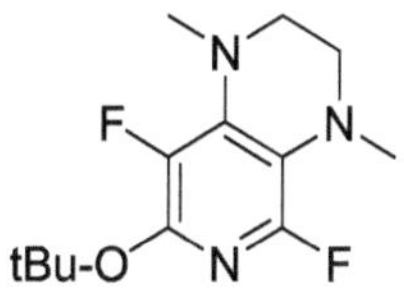 **464e,** 66%
PhOK/Microwaves, THF, 150˚C, 1 h	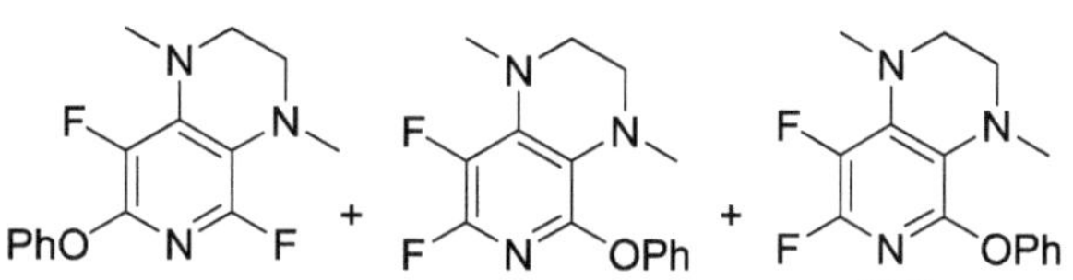 **464f** **464g** **464h** 65%, 4.9:1:1.2
EtNHLi/THF, 90˚C	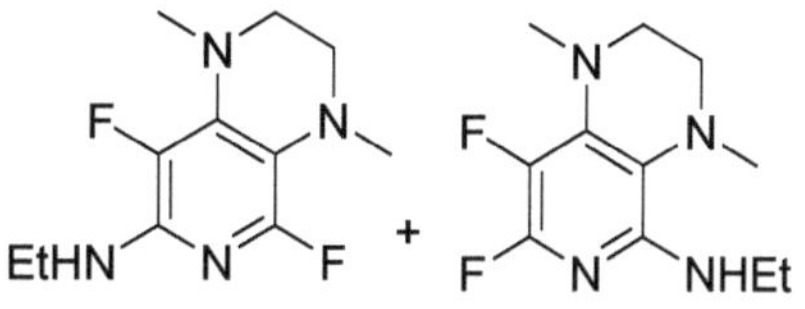 **464i** **464j** 21%, 1.6:1
Et_2NLi/ THF, 90˚C	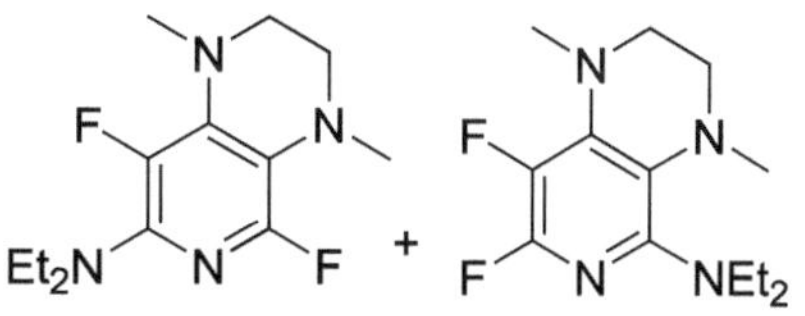 **464k** **464l** 26%, 4:1
PhSLi/ Microwaves, THF, 150˚C, 1 h	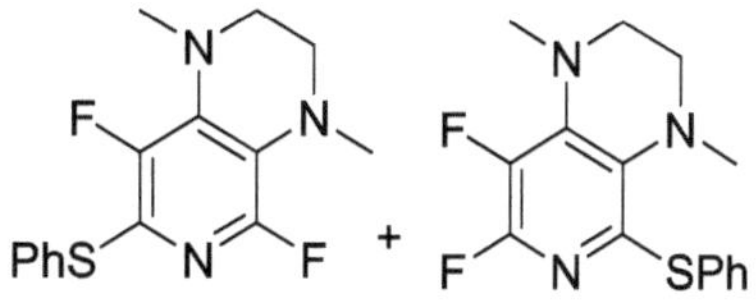 **464m** **464n** 10%, 1:1

Table 2-3. Nucleophilic substitution reactions of 464a with nucleophiles.

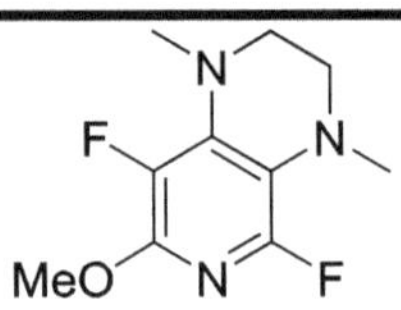

Nucleophile/conditions	Product(s)
EtONa/EtOH, 90°C	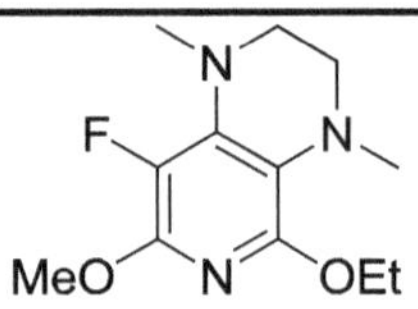 **465a**, 77%
Et$_2$NLi/THF, 90°C	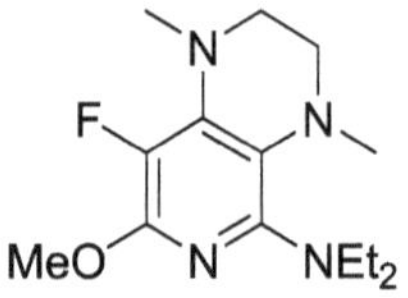 **465b**, 64%
n-BuLi/THF, 90°C	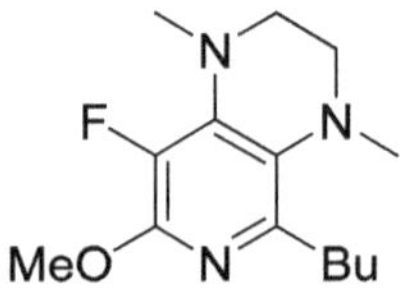 **465c**, 31%
Et$_2$NLi/ THF, 90°C	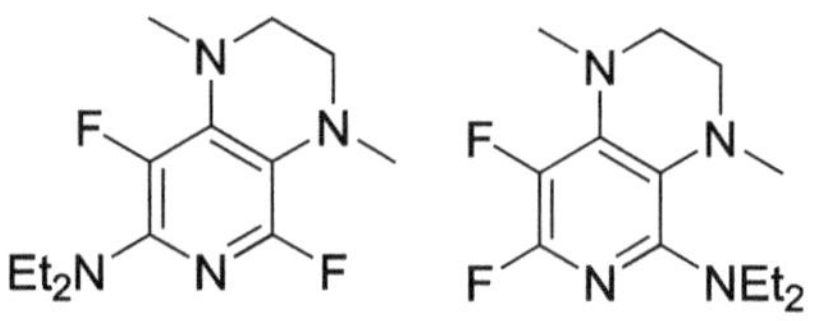 **465d** 26%, 4:1 **465e**

Phenylsulphonyl group of compounds **24** leades to enhancement the reactivity of pyridine ring toward nucleophilic attack. Its reaction with 1,2-diamines produced tetrahydropyrido[2,3-*b*]pyrazine systems **467** and **468** (Table **2-4**), and with *N,N'*-dimethylpropane-1,3-diamine formed tetrahydro-1H-pyrido[2,3-*b*] [1, 4]diazepine

470 (Scheme 2 - 173) [142].

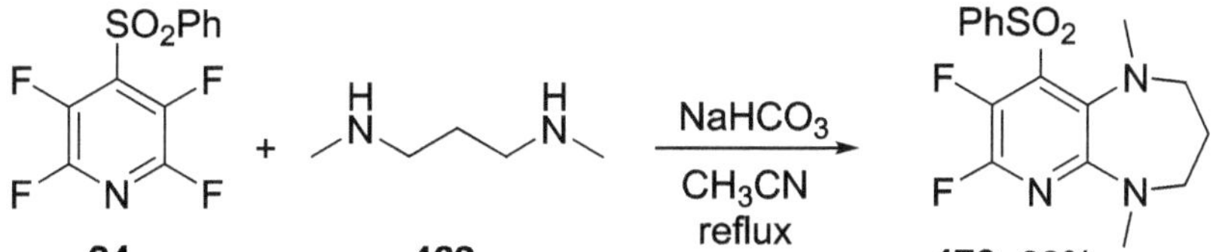

Scheme 2-173. Reaction of **24** with *N,N'*-dimethylpropane-1,3-diamine **469**.

Table 2-4. Reaction of 4-phenylsulphonyltetraflouropyridine 24 with 1,2-diamines.

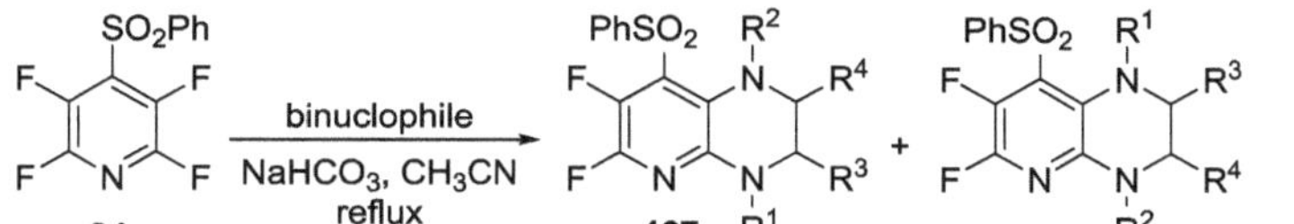

Binucleophile	product	Binucleophile	product
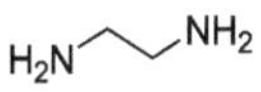 H_2N—NH_2 **377ba**	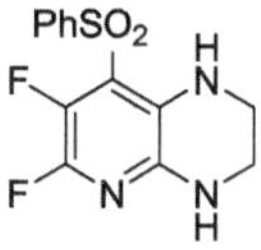 **467a**, 92%	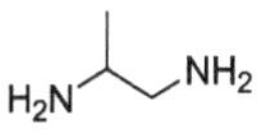 H_2N—NH_2 **466b**	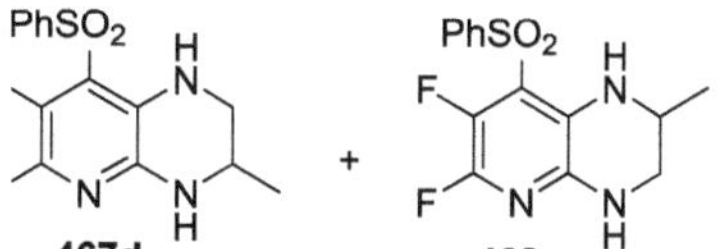 **467d** 85% ratio 1.3:1 **468a**
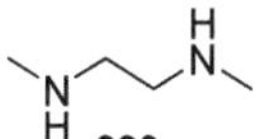 **380ga**	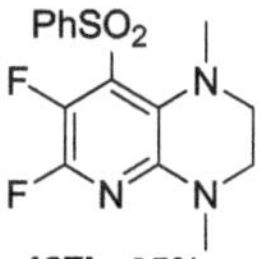 **467b**, 65%	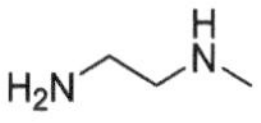 H_2N—**466c**	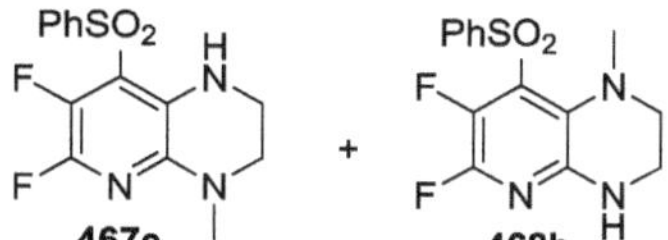 **467e** 68% ratio 4.3:1 **468b**
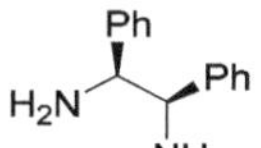 Ph, Ph, H_2N, NH_2 **467c**	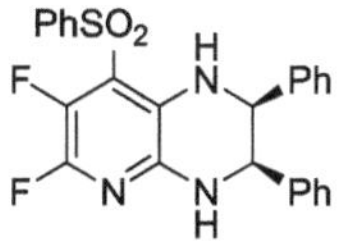 **465c**, 34%		

Phenylsulphonyl group in compounds **467a** and **467b** have been replaced on reaction with lithium diethylamide and sodium thiophenoxide, respectively (Schemes 2 - 174 and 2 - 175) [142]. Acetylation of piperazine ring in **471a** carried out in *N*-1 than pyridine nitrogen because of more nucleophilicity of this site than *N*-4 (Scheme 2 - 176) [142].

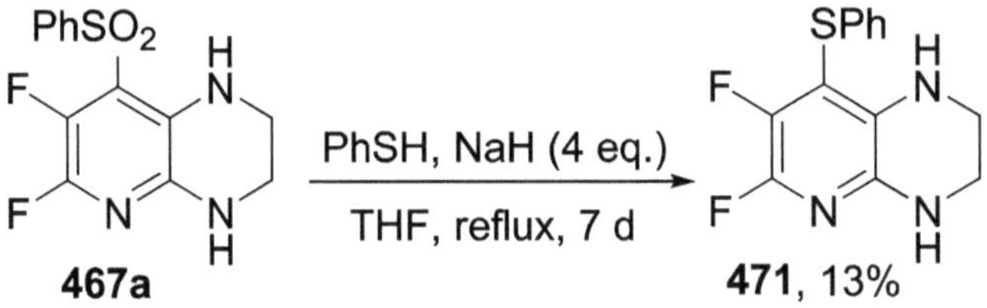

Scheme 2-174. Reaction of **467a** with PhSH.

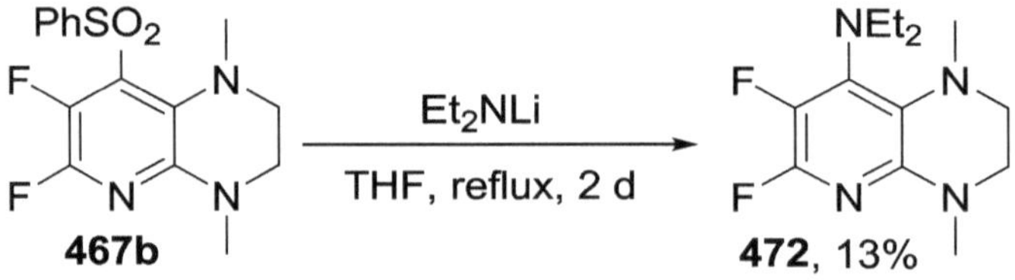

Scheme 2-175. Reaction of **467b** with Et$_2$NLi.

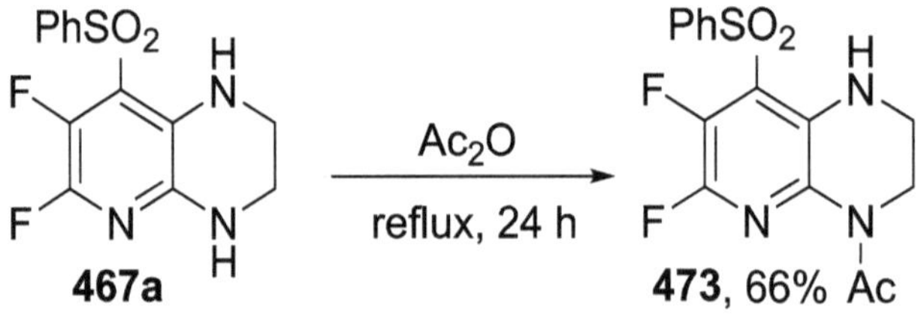

Scheme 2-176. Acetylation of **467a** with acetic anhydride.

Perfluoropyridines with electron withdrawing groups or hydrogen substituent located at four position caused more efficient synthesis of polyfunctional ring-fused systems, while present of electron releasing group at the 4-position of pyridine made difficult formation of ring-fused system (Scheme 2 - 177) [145].

Reaction 4-substituted tetrafluoropyridines with bifunctional *N* and *O*-centered nucleophiles produced pyridooxazine **483** and pyridobenzoxazine derivative **485a** (Schemes 2 - 178 and 2 - 179) [146]. Reaction of *N*-methylethanolamine with tetrafluoropyridine derivatives **24** and **27** carried out firstly by attack of *N* atom to the 2-position and followed by attack of *O* atom to the 3-position of pyridine ring.

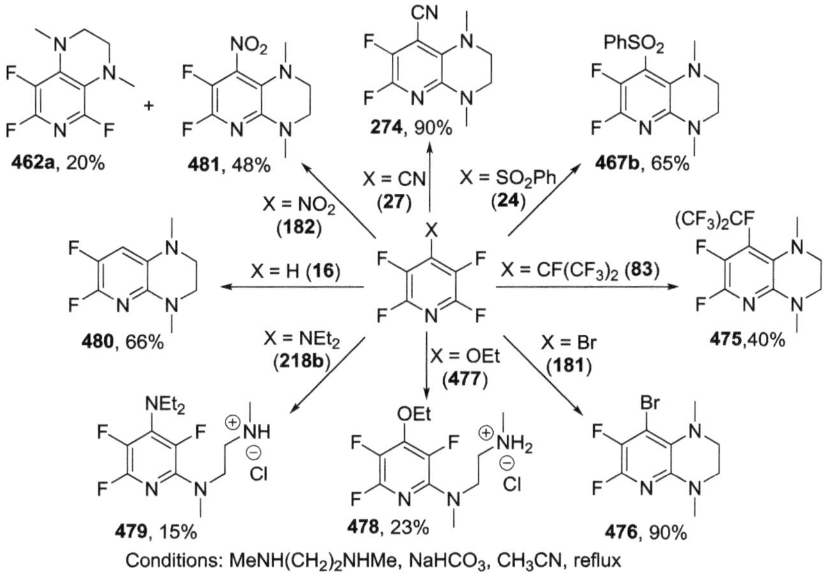

Conditions: MeNH(CH$_2$)$_2$NHMe, NaHCO$_3$, CH$_3$CN, reflux

Scheme 2-177. Reaction of 4-substituted tetrafluoropyridines with bidentate nucleophiles.

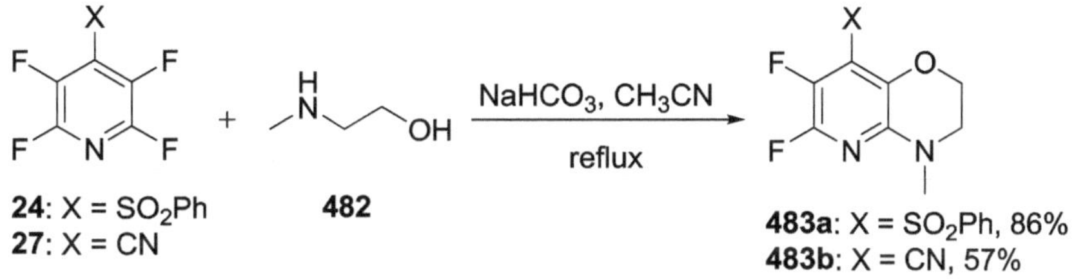

Scheme 2-178. Reaction 4-substituted tetrafluoropyridines with *N*-methylethanolamine **482**.

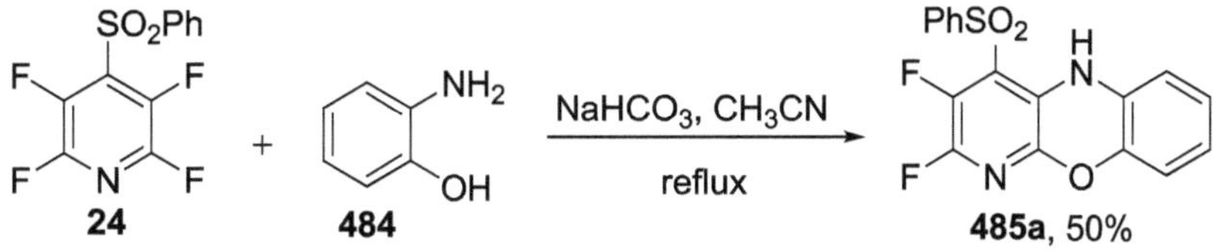

Scheme 2-179. Reaction 4-phenylsulphonyltetrafluoropyridine **24** with 2-aminophenol **484**.

Phenylsulphonyl group is strong electron withdrawing group and substitution it on pentafluoropyridine helps to maintain the reactivity of pyridine ring toward further nucleophilic substitution reactions. Regioselectivity of 4-phenylsulphonyl terafluoropyridine, obtained from reaction of sodium benzenesulphinate with pentafluoropyridine [18], achieved by reaction with unequal bifunctional nucleophiles [147]. Tetrahydropyrido[2,3-*b*]oxazine, thiazine and pyrazine systems produced by reaction of 4-phenylsulphonylterafluoropyridine with these nucleophiles (Scheme 2 - 180).

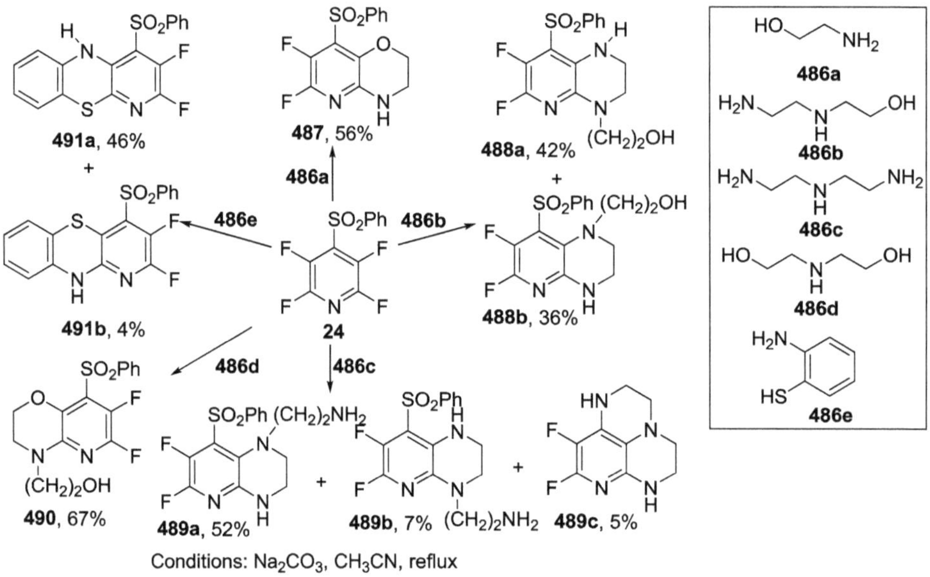

Conditions: Na_2CO_3, CH_3CN, reflux

Scheme 2-180. Synthesis of tetrahydropyrido[2,3-b]oxazine, thiazine and pyrazine systems.

Order reactivity of pentafluoropyridine toward nucleophilic attack followed the sequence 4-F > 2-F > 3-F. However, this may be affected by nature of each substituent once attached to the heterocyclic ring and the nature of the attacking nucleophile. On the other hand, this site-reactivity order may be changed by reaction of bidentate nucleophiles with pentafluoropyridine. Effect of 4-position substituent evaluated by reaction of 4-substituted tetrafluoropyridines with bifunctional *N*-nucleophiles [145]. Reaction of pentafluoropyridine with aromatic diols produced trifluorobenzo [5, 6] [1, 4]dioxino derivatives, whereas, its reaction with aromatic diamines gave bridged bispyridyl systems as major product (Scheme 2 - 181) [144].

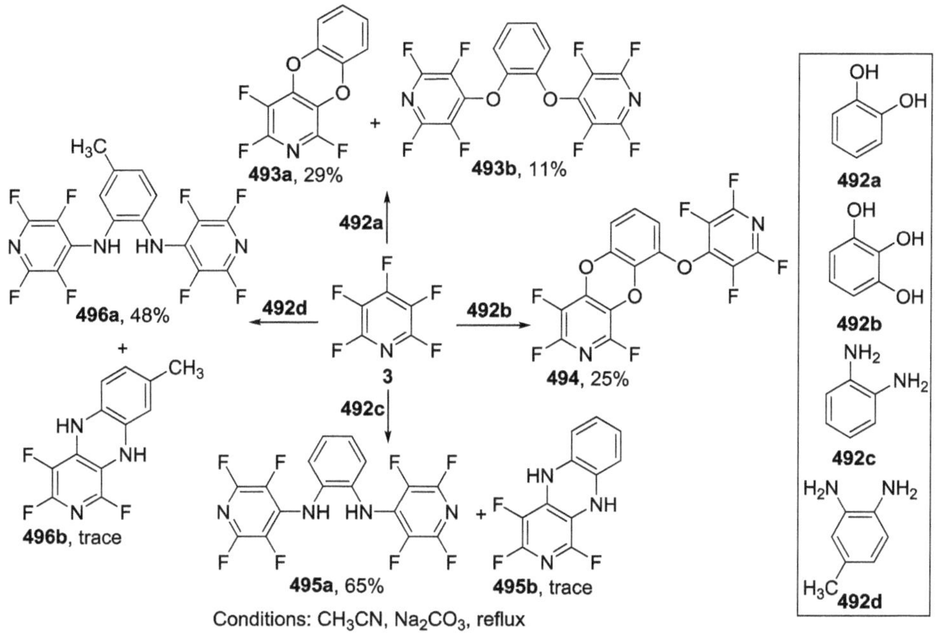

Scheme 2-181. Reaction of pentafluoropyridine **3** with aromatic diolas and diamines.

Tricyclic difluoro-4-phenylsulfonylbenzo [5, 6] [1, 4] dioxino[2,3-b]pyridine, difluoro4-benzenesulfonyl-5, 10-dihydro-pyrido[2,3-b]quinoxaline scaffolds synthesized by the reaction of 4-phenylsulphonyltetrafluoropyridine **24** with aromatic diols and diamines (Scheme 2 - 182) [144].

Reaction of pentafluoropyridine **3** with benzamidine hydrochloride produced imidazopyridine **506** in two steps, whereas tricyclic system **509** produced in one-step from reaction of pentafluoropyridine **3** with 2-iminopiperidine (Scheme 2 - 183) [148]. Reaction of pentafluoropyridine with acetamidine formed amidine **507**, followed by losing of acetonitrile in the presence of various bases and give 4-aminotetrafluoropyridine instead of ring formation (Scheme 2 - 183) [148]. In addition, formimidamide hydrochloride in reaction with pentafluoropyridine produced 4-aminotetrafluoropyridine and amidine **508**. The postulated mechanism leads to **13** is shown in Scheme 2 - 184 that involves elimination of acetonitrile and hydrogen cyanide from the amidine substituent, respectively.

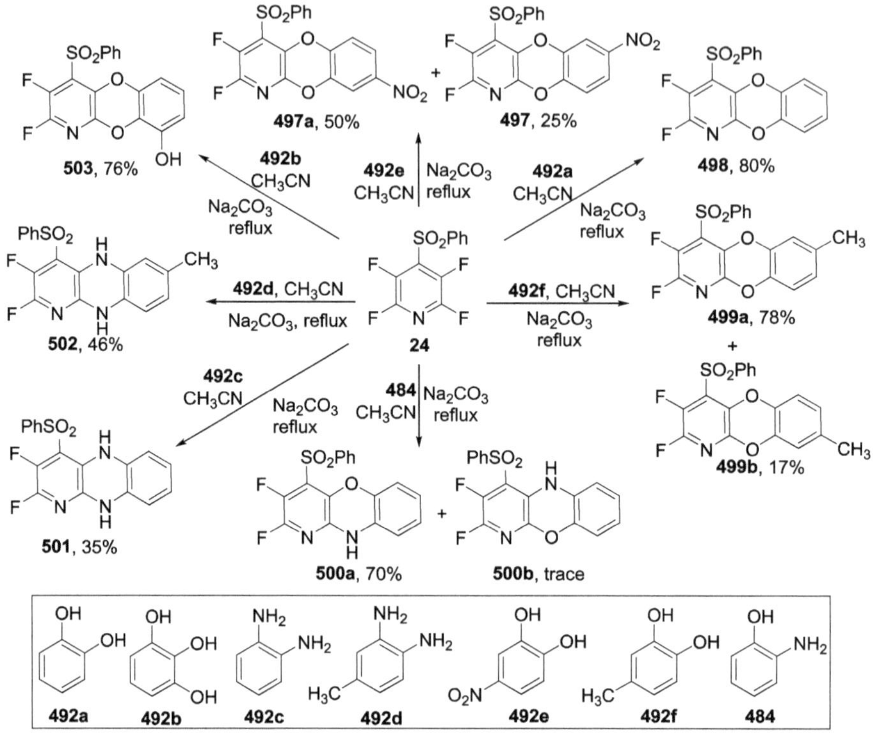

Scheme 2-182. Reaction of 4-phenylsulphonyl tetrafluoropyridine **24** with aromatic diols and diamines.

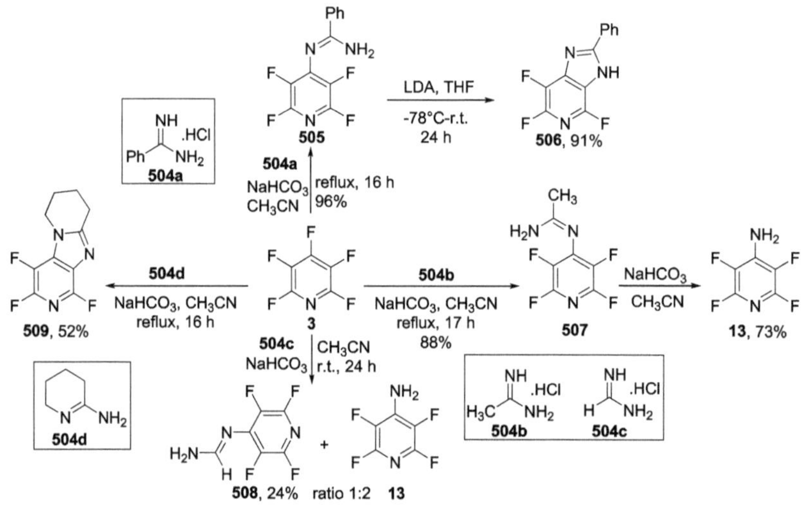

Scheme 2-183. Reaction of pentafluoropyridine **3** with amidines **504**.

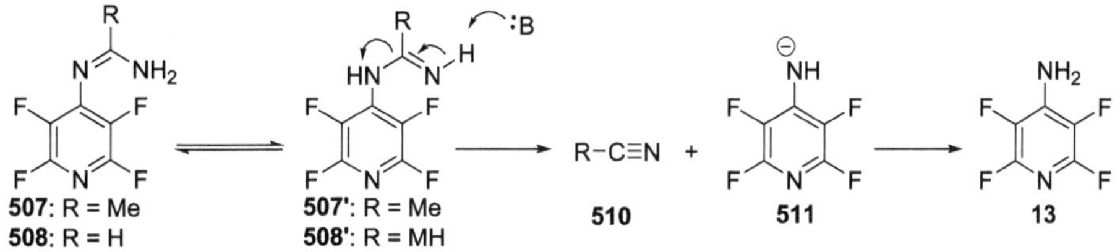

Scheme 2-184. The postulated mechanism for the elimination process.

Imidazole system **506** is methylated at *N*-atom by MeI. In addition, fluorine atom located at the 2-position of pyridine is replaced in reaction with *N*-methyl benzylamine (Scheme 2 - 185) [148].

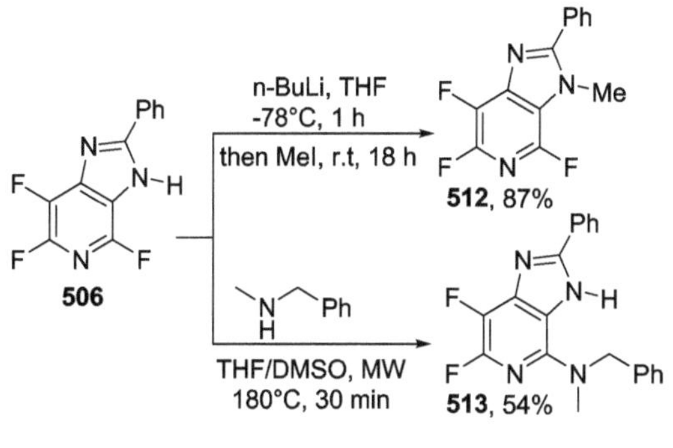

Scheme 2-185. Reaction of compound **248** with *n*-BuLi and *N*-methyl benzylamine.

Ring-fused systems **514a** and **514b** have been produced on reaction of 4-phenylsulphonyltetrafluoropyridine **24** with benzamidine and acetamidine hydrochloride (Scheme 2 - 186) [148].

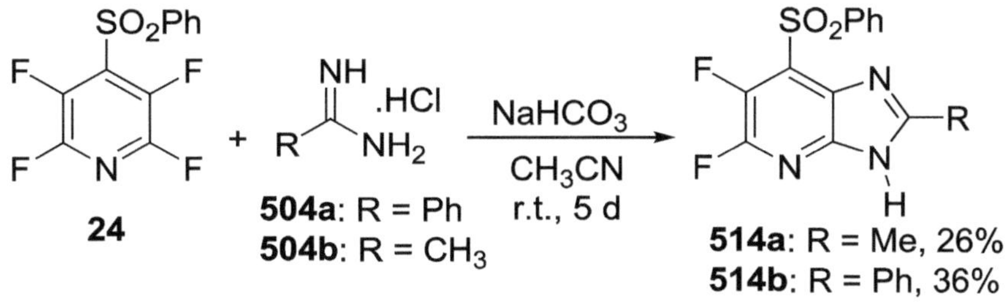

Scheme 2-186. Reaction of 4-phenylsulphonyltetrafluoropyridine **24** with amidines.

Reaction of 4-cyanotetrafluoropyridine with benzamidine and acetamidine hydrochloride leaded to cyclic and acyclic products (Scheme 2 - 187) [148].

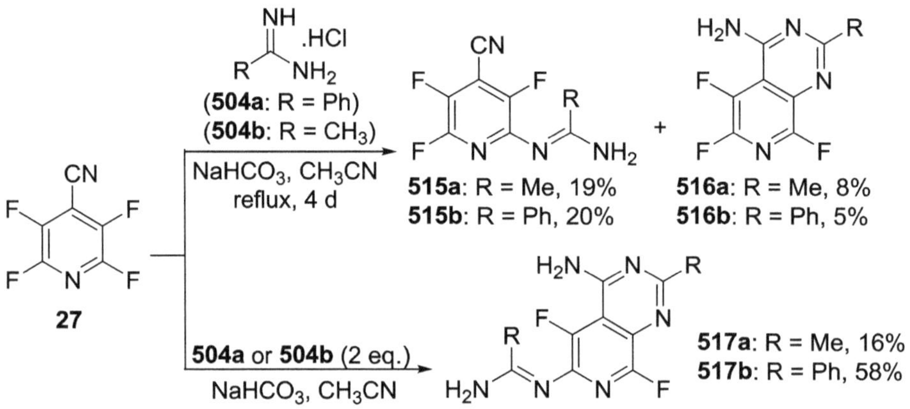

Scheme 2-187. Reaction of 4-cyanotetrafluoropyridine **27** with amidines.

Substituted imidazopyridines **518** have been efficiently synthesized from the reaction of 4-Phenylsulfonyltetrafluoropyridine with *N*-arlyamidines *via* an intramolecular neuclophilic substation reaction, while uncyclized product **519** is obtained using amidine **368e** (Scheme 2 - 188) [116].

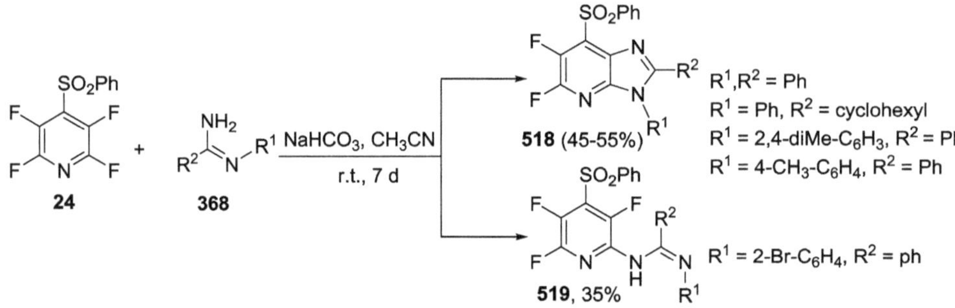

Scheme 2-188. Reaction of 4-phenylsulphonyltetrafluoropyridine **24** with various *N*-aryl amidines **368**.

Fluorothiazolopyridines have obtained from the reaction of pentafluoropyridine **3** and 4-phenylsulphonyltetrafluoropyridine **24** with bifunctional *S*- and *N*-centered nucleophiles (Schemes 2 - 189 and 2 - 190) [149].

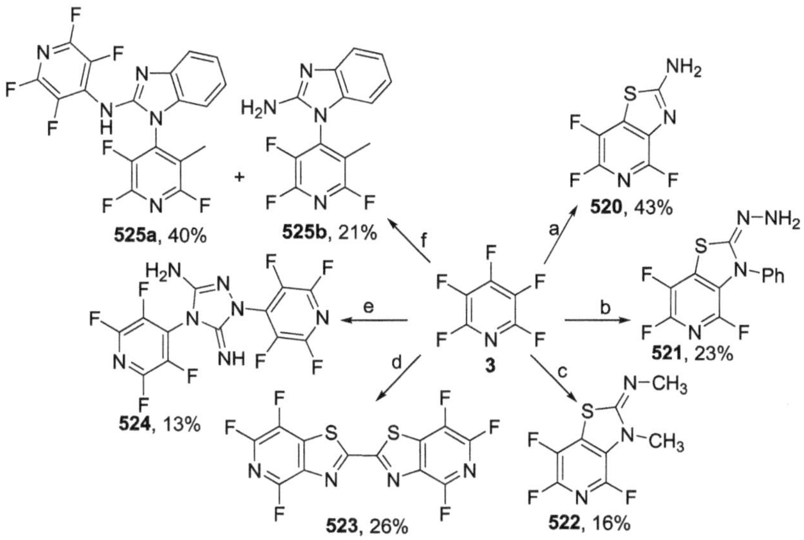

a) thiourea, Na_2CO_3, DMSO, 130°C, 48 h; b) 4-phenylthiosemicarbazide, Na_2CO_3, DMSO, 130°C, 48 h; c) N,N'-dimethyl-thiourea, Na_2CO_3, DMSO, 130°C, 48 h; d) ethanebis(thioamide), Na_2CO_3, DMSO, 130°C, 38 h; e) 1H-1,2,4-triazole-3,5-diamine, Na_2CO_3, CH_3CN, reflux, 8 h; f) 2-aminobenzoimid-azole, Na_2CO_3, CH_3CN, reflux, 8 h

Scheme 2-189. Reaction of pentafluoropyridine **3** with bidentate *S* and *N*-centered nucleophiles.

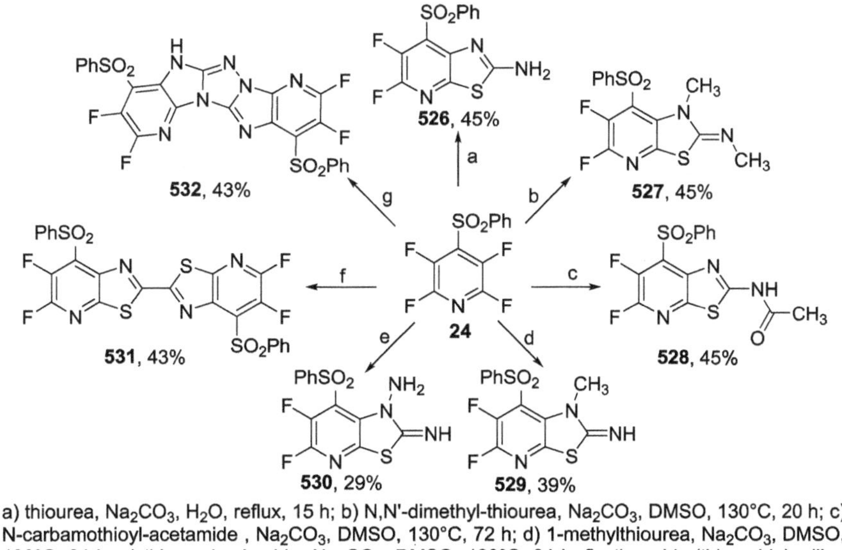

a) thiourea, Na_2CO_3, H_2O, reflux, 15 h; b) N,N'-dimethyl-thiourea, Na_2CO_3, DMSO, 130°C, 20 h; c) N-carbamothioyl-acetamide , Na_2CO_3, DMSO, 130°C, 72 h; d) 1-methylthiourea, Na_2CO_3, DMSO, 130°C, 24 h; e) thiosemicarbazide, Na_2CO_3, DMSO, 130°C, 24 h; f) ethanebis (thioamide), silica gel-KF, Na_2CO_3, CH_3CN, reflux, 48 h; g) 1H-1,2,4-triazole-3,5-diamine, K_2CO_3, DMF, 120°C, 7 d.

Scheme 2-190. Reaction of **24** with bidentate *S*- and *N*-centered nucleophiles.

Diaminodihydro substituted pyridine derivatives react chemoselectivity with pentafluoropyridine and produced dipyrido[1,2-b:30,40-e] [1, 2, 4] triazine systems **534** as major product along with forming uncyclized products **535** in low yields or trace (Scheme 2 - 191) [150].

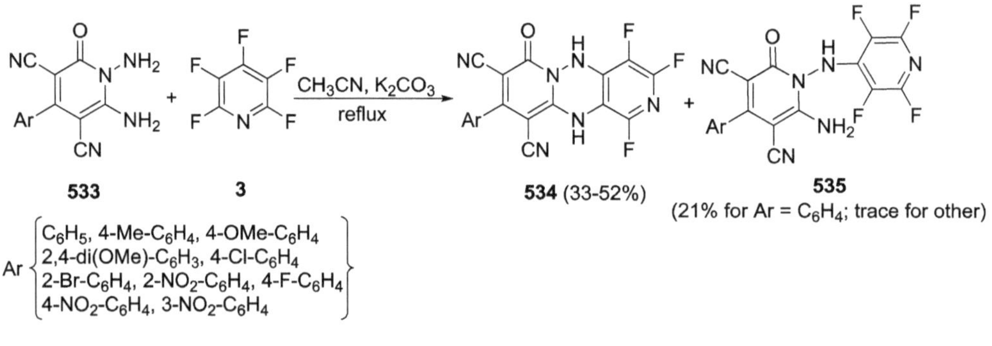

Scheme 2-191. Reaction of diamino-dihydro substituted pyridines **533** with pentafluoropyridine **3**.

6. ORGANOMETALLIC COMPOUNDS OF PERFLUORO-HETEROAROMATICS

The base method for introduction of allylic group on perfluoroheteroaromatics is the reaction of allylhalides with organometallic perfluoroheteroaromatics or allylmagnesium halides with perfluoroheteroaromatics [151, 152]. Mainly, reactions are involving of magnesium and lithium organometallic compounds in etheric solvents, but reaction of zinc perfluoroheteroaromatics with allyl chlorides and bromides carried out in DMF [153, 154].

Pentafluoropyridine on reaction with zinc powder at the presence of $SnCl_2$ as catalyst produced tetrafluoropyridine-4-ylzinc chloride **536** in high yield, which as nucleophile can be attack to allylchloride and produce 4-allyl tetrafluoropyridine **537** (Scheme 2 - 192) [155].

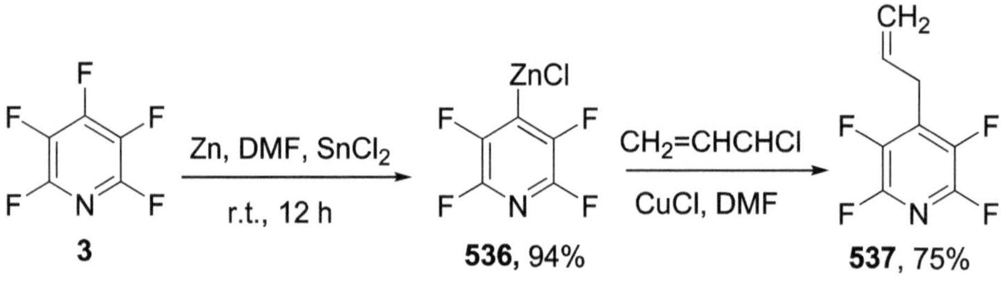

Scheme 2-192. Synthesis of 4-allyl tetrafluoropyridine **537**.

Synthesis of perfluoroarylcopper reagents carried out *via* metathesis of the corresponding perfluoroaryllithium or perfluoroarylmagnesium compounds with copper halides at low temperature [156 - 158]. This method is limited by the thermal stability of perfluoroaryl-magnesium or -lithium reagents. A route for synthesis of 4-tetrafluoropyridylcopper **539** reagent is reaction of 4-tetrafluoropyridylmagnesium bromide **538** with CuBr in THF as solvent (Scheme 2 - 193) [159].

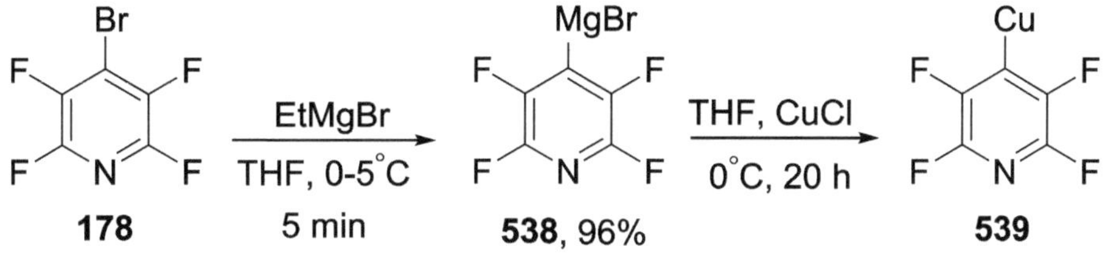

Scheme 2-193. Synthesis of 4-tetrafluoropyridylcopper reagent **539**.

4-tetrafluoropyridyl-cadmium and -zinc reagents are more stable than the lithium and Grignard reagents [160]. These reagents prepared from the reaction of 4-iodo or 4-bromotetrafluoropyridine with cadmium or zinc powder. These reagents undergo metathesis with CuBr and produced 4-tetrafluoropyridylcopper **539** reagent (Scheme 2 - 194) [161]. Copper reagent coupled easily with terminal vinyl iodides, aryl iodides, acid chlorides and allyl halides at room temperature (Scheme 2 - 195) [161].

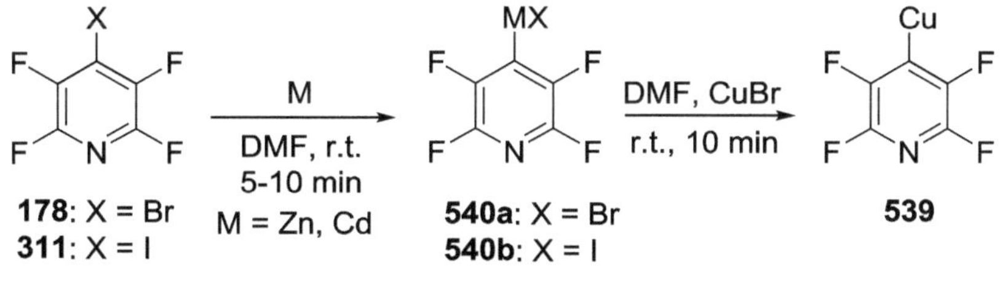

Scheme 2-194. Synthesis of 4-tetrafluoropyridylcopper reagent **539**.

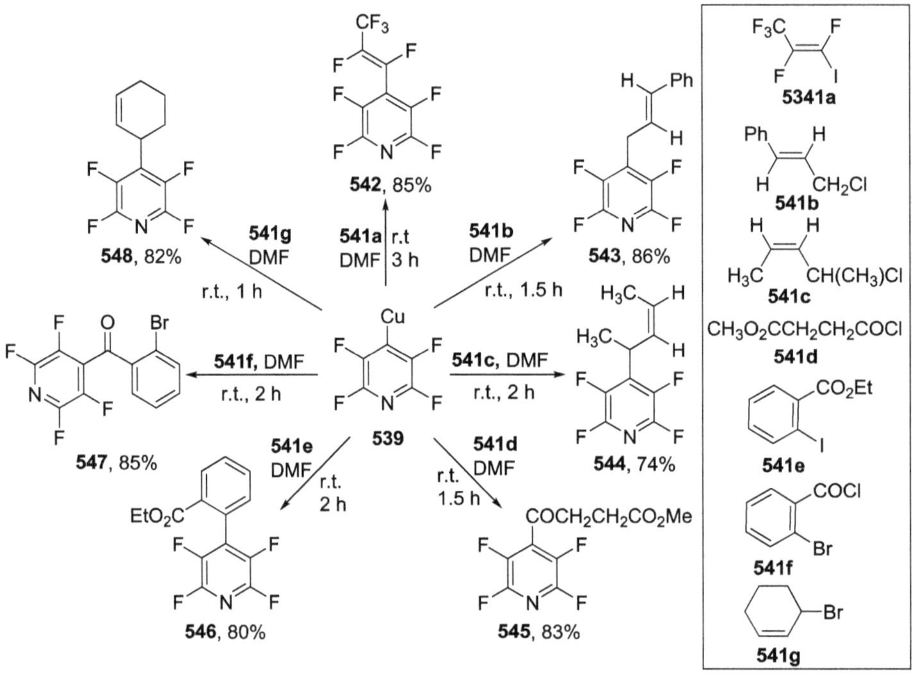

Scheme 2-195. Reactions of 4-tetrafluoropyridylcopper reagent **539**.

Functionalized fluorinated organic compounds have great interest in organic synthesis. An efficient method for the preparation them is the transformation of perfluoroarenes coupling reactions [162 - 167]. Tetrafluoro-4-phenylpyridine **14** and tetrafluoro-2-phenylpyridine **550** have been obtained on reaction of pentafluoropyridine with $ZnPh_2$ with using palladium as a cross-coupling catalyst (Scheme 2 - 196) [168].

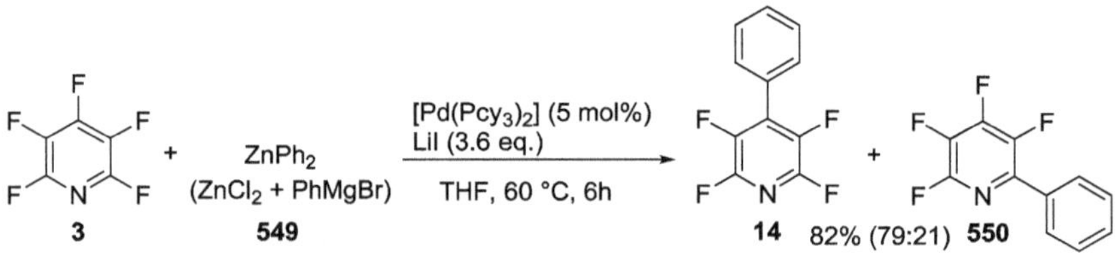

Scheme 2-196. Palladium(0)-catalyzed coupling reaction of pentafluoropyridine **3** with $ZnPh_2$ **549**.

Tetrafluoro-3-lithiopyridine, prepared form the reaction of **324** with *n*-BuLi, as a nucleophile could be added to electrophilic types and formed various substituted perfluoropyridine derivatives (Table **2-5**) [106].

Table 2-5. Reaction of tetrafluoro-3-lithiopyridine 551 with various electriphiles.

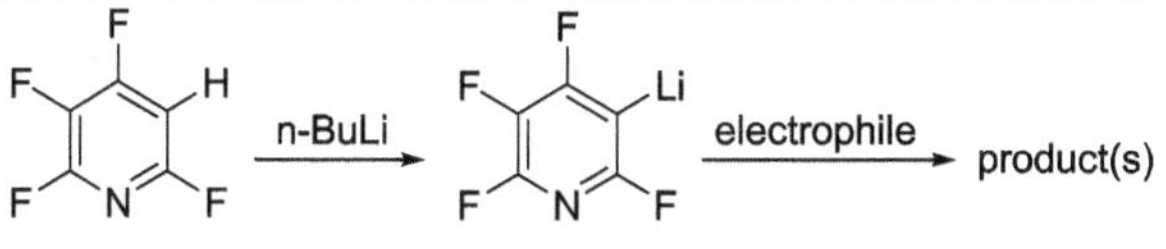

Entry	Condition	552/Yield
1	Et$_2$O, n-BuLi, -78 °C, 1 h; then CO$_2$, -55 °C, 2 h	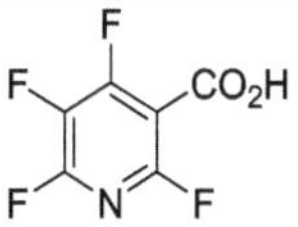 **552a**, 89.1%
2	Et$_2$O, n-BuLi, -70 °C, 40 min; then Me$_3$SiCl, -70 °C, 2 h	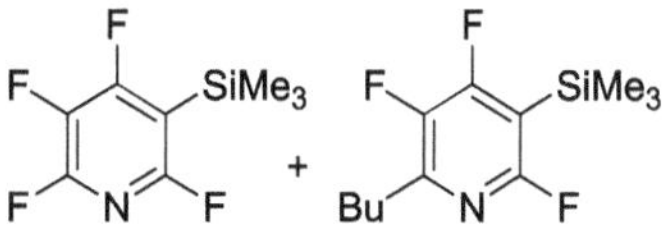 **552b**, 39% + **552c**, 11.5%
3	Et$_2$O, n-BuLi, -78 °C; then -70 °C, 90 min; then Bu$_3$SnCl, -70 °C, 2 h	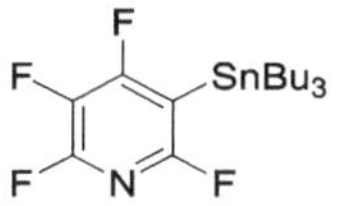 **552d**, 73.3%
4	Et$_2$O, n-BuLi, -78 °C, 30 min; then I$_2$, -78 °C, 30 min	**552e**, 52.6%
5	Et$_2$O, n-BuLi, -78 °C, 30 min; then N-Methylformanilide, -78 °C, 2 h	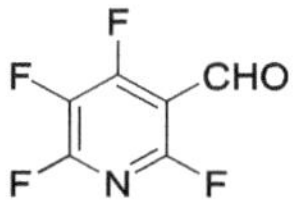 **552f**, 84.3%
6	Et$_2$O, n-BuLi, -78 °C, 30 min; then NOCl, -78 °C, 2 h	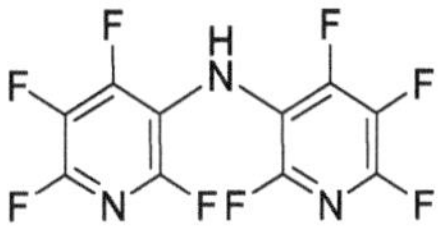 **552g**, 63%

(Table 2-5) cont.....

7	Et$_2$O, n-BuLi, -78 °C, 30 min; then PhCHO, -78 °C, 30 min; then r.t., 1 h	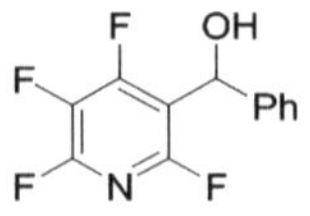 **552h**, 70.7%
8	Et$_2$O, n-BuLi, -78 °C, 30 min; then CH$_3$COCl, -70 °C, 30 min	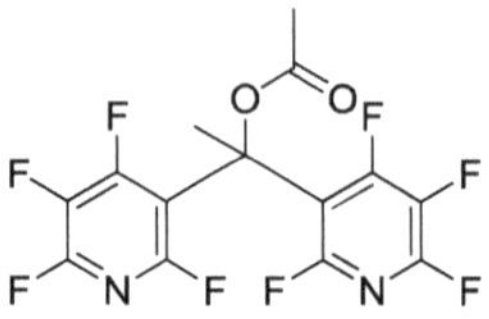 **552i**, 80.8%
9	Et$_2$O, n-BuLi, -78 °C, 30 min; then TFAA, -70 °C, 30 min; then r.t., 1h	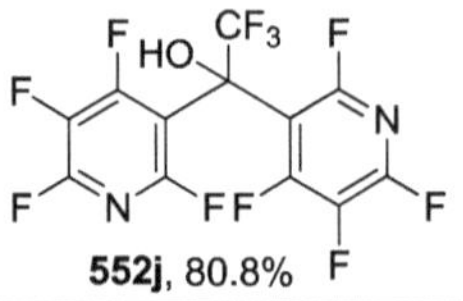 **552j**, 80.8%

Tetrafluoro-3-lithiopyridine in reaction with CO$_2$ and NH$_3$ produced directly 4-amino-2,5,6-trifluoronicotinic acid **553** (Scheme 2 - 197) [106]. This compound underwent Curtius reaction on treatment with diphenyl phosphorazidate (DPPA) and produced 3-deaza-2,3,6-trifluoro-8-hydroxypurine **554** (Scheme Scheme 2 - 197).

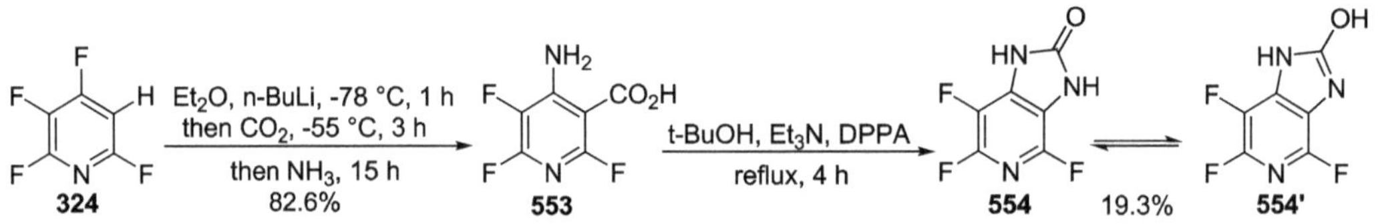

Scheme 2-197. Preparation of 3-deaza-2,3,6-trifluoro-8-hydroxypurine **554** using tetrafluoro-3-lithiopyridine.

2,3,5,6-Tetrafluoropyridine on treatment with *n*-BuLi converted to tetrafluoro-4-lithiopyridine, which in the presence of ethyl chloroformate produced ethyl tetrafluoroisonicotinate **555** (Scheme **2 - 198**) [106].

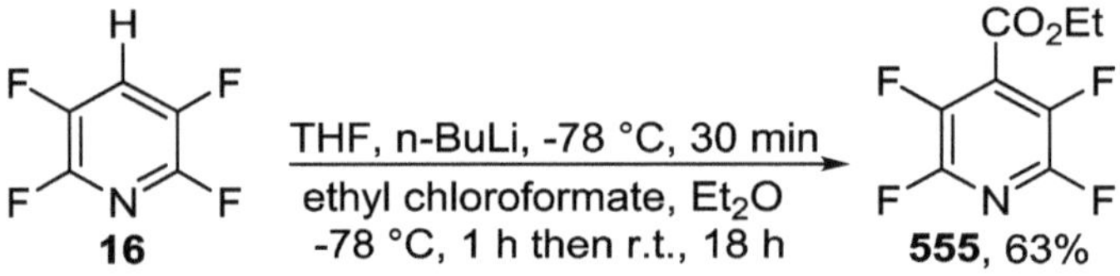

Scheme 2-198. Preparation of ethyl tetrafluoroisonicotinate **555** from 2,3,5,6-tetrafluoropyridine **16**.

The tetrafluoropyridyl group has attracted considerable interest in metal chemistry [169]. 4-Tetrafluoropyridyl silver (I) is versatile tool for redox transmetallations. AgC_5F_4N **556** has been obtained *via* $Me_3SiC_5F_4N$ **315** and AgF in nearly quantitative yield (Scheme 2 - 199) [169]. AgC_5F_4N **556** has been shown good oxidizing abilities in reaction with elemental Zn, Cd, Hg, Ga, In, Sn, Bi, Sb, As, Te and Se [169 - 171]. Redox transmetallations of AgC_5F_4N and these elements yielded the corresponding 4-tetrafluoropyridyl elements (Scheme 2 - 200). The reaction of AgC_5F_4N **556** and bis(triphenylphosphoranyliden)ammonium chloride, [PNP]Cl **565**, in a stoichiometric ratio of 2:1 gave crystalline $[PNP][Ag(C_5F_4N)_2]$ **566** (Scheme 2 - 201) [169].

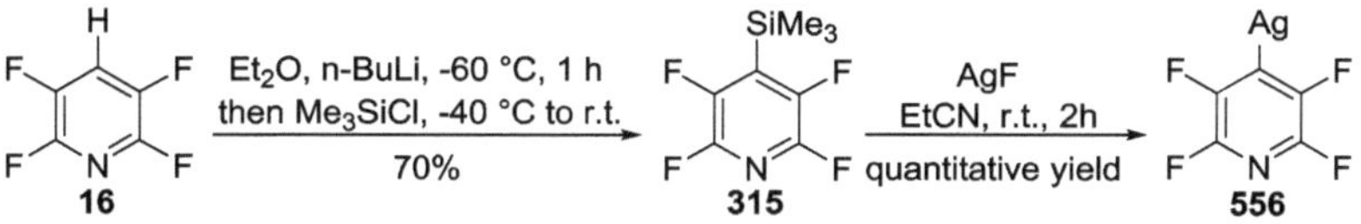

Scheme 2-199. Synthesis of AgC_5F_4N **556**.

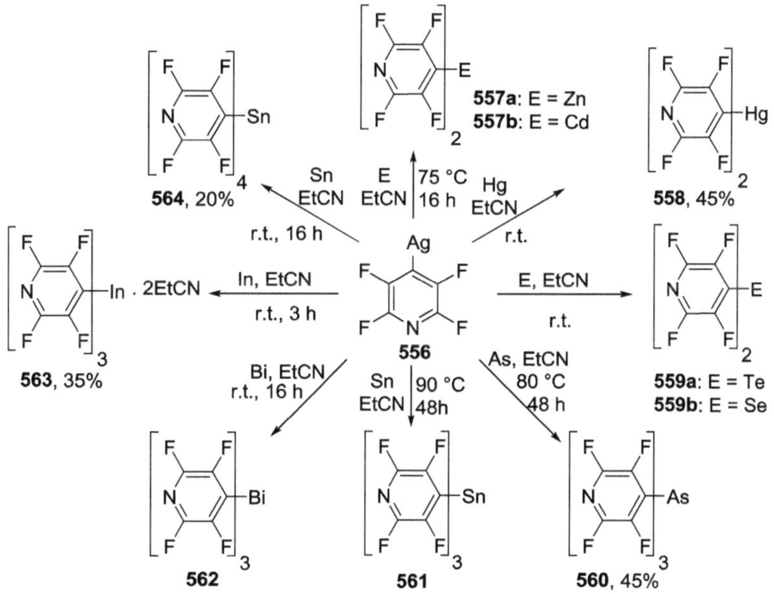

Scheme 2-200. Reaction of AgC_5F_4N **556** with various metals.

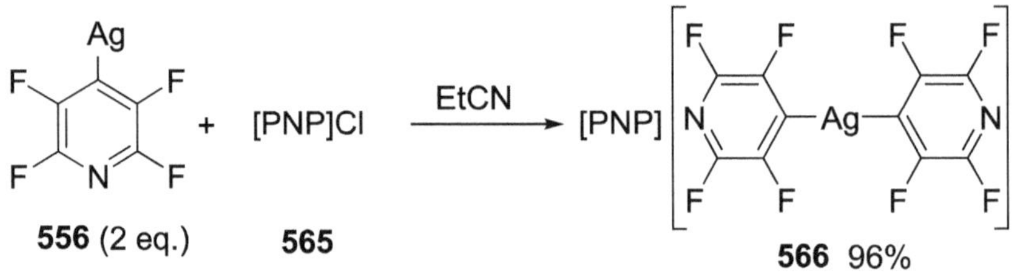

Scheme 2-201. Preparation of [PNP][Ag(C$_5$F$_4$N)$_2$] **566**.

In last two decades, C-F bond activation has been very considered [172 - 174]. C-F bond of pentafluoropyridine activated selectively at the 2-position by Ni reagent **567** in the presence of PEt$_3$ [175], followed by reaction with tributyl(vinyl)stannane and gave **569**. Repetition this process leaded to formation of compound **571** (Scheme 2 - 202) [176]. In addition, perfluoropyridines **3** and **16** converted to 2-vinylperfluoropyridines **572a** and **572b** on reaction with tributyl(vinyl)stannane in the presence of Ni reagent **567** (Scheme 2 - 203) [176].

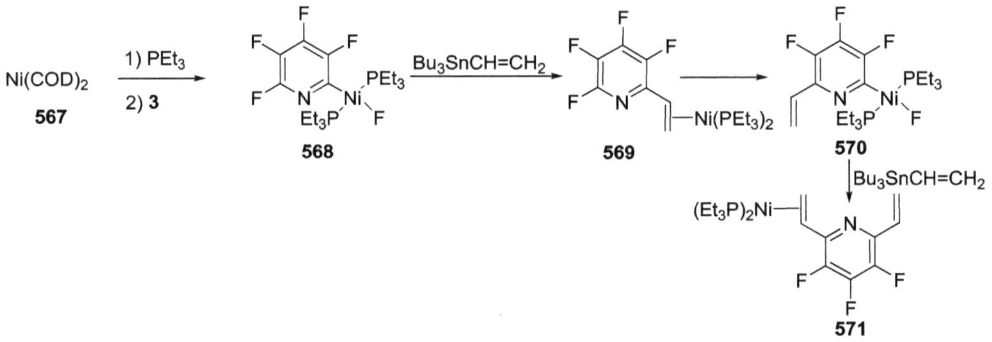

Scheme 2-202. Catalytic conversion of pentafluoropyridine **3** to 2-vinyl derivative **571**.

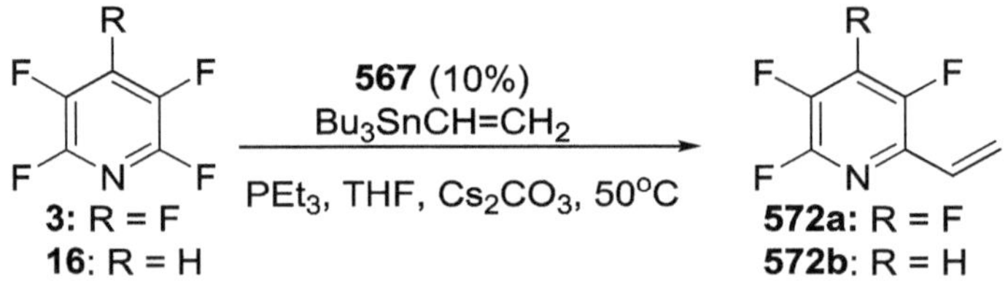

Scheme 2-203. Catalytic conversion of perfluoropyridines **3** to 2-vinyl derivatives **572**.

Hydrodefluorination reactions are common routes to access fluoroorganic compounds *via* transition metal mediated C–F activation, for example the replacement of a C–F by a C–H bond [47, 177]. Hydrogen sources can be boranes, alanes, silanes, and dihydrogen. The conversions are thermodynamically favourable due to the strength of the E–F bonds (E = H, Al, Si, B) which are formed [178]. Palladium selectively activated 4-position C-F bond of pentafluoropyridine and followed *via* replacement of F by H to obtained tetrafluoropyridine **16** (Scheme 2 - 204) [179].

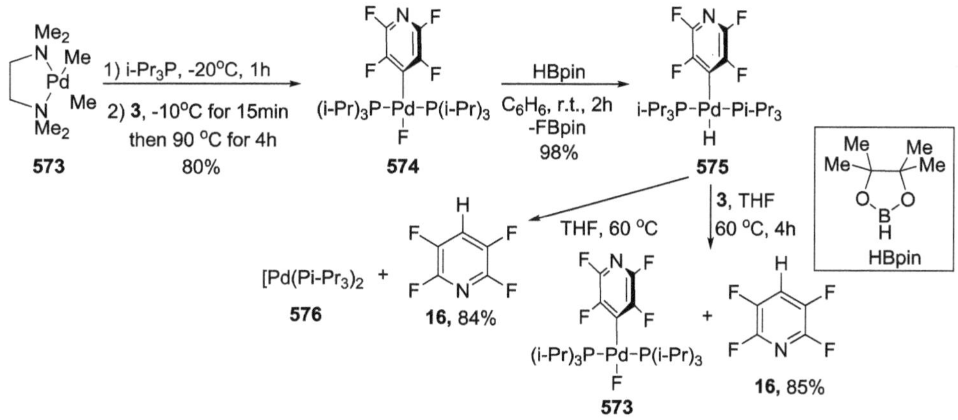

Scheme 2-204. Selective conversion of pentafluoropyridine **3** to tetrafluoropyridine **16** by Pd catalyst.

Hydrodefluorination of pentafluoropyridine by bifunctional C–N chelating amido complex **577a** as transfer hydrogenation catalyst in the presence of 2-propanol gave 2,3,5,6-tetrafluoropyridine in 94% yield (Scheme 2 - 205) [180]. The great outcome obtained using catalyst **577b** and **577c** in the presence of formate salt without 2-propanol (Scheme 2 - 206).

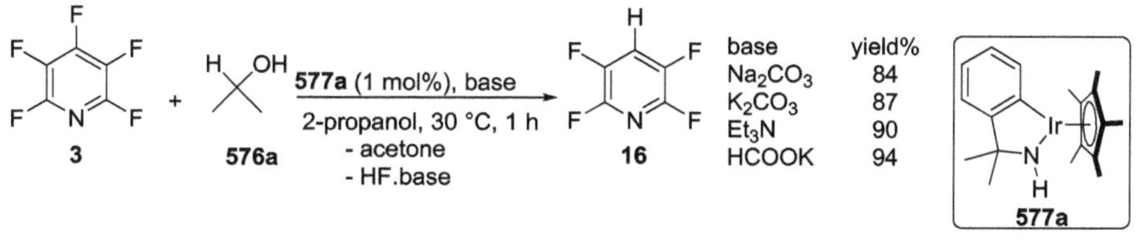

Scheme 2-205. Catalytic hydrodefluorination of pentafluoropyridine **3** using 2-propanol **576a**.

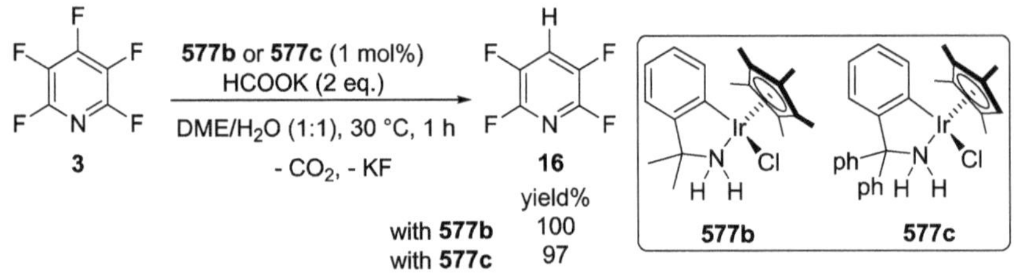

Scheme 2-206. Catalytic hydrodefluorination of pentafluoropyridine **3** using potassium formate.

The successful selective hydrodefluorination of pentafluoropyridine has been achieved using cobalt catalyst supported by trimethylphosphine and with sodium formate as a reducing agent in acetonitrile (Scheme 2 - 207) [181].

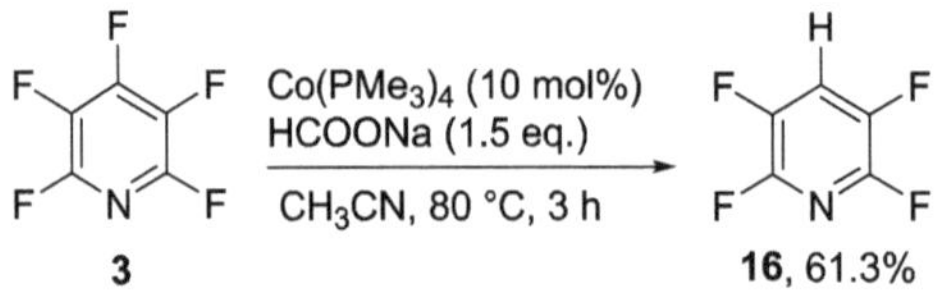

Scheme 2-207. Cobalt-catalyzed hydrodefluorination of pentafluoropyridine **3**.

C−F bond of pentafluoropyridine and 2,3,5,6-tetrafluoropyridine can be activate by photolysis of Tp′Rh(PMe$_3$)H$_2$ or thermal reaction with Tp′Rh(PMe$_3$)(CH$_3$)H (Scheme 2 - 208) [182]. C−F activation of pentafluoropyridine has been occured selectively at the *ortho* position and two conformers observed. The reaction of 2,3,5,6-tetrafluoropyridine has been generated a mixture of C−H and C−F bond activation products.

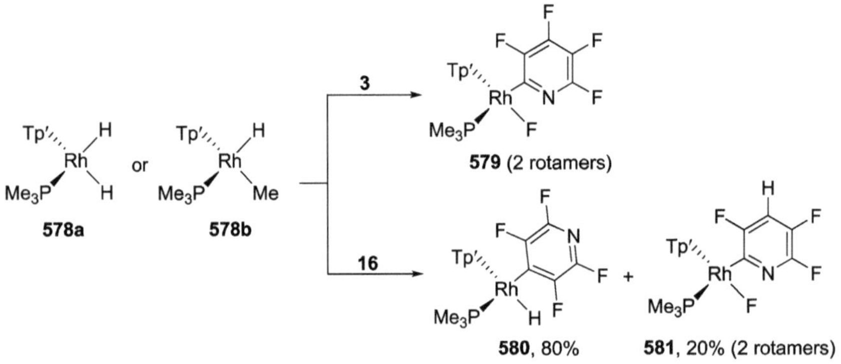

Scheme 2-208. C-F bond activation of perfluoropyridines **3** and **16** using Rh catalyst.

The *para* fluorine atom of the pentafluoropyridine is easily activated by treatment with LPbNMe$_2$**582** and gives LPbF **583** together 4-dimethylaminotetra-fluoropyridine (Scheme 2 - 209) [183]. The stable LPbF **583** can be served as a nucleophilic reagent. Its reaction with L^{1}SiCl(BH$_3$) **584** has been produced L^{1}SiF(BH$_3$) **585** and LPbCl **586** (Scheme 2 - 210).

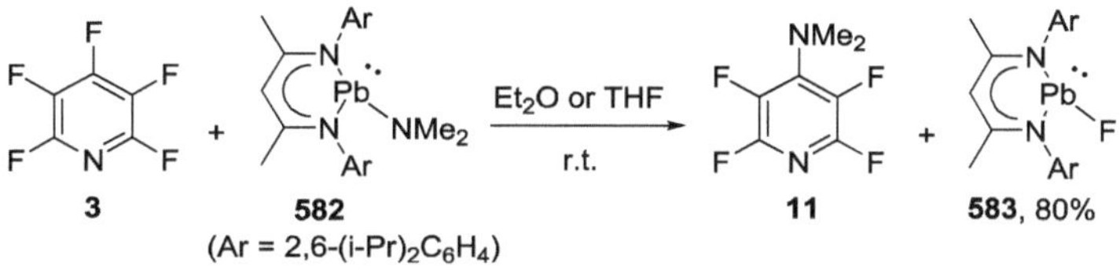

Scheme 2-209. Synthesis of *β*-diketiminatolead (II) monofluoride **583**.

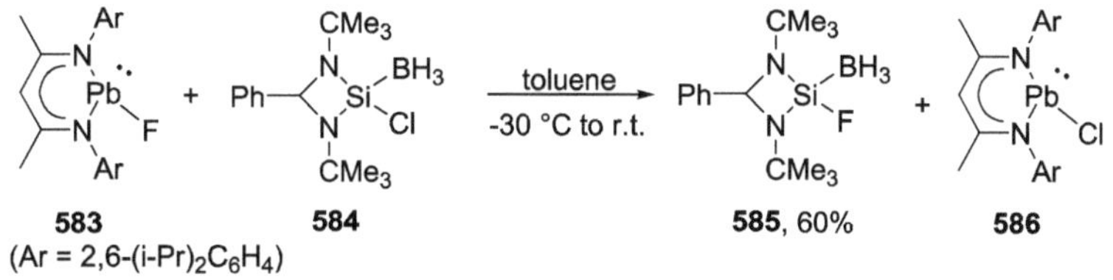

Scheme 2-210. Synthesis of organosilicon(II) monofluoride **585**.

Dialkylamino functionalized group 14 metalylenes (Si, Ge, Sn) in the +2 oxidation state have been shown different modes of reactivity on reaction with pentafluoropyridine, depending on the basicity of the substituent on the metal and the metal atom [54]. Pentafluoropyridine has been underwent oxidative addition reaction on treatment with metalylenes LSiNMe$_2$ and LGeNiPr$_2$, whereas substitution of the NMe$_2$ group occured at the *para* fluorine of pentafluoropyridine by using metalylene LSnNMe$_2$ (Scheme 2 - 211) [54].

Diphosphine **593** in reaction with pentafluoropyridine can be replaced at 4-position C-F bond of pyridine ring and results in the formation of tetrafluoropyridyl-substituted diphosphine **596** (Scheme 2 - 212) [184]. Diphosphine **596** has been linked to a Cp* ligand in a cationic rhodium (III) complex by intramolecular dehydrofluorinative carbon-carbon coupling and gave cationic complexes **598** and **599** (Scheme 2 - 213) [184]. Complex **598** underwent of proton sponge and gave cationic complex **600** (Scheme 2 - 213). Also, complex **600** has been obtained on refluxing mixture of diphosphine **596** and rhodium (III) complex **597** in benzene in the presence of NaBF$_4$ (Scheme 2 - 213).

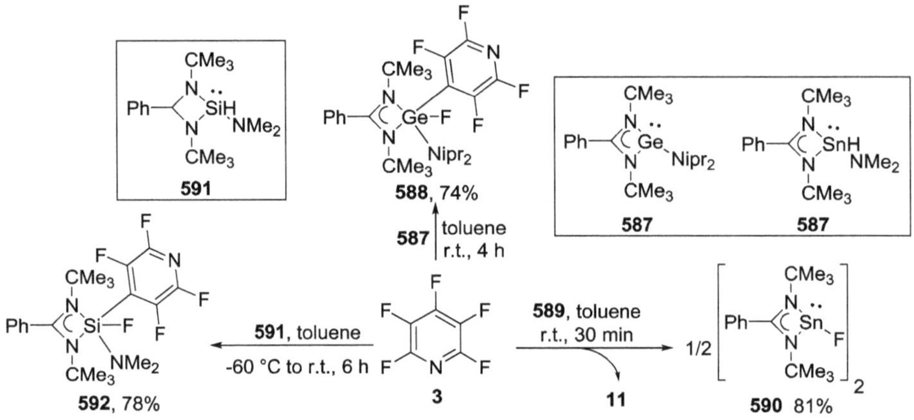

Scheme 2-211. The reaction of metalylenes LGeNiPr$_2$, LSiNMe$_2$, and LSnNMe$_2$ with pentafluoropyridine **3**.

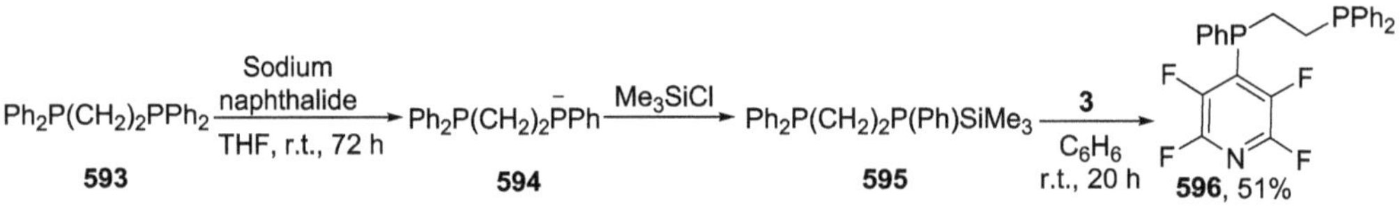

Scheme 2-212. Synthesis of Ph$_2$PCH$_2$CH$_2$PPh(C$_5$F$_4$N) **596**.

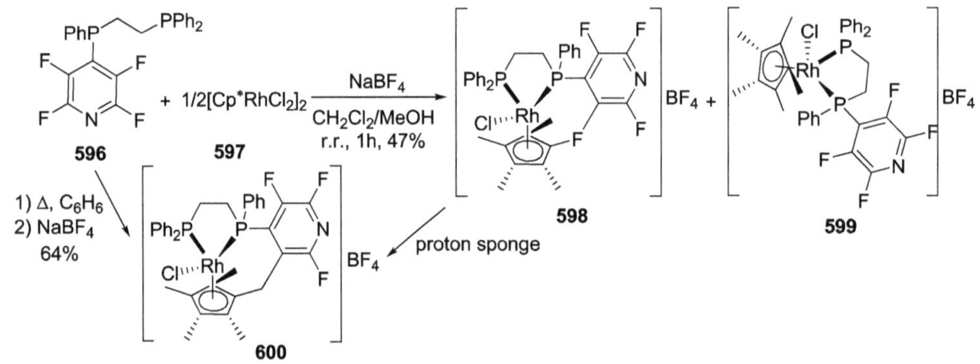

Scheme 2-213. Reaction of Ph$_2$PCH$_2$CH$_2$PPh(C$_5$F$_4$N) **596** with [Cp*RhCl$_2$]$_2$ **597**.

16-electron rhodium(I)–boryl complex **601** is activated selectively C-F bond of pentafluoropyridine at 2-position in the presence of B$_2$pin$_2$ and produced perfluoropyridyl boronate ester **602** (Scheme 2 - 214) [185]. The calculation suggested that C-F activation proceeds *via* boryl-assisted pathway that involves direct transfer of fluorine onto the boron center *via* four-membered transition state **603** (Scheme 2 - 215).

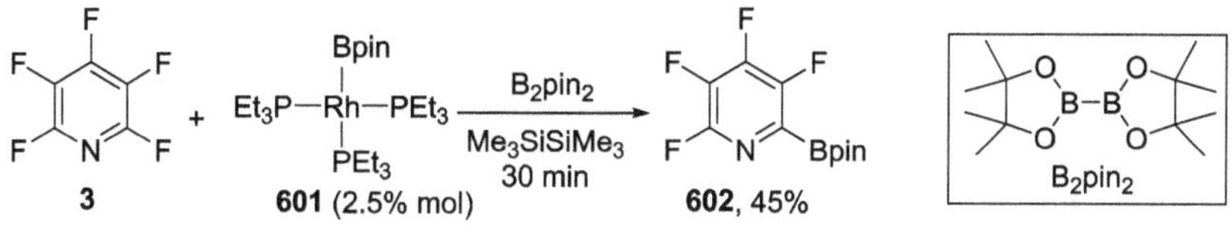

Scheme 2-214. Scheme. Catalytic formation of a perfluoropyridyl boronate ester **602**.

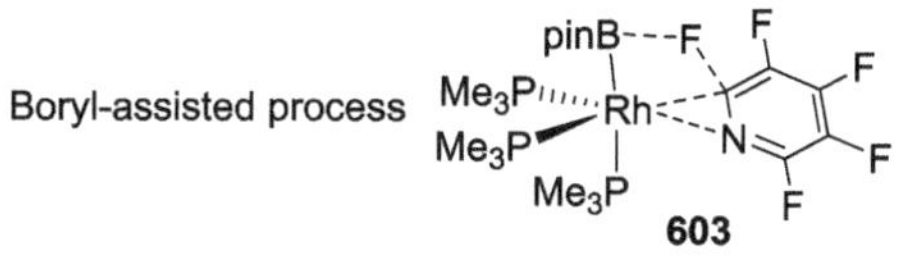

Scheme 2-215. Computed transition state for C-F activation of **3** by [Rh(Bpin)(PMe$_3$)$_3$] **601**.

Complexes **604a** and **604b** treated stoichiometrically with **602** in the presence of CsF and gave the cross-coupling products **605a** and **605b** in high yield (scheme 2 - 216) [186], which resembles a transmetallation and a subsequent reductive elimination. Also, the cross-coupling products **605a**, and **605b** formed by a catalytic reaction of **606a** and **606b** with **602** in the presence of **604a** and **604b** (Scheme 2 - 217) [186].

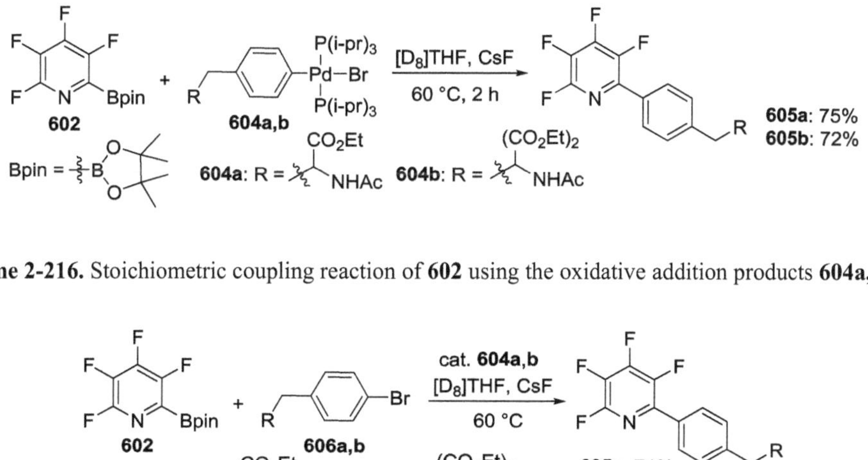

Scheme 2-216. Stoichiometric coupling reaction of **602** using the oxidative addition products **604a,b**.

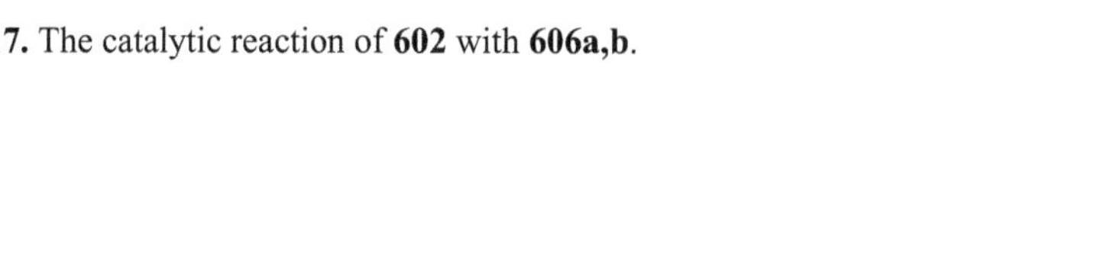

Scheme 2-217. The catalytic reaction of **602** with **606a,b**.

Furthermore, compound **605b** is produced in an independent reaction from boronate [NMe4][BF(2-C5NF4)(pin)] **607**, which is formed by treatment of **602** with NMe$_4$F, with **604b** or **608** (Scheme 2 - 218) [186].

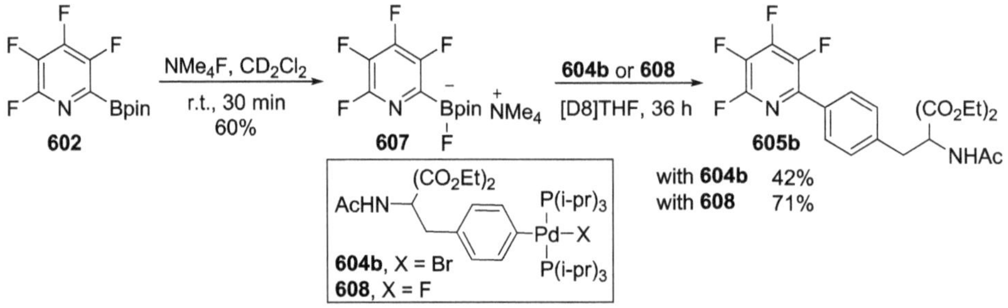

Scheme 2-218. Synthesis of compound **605b** using **608**.

The reaction of [Ni(COD)$_2$] (COD = 1,5-cyclooctadiene) in the presence of i-pr$_2$PCH$_2$CH$_2$OMe with pentafluoropyridine leades to a C-F activation at both 2- and 4-positions and produced complexes **609** and **610** in a ratio 8:1 (Scheme 2 - 219), while in the presence of i-pr$_2$PCH$_2$CH$_2$NMe$_2$ mainly C-F activation occurs at 4-position of pyridine ring (Scheme 2 - 219) [52]. C-F activation of tetrafluoropyridine **16** using [Ni(COD)$_2$] in the presence both of i-pr$_2$PCH$_2$CH$_2$OMe and i-pr$_2$PCH$_2$CH$_2$NMe$_2$ occurs at 2-position of pyridine ring (Schemes 2 - 220) [52].

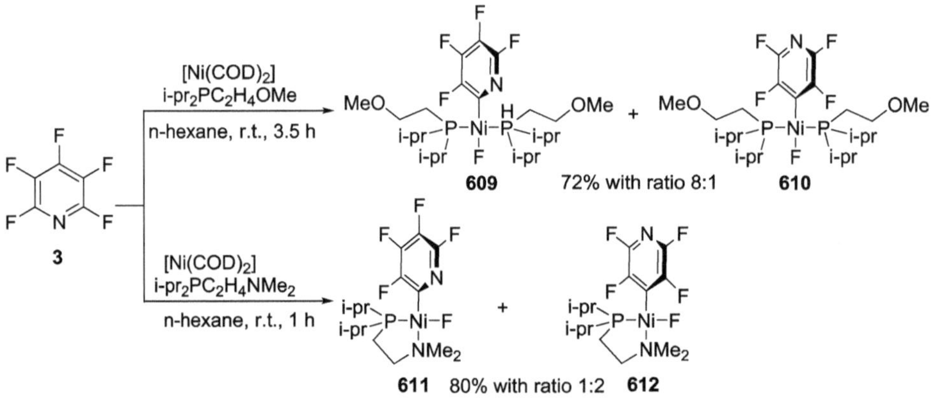

Scheme 2-219. C–F activation of perfluoropyridines **3** [Ni(COD)$_2$]/i-pr$_2$PCH$_2$CH$_2$OMe and [Ni(COD)$_2$]/i-pr$_2$PCH$_2$CH$_2$NMe$_2$.

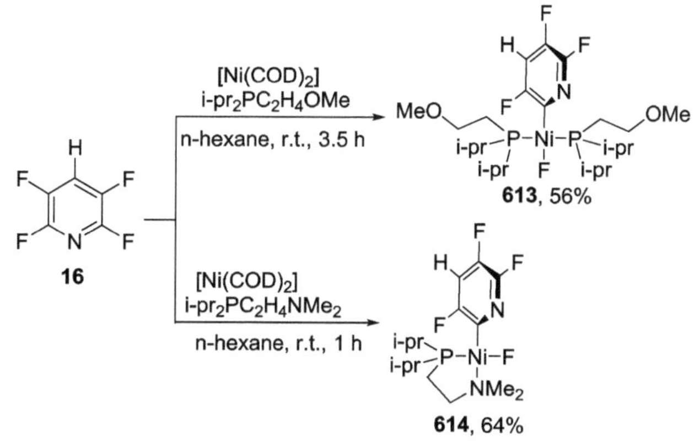

Scheme 2-220. C–F activation of **16** using [Ni(COD)$_2$]/i-pr$_2$PCH$_2$CH$_2$OMe and [Ni(COD)2]/i-pr$_2$PCH$_2$CH$_2$NMe$_2$.

Treatment of pentafluoropyridine with phenylboronic acid in the presence of 5 mol% of a mixture of complexes **609** and **610** (ratio 8:1) gives C–C coupling products 3,4,5-trifluoro-2,6-biphenylpyridine and 3,5-difluoro-2,4-6-triphenylpyridine (Scheme 2 - 221) [52]. In contrast to the reaction above, only 3,5-difluoro-2,4,6-triphenylpyridine formed using complexes **612** and **613** (ratio 1:2) (Scheme 2 - 221). Cross-coupling reaction of 2,3,5,6-tetrafluoropyridine with boronic acids in the presence of 5 mol% **611** or **614** afforded 3,5-difluoro-2-6-di(aryl)pyridines **617a-d** with high regioselectively (Scheme 2 - 222).

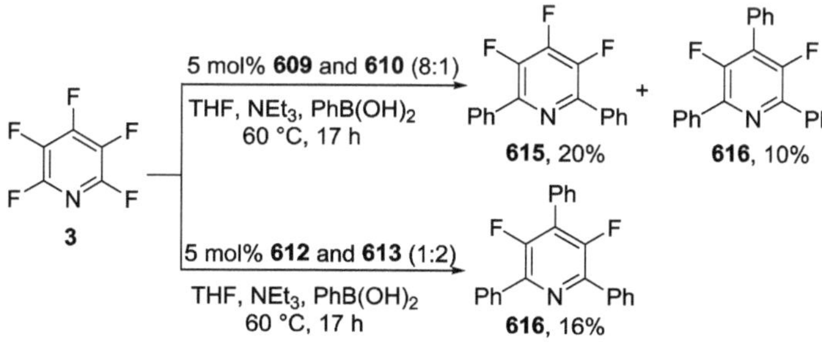

Scheme 2-221. Catalytic cross-coupling reactions of pentafluoropyridine **3**.

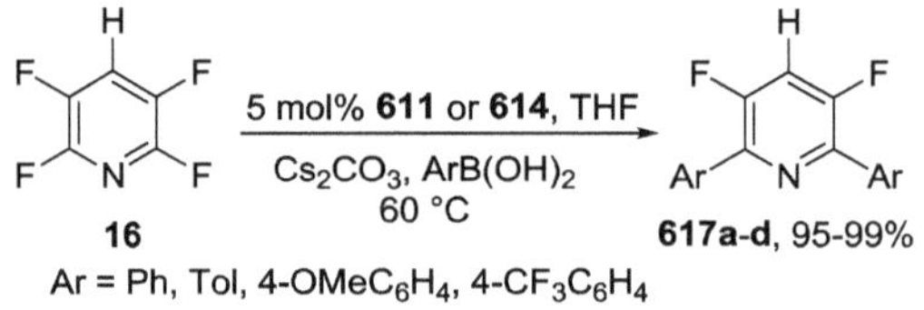

Scheme 2-222. Catalytic cross-coupling reactions of tetrafluoropyridine **16**.

Treatment of the complex trans-[NiF(2-C_5F_4N)(PEt$_3$)$_2$], which was obtained by reaction of Ni(COD)$_2$ with PEt$_3$ and pentafluoropyridine [187], with Me$_3$SiOTf produced the air-stable triflate complex trans-[Ni(OTf)(2-C_5F_4N)(PEt$_3$)$_2$] **618** (Scheme 2 - 223) [188]. Also, this complex was obtained by stepwise treatment of a hexane solution of [Ni(PEt$_3$)$_2$(COD)] with C_5F_5N and Me$_3$SiOTf without isolation of complex **568** [188]. OTf group of complex **618** can be replaced with nucleophiles such as phenoxy. Fluorine atom attached to Ni in complex **568** substituted with phenyl and methyl on reaction with PhLi and Me$_2$Zn, respectively (Scheme 2 - 223). Mainly, pentafluoropyridine substituted at *para* the position by either electrophilic or nucleophilic substitution, so it is very difficult to prepare 2-substituted tetrafluoropyridines. However, these nickel compounds are rare examples of 2-psition metal coordinated tafluoropyridines. Complex **620** in reaction with CO and air produced 2-acetyl and 2-methytetrafluoropyrine, respectively (Scheme 2 - 223) [188].

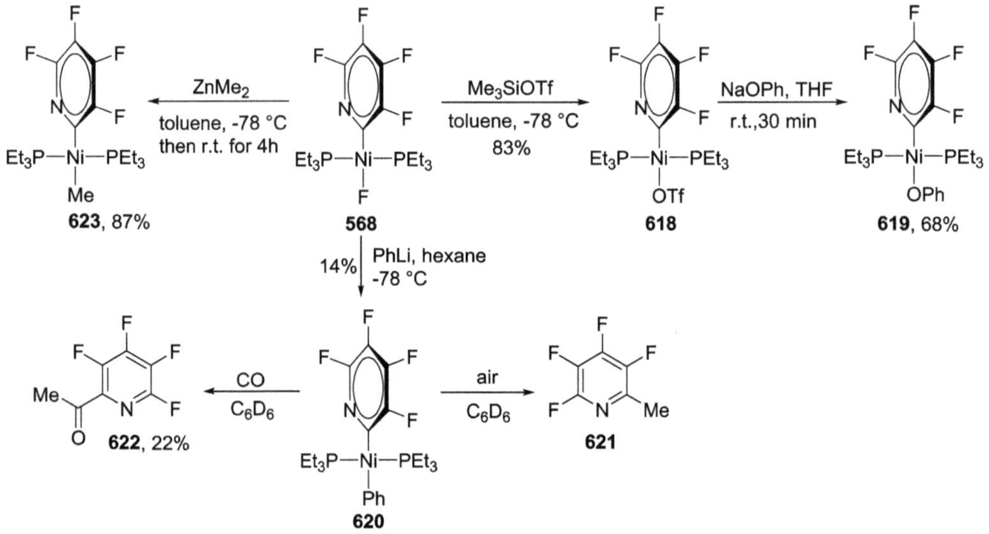

Scheme 2-223. Reactions of nickel tetrafluoropyridyl complexes **568**.

7. PHOTOCHEMICAL REACTIONS OF FLUORINATED PYRIDINES

C–F functionalizations to C–C bonds are challenging synthetic transformations due to C–F bonds are significantly strong, short and not polarizable. Alkylation of pentafluoropyridine has been successfully performed with various alkenes using fac-Ir(ppy)$_3$ in the presence of Blue LED's, while the C-F Alkylation occurs selectively at 4-F bond of pyridine rings (Table **2-6**) [189].

Table 2-6. The photocatalytic C-F alkylation of pentafluoropyridine 3 using fac-Ir(ppy)$_3$.

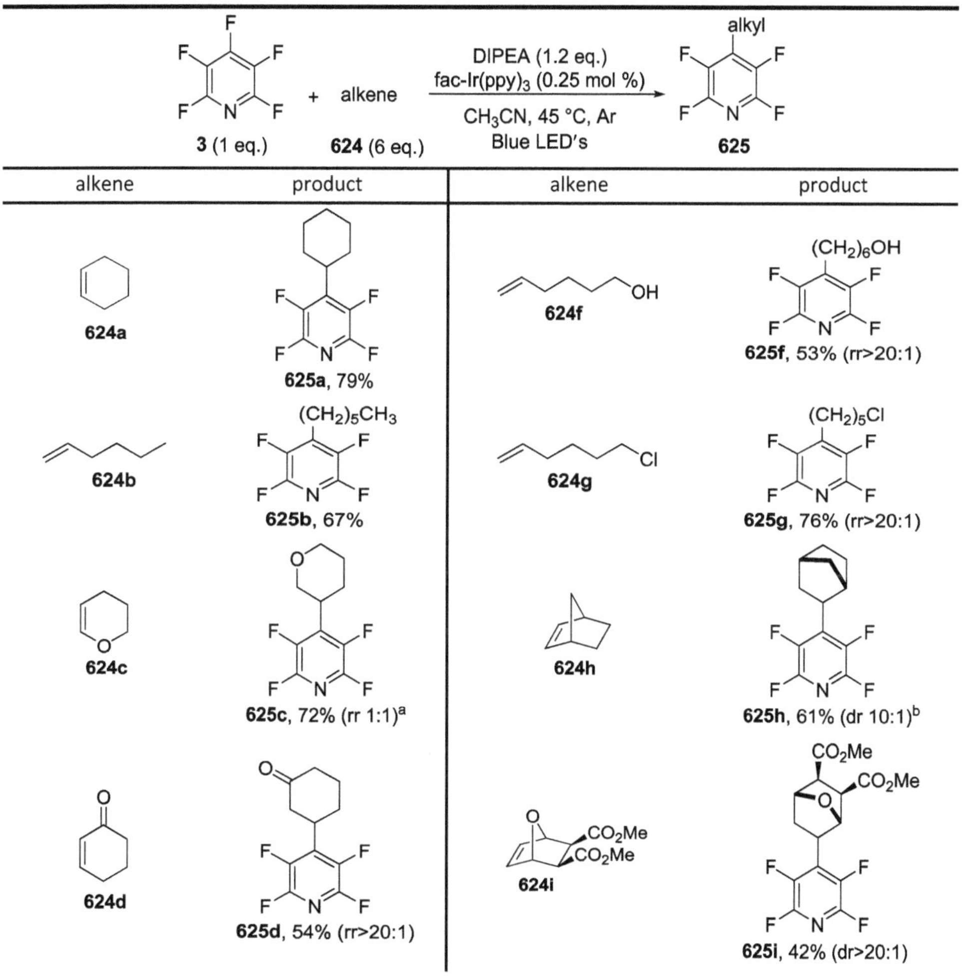

Reaction scheme: **3** (1 eq.) + alkene **624** (6 eq.) → **625**, with DIPEA (1.2 eq.), fac-Ir(ppy)$_3$ (0.25 mol %), CH$_3$CN, 45 °C, Ar, Blue LED's.

alkene	product	alkene	product
624a	**625a**, 79%	**624f**	**625f**, 53% (rr>20:1)
624b	**625b**, 67%	**624g**	**625g**, 76% (rr>20:1)
624c	**625c**, 72% (rr 1:1)[a]	**624h**	**625h**, 61% (dr 10:1)[b]
624d	**625d**, 54% (rr>20:1)	**624i**	**625i**, 42% (dr>20:1)

(Table 2-6) cont.....

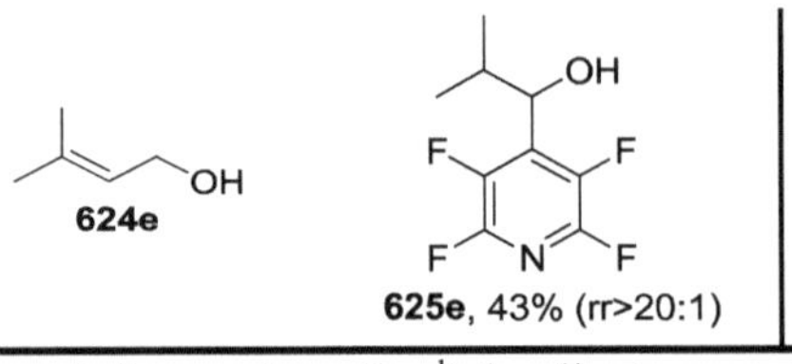

624e	**625e**, 43% (rr>20:1)

[a] rr: regioisomeric ratio; [b] dr: diastereomeric ratio

Tetrafluoropyridine **354** underwent the photocatalytic C-F alkylation at 2-F bond of pyridine ring on reaction with alkenes **624h** and **624i** and produced compoundes **626** and **627**, respectively (Scheme 2-**224**) [189]. Compound **627** converted to difluoropyridine **628** *via* hydrodefluorination by Ir(ppy)$_3$.

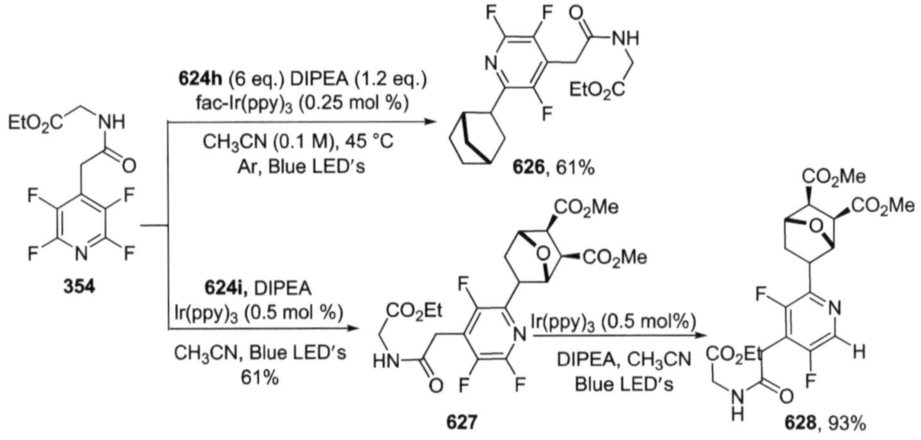

Scheme 2-224. The photocatalytic C-F alkylation of **354** using fac-Ir(ppy)$_3$ followed hydrodefluorination reaction.

The photocatalytic alkylation of 3-chlorotetrafluoropyridine occurs selectively at C-Cl bond (Scheme 2 - 225) [189]. Similarly, compound **630** underwent C-Cl alkylation and produced derivative **632**, which gives product **633** on hydrodefluorination by Ir(ppy)$_3$ (Scheme 2 - 226).

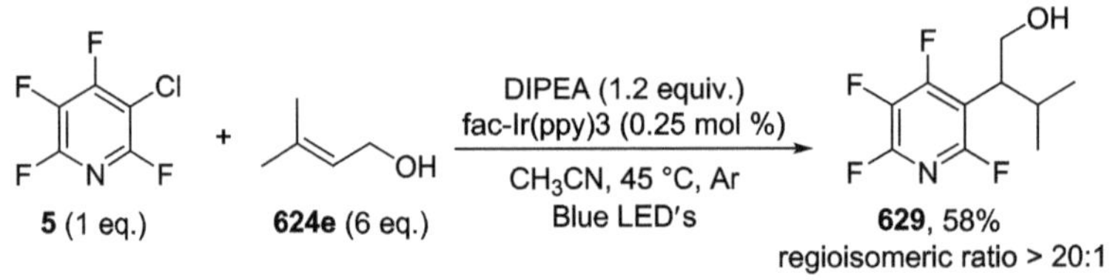

Scheme 2-225. The photocatalytic C-F alkylation of 3-chlorotetrafluoropyridine **5** using fac-Ir(ppy)3.

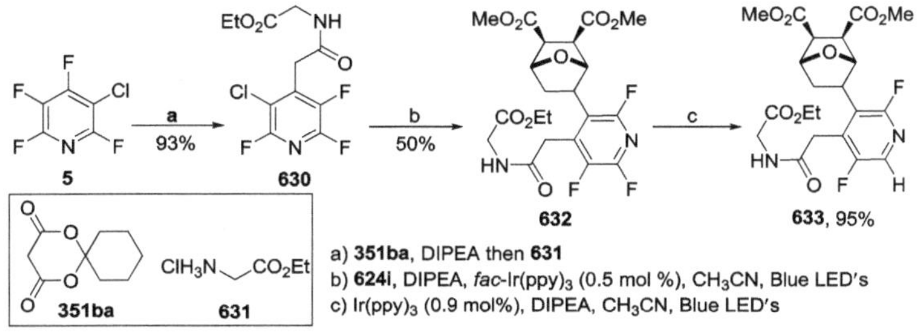

a) **351ba**, DIPEA then **631**
b) **624i**, DIPEA, *fac*-Ir(ppy)₃ (0.5 mol %), CH₃CN, Blue LED's
c) Ir(ppy)₃ (0.9 mol%), DIPEA, CH₃CN, Blue LED's

Scheme 2-226. The photocatalytic C-F alkylation of compound **630** using fac-Ir(ppy)₃ followed hydrodefluorination reaction.

Fluorinated biaryls are an important class of molecules with many examples in agrochemicals [190], functional materials [191 - 194], and drugs [195, 196]. The photocatalytic coupling *via* direct functionalization of the C−F bond of pentafluoropyridine and C−H bond of the arene has been leaded to multifluorinated biaryls (Scheme 2 - 227) [197]. The perfluoropyridyl radical generated by the photocatalyst fac-Ir (ppy)₃, blue light, and an amine has been utilized to form a new C−C bond *via* dual C−F, C−H functionalization.

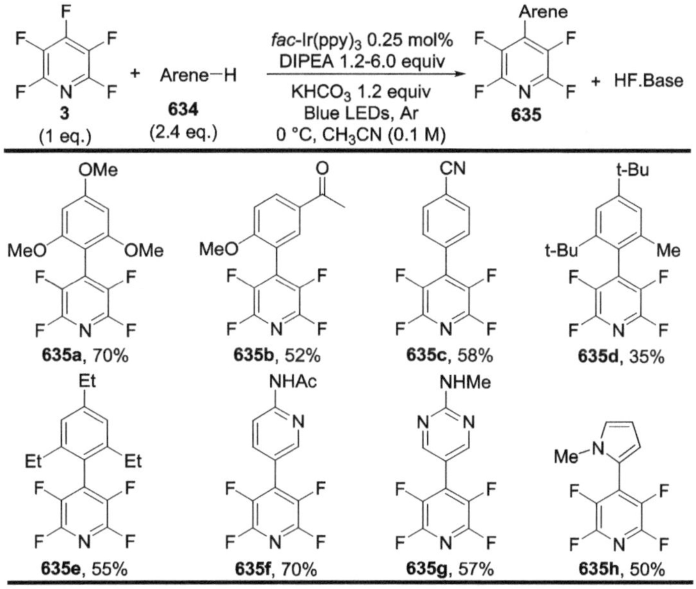

Scheme 2-227. Photocatalytic coupling of pentafluoropyridine **3** with arenes **634**.

Photocatalytic arylation of compound **630** occurred at C-Cl bond and gives asymmetric molecule **636**. In fallowing, this compound reduced at 6-position of pyridine ring to generated hard-to-access difluorinated heteroarene **637** (Scheme 2

- 228) [197].

CO_2Et
NH
O
F
Cl
F
N
F
630
1,3,5-trimethoxybenzene
fac-Ir(ppy)$_3$ 0.25 mol%
DIPEA, CH_3CN
Bluw LEDs, Ar, 0 °C
48%
MeO
OMe
OMe
636
fac-Ir(ppy)$_3$ 0.25 mol%
DIPEA, CH_3CN
Bluw LEDs, Ar,45 °C
637, 81%, rr = 2:1

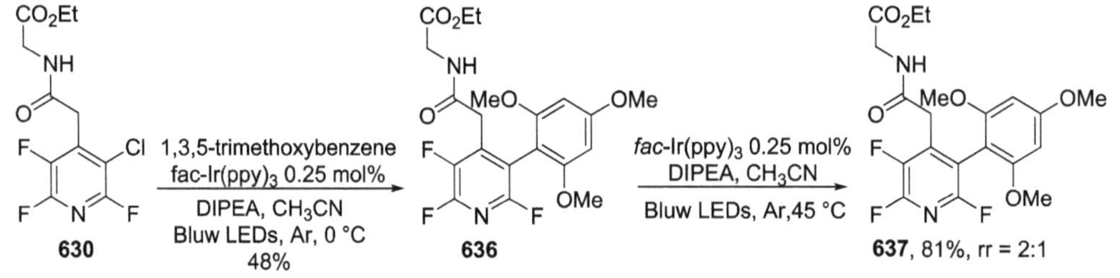

Scheme 2-228. Functionalization of 3-chlorotrifluoropyridine 630 to access perfluorinated biaryls.

Photocatalytic hydrodefluorination of various 4-substituted perfluoropyridines at the presence of fac-Ir(ppy)$_3$ and blue LEDs has been occurred regioselectively at 3-position of pyridine ring (Scheme 2 - 229 to 2-232) [62].

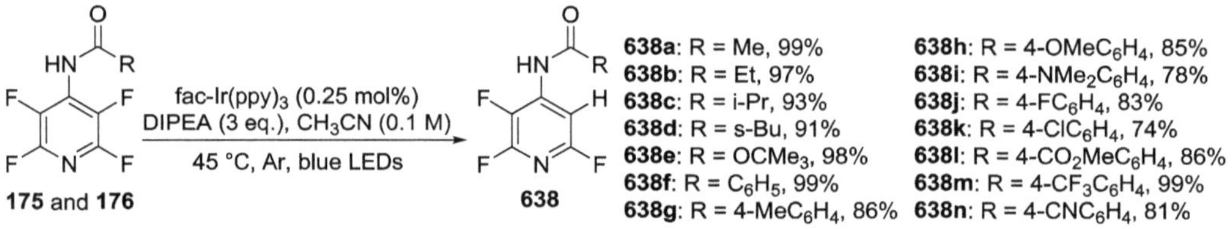

O
HN
R
F
N
175 and 176
fac-Ir(ppy)$_3$ (0.25 mol%)
DIPEA (3 eq.), CH_3CN (0.1 M)
45 °C, Ar, blue LEDs
H
638
638a: R = Me, 99%
638b: R = Et, 97%
638c: R = i-Pr, 93%
638d: R = s-Bu, 91%
638e: R = $OCMe_3$, 98%
638f: R = C_6H_5, 99%
638g: R = 4-MeC_6H_4, 86%
638h: R = 4-$OMeC_6H_4$, 85%
638i: R = 4-$NMe_2C_6H_4$, 78%
638j: R = 4-FC_6H_4, 83%
638k: R = 4-ClC_6H_4, 74%
638l: R = 4-$CO_2MeC_6H_4$, 86%
638m: R = 4-$CF_3C_6H_4$, 99%
638n: R = 4-CNC_6H_4, 81%

Scheme 2-229. Selective reduction of 4-(*N*-acylated)tetrafluoropyridines **175** and **176** using fac-Ir(ppy)$_3$ and blue LEDs.

HN
Ar
F
N
189
fac-Ir(ppy)$_3$ (0.25 mol%)
DIPEA (3 eq.), CH_3CN (0.1 M)
45 °C, Ar, blue LEDs
H
639
639a: Ar = C_6H_5, 76%
639b: Ar = 4-MeC_6H_4, 79%
639c: Ar = 4-$OMeC_6H_4$, 41%
639d: Ar = 2-MeC_6H_4, 68%
639e: Ar = 4-FC_6H_4, 69%
639f: R = 2-pyridyl, 71%

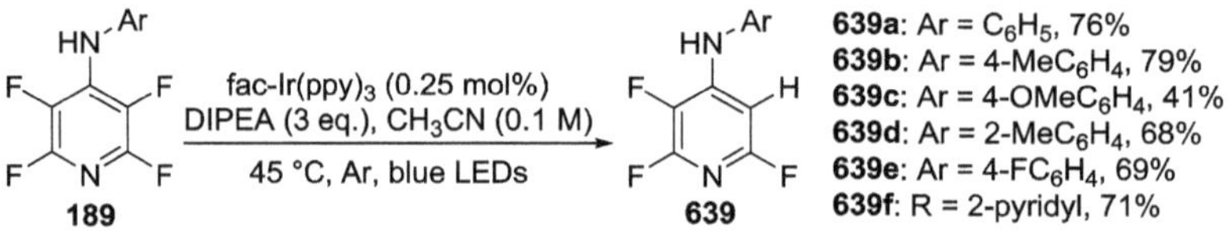

Scheme 2-230. Selective reduction of 4-arylaminotetrafluoropyridines **189** using fac-Ir(ppy)$_3$ and blue LEDs.

O
NHR
F
N
354 and 356
fac-Ir(ppy)$_3$ (0.25 mol%)
DIPEA (3 eq.), CH_3CN (0.1 M)
45 °C, Ar, blue LEDs
H
640
640a: R = CO_2Et, 82%
640b: R = C_6H_5, 81%
640c: R = 4-$OMeC_6H_4$, 65%
640d: R = 4-CNC_6H_4, 75%
640e: R = 2-pyrimidyl, 93%
640f: R = 2-benzothiazolyl, 89%

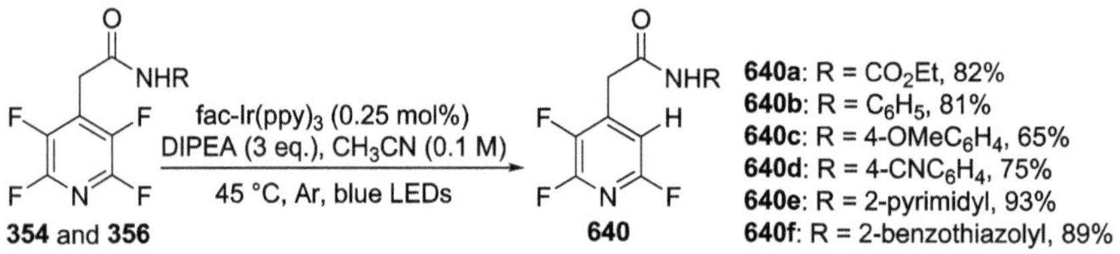

Scheme 2-231. Selective reduction of 4-acetamidotetrafluoropyridines **354** and **356** using fac-Ir(ppy)$_3$ and blue LEDs.

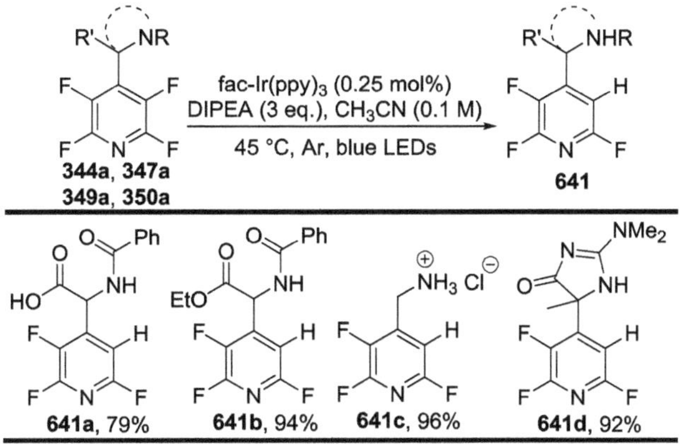

Scheme 2-232. Selective reduction of **344a, 347a, 349a** and **350a** using fac-Ir(ppy)$_3$ and blue LEDs.

Alkenylation of pentafluoropyridine has been well down using photocatalyst and blue LEDs [198]. The structure of photocatalyst used to control the rate of the energy transfer, provided a mechanistic handle over two processes. With use of fac-Ir(Fppy)$_3$ as photocatalyst, Z-isomer obtained as major product (Schemes **2 - 233** and **2 - 234**). Whereas, by utilizing fac-Ir(t-Buppy)$_3$, which has a large volume, E-isomer mainly obtained (Scheme 2 - 235).

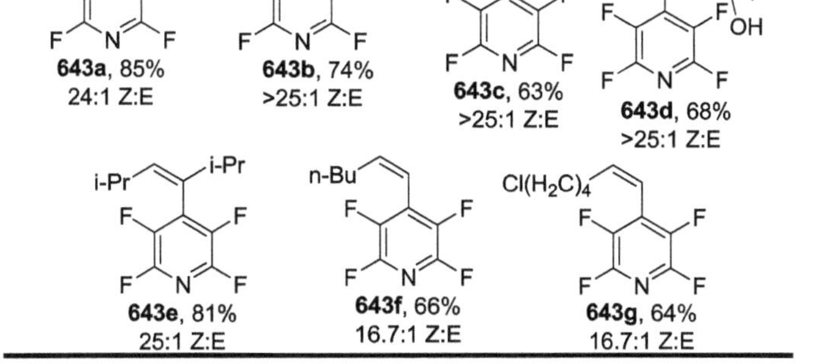

Scheme 2-233. Photocatalytic Z-alkenylation of pentafluoropyrdine **3**.

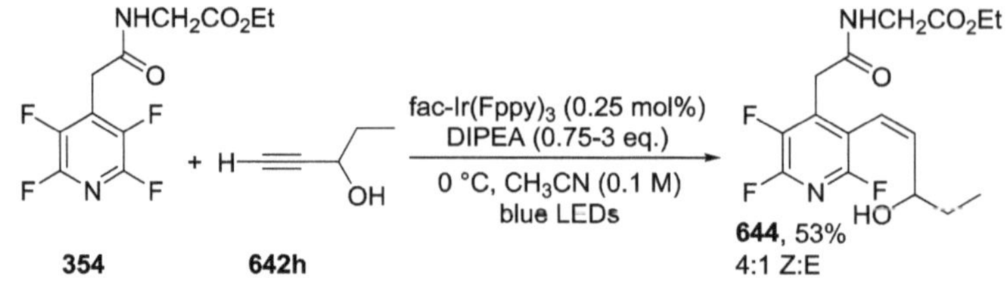

Scheme 2-234. Photocatalytic Z-alkenylation of tetrafluoropyridine **354**.

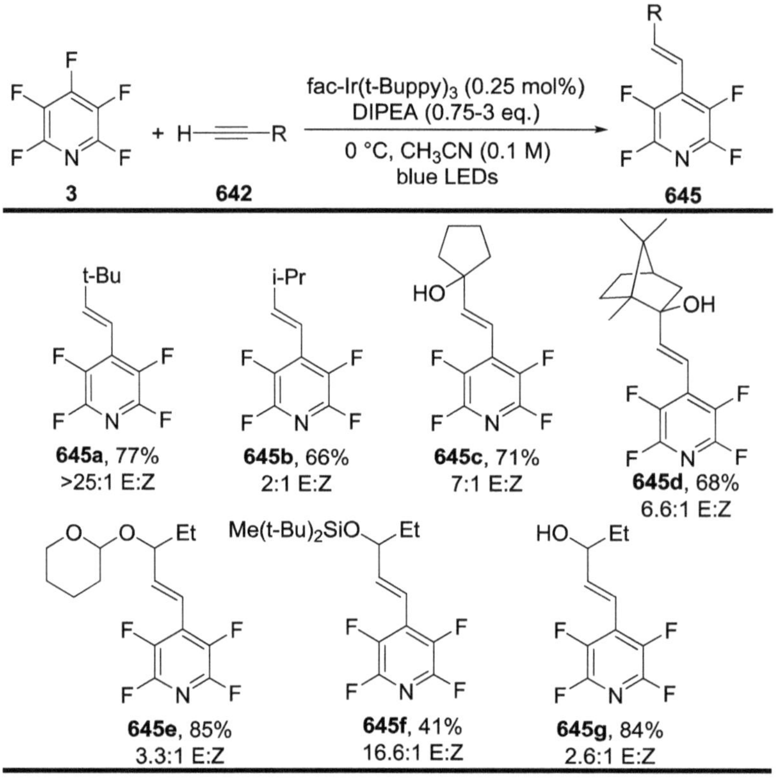

Scheme 2-235. Photocatalytic E-alkenylation of pentafluoropyrdine **3**.

The photochemical transformations and cycloaddition reactions of heteroaromatic molecules have received much less attention than aromatic molecules. [2+2] photoaddition of cyclopentene or cycloheptene to pentafluoropyridine in cyclohexane proceeds regiospecifically at 3- and 4-positions of pyridine ring (Scheme 2-236a) [199]. In the same paper, the photochemical addition of cycloalkenes to pentafluoropyridine have been reported [200]. Based on mixture of endo and exo products formed *via* [2 + 2] addition at C-3 and -4 and [4 + 2] addition at C-2 and -5 of pentafluoropyridine [200]. The study of their stereochemistry suggested that endo addition of cyclo-pentene and -octene, and exo-addition of cyclohexene, is favoured for [2+ 2] addition (Scheme **2-236b**).

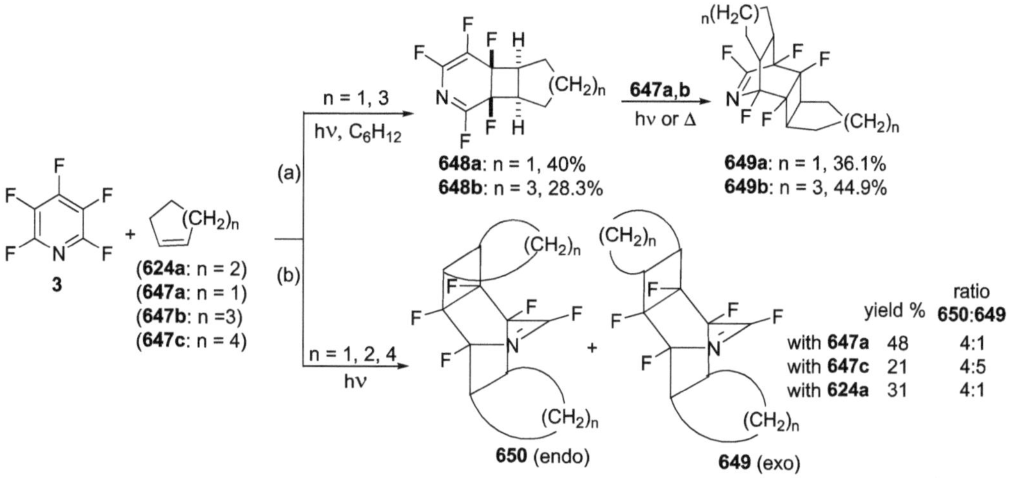

Scheme 2-236. Photochemical addition of cycloalkenes **624a** and **647a-c** to pentafluoropyridine **3**.

Photochemical addition of ethylene to pentafluoropyridine gives 1,2,4,5,6-pentafluoro-3-azabicyclo[4.2.0]octa-2,4-diene **651** and 1,2,5,6,8-pentafluoro-7-azatricyclo[4.2.2.0^{2,5}]dec-7-ene **652**, which later slowly formed thermally from **651** (Scheme 2 - 237) [201].

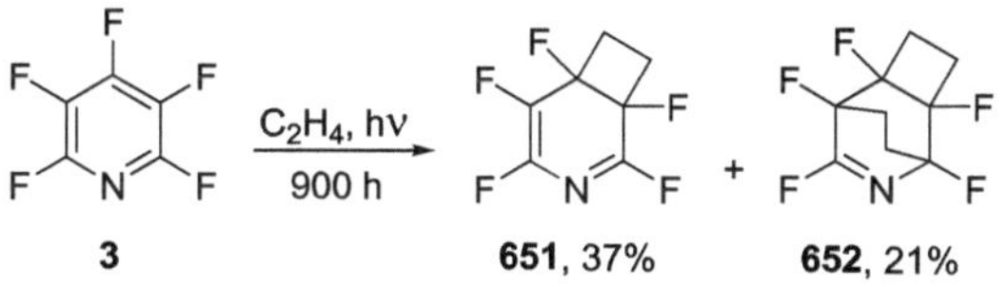

Scheme 2-237. Irradiation of pentafluoropyridine **3** with Ethylene.

But-2-yne photochemically added to pentafluoropyridine and gave products **653** and **654** *via* a 1:1 adduct, and compound **655** *via* a 1:2 adduct (Scheme 2 - 238). The later on hydrolysis has been formed compound **656** in high yield (Scheme 2 - 239) [202].

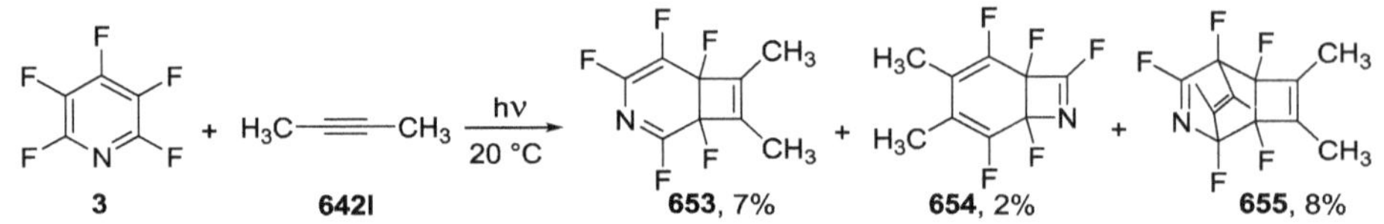

3 **642l** **653**, 7% **654**, 2% **655**, 8%

Scheme 2-238. Photochemical addition of but-2-yne **624l** to pentafluoropyridine **3**.

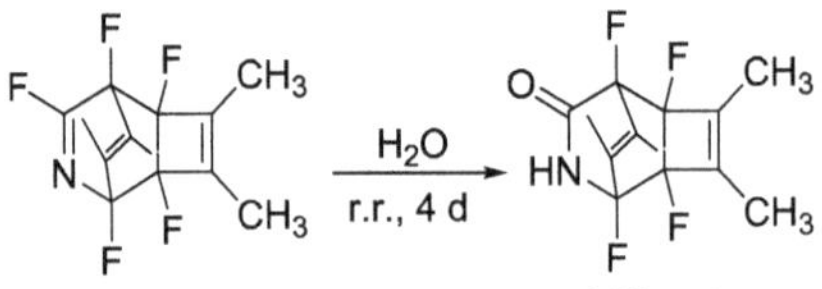

655 **656**, 92%

Scheme 2-239. Hydrolysis of compound **655**.

Irradiation of pentafluoropyridine **3** and 1-phenyl-2-alkylacetylenes **642m** and **642n** in cyclohexane under irradiation underwent regiospecific 2+2 photocycloaddition and produced 3-aza-bicyclo[4.2.0]octa-2,4,7-triene derivatives **657** (Scheme 2 - 240) and **660** (Scheme 2 - 241), respectively, which further phototransformed to 7-aza-trlcycio[4.2.0.00^{2,5}]octa-3,7-diene derivatives **658** (Scheme 2 - 240) and **661** (Scheme 2 - 241), respectively [203]. Further phototransformation of the tricyclic systems **658** and **661** have been produced compounds **659** (Scheme 2 - 240) and **662** (Scheme 2 - 241), respectively.

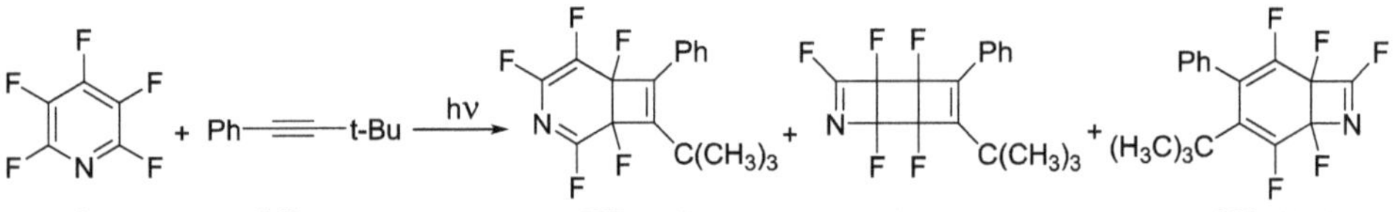

3 **642m** **657**, 14% **658**, 12% **659**, 33.6%

Scheme 2-240. Irradiation of pentafluoropyridine **3** with 1-phenyl-2-tert-butylacetylene **642m**.

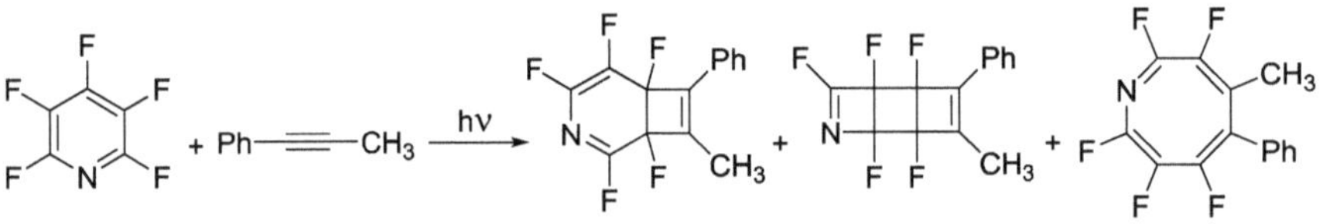

3 **642n** **660**, 13% **661**, 23% **662**, 20%

Scheme 2-241. Irradiation of pentafluoropyridine **3** with 1-Phenylpropyne **642n**.

Pentafluoropyridine on irradiation in the presence of $CpRh(PMe_3)(C_2H_4)$ ($Cp =\eta^5$-C_5H_5) has been coordinated in an η^2-C,C mode, while 2,3,5,6-tetrafluoropyridine yielded C–H oxidative addition product (Scheme 2 - 242) [204]. The 4-substituted tetrafluoropyridines containing an NMe_2 or OMe group have been formed metallacycle products *via* combined C–H and C–F bond activation with HF elimination [204].

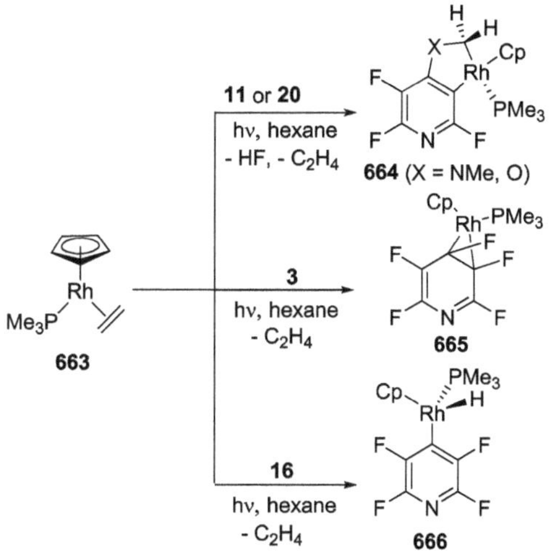

Scheme 2-242. Photochemical reactions of fluorinated pyridines with $CpRh(PMe_3)(C_2H_4)$ **663**.

Irradiation of primary hydroxy alkane solutions of pentafluoropyridine in the presence of benzophenone lead to regiospecific substitution at the 4-position of pyridine ring and 2,3,5,6-tetrafluoro-4-(1-hydroxyalkyl)pyridine **470a-e** compounds are formed (Scheme 2 - 243) [205]. Also, 1,1,2,2-tetraphenyl-1-2-dihydroxyethane has been obtained as second product. 2,3,5,6-tetrafluoro-4-(1-hydroxyalkyl)pyridine has been obtained in high yield by using ethanol and 1-propanol. 4-substituted products have been obtained in low yield in the presence of 2-propanol and cyclohexanol [205].

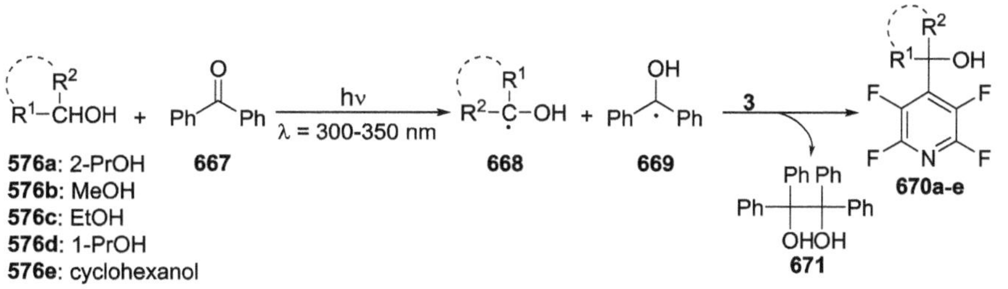

Scheme 2-243. Regiospecific synthesis of 2,3,5,6-tetrafluoro-4-(1-hydroxyalkyl)pyridine **670a-e**.

p- and *m*-amide isomers **171a** and **171b** underwent alkylation reaction in the presence of 1,4-cyclohexadiene (1,4-CHD) *via* photochemical reaction (Schemes 2 - 244 and 2 - 245), while the o-isomer only underwent an intramolecular reaction and formed **674** and **675** (Scheme 2 - 246) [60]. Postulated mechanism for formation **674** and **675** is shown in Scheme 2 - 247. Proposed mechanism of photocycloaddition of *m*- and *p*-isomers with 1,4-CHD represented in scheme 2 - 248.

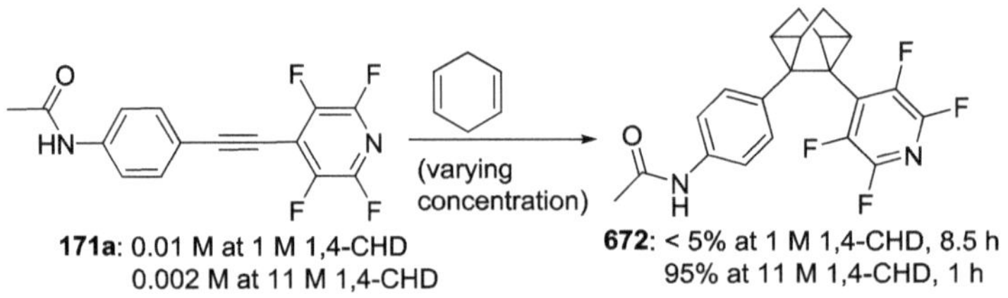

Scheme 2-244. Photocycloaddition of *p*-amido isomer **171a** with 1,4-CHD.

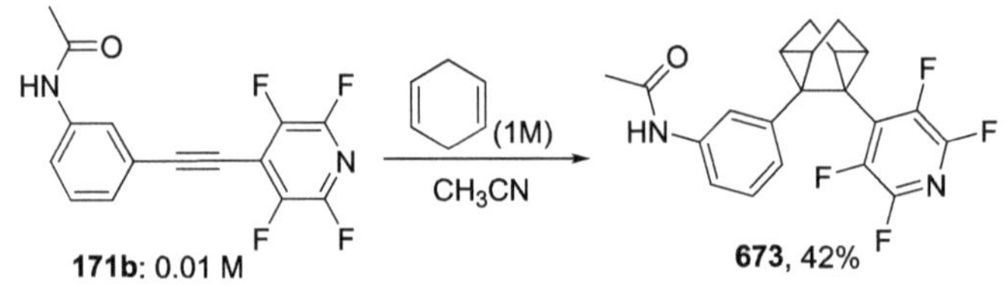

Scheme 2-245. Photocycloaddition of *m*-amido isomer **171b** with 1,4-CHD.

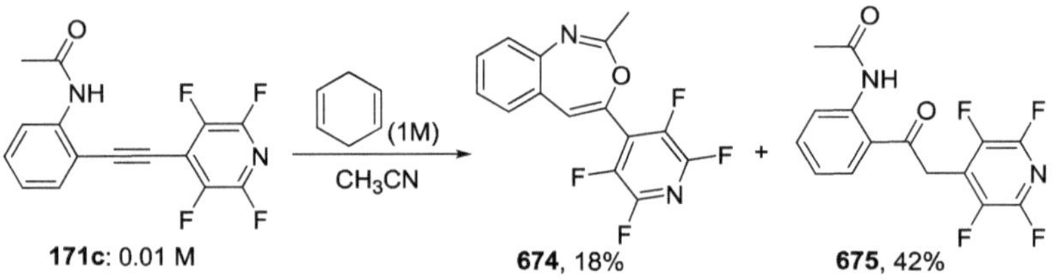

Scheme 2-246. Photocycloaddition of *o*-amido isomer **171c** with 1,4-CHD.

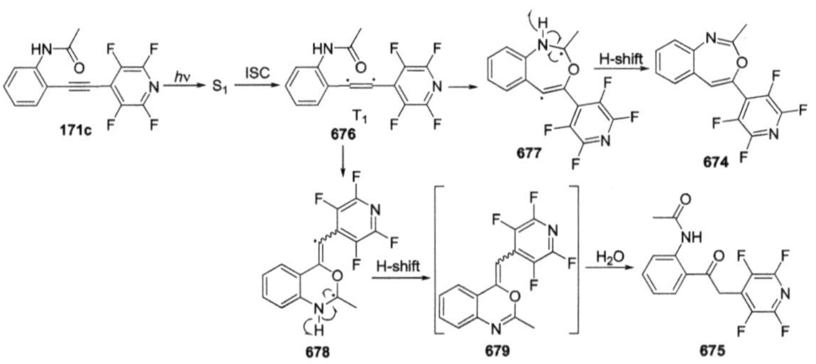

Scheme 2-247. Possible mechanism for photochemical formation of **674** and **675**.

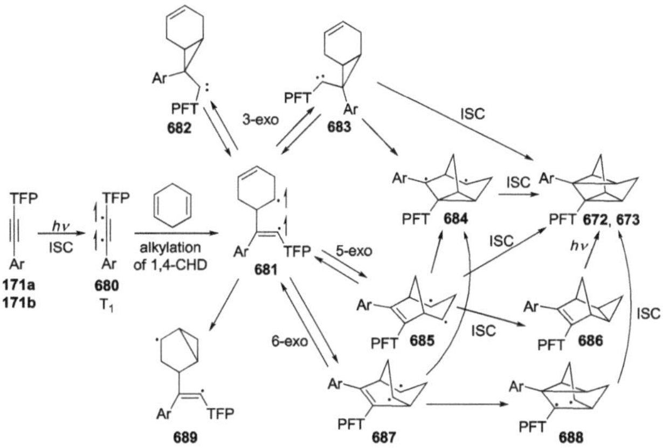

Scheme 2-248. Proposed mechanism of photocycloaddition of **171a** and **171b** with 1,4-CHD.

The tetrafluoropyridine-substituted enediynes **690** prepared readily using reaction of bis(trimethylsilylethynyl)benzenes with pentafluoropyridine [206]. These compounds underwent photochemical transformation into a mixture of isomeric indenes **691** and **692** upon UV irradiation (320 nm) in the presence of 1,4-cyclohexadiene in acetonitrile (Scheme 2 - 249) [206]. The formation of products has been explained by 5-exo-dig C1-C5 cyclization with formation of a fulvene intermediate **696**. The reaction involved photoinduced electron transfer (PET) from 1,4-cyclohexadiene to the singlet excited states of the enediynes (Scheme 2 - 250). PET affected by the presence of strongly electron-withdrawing tetrafluoropyridine substituents.

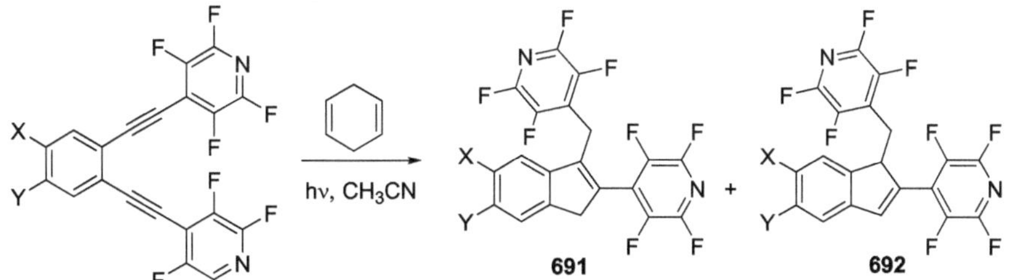

	691	692
X = Y = H	22%	trace
X = Y = Me	17%	trace
X = Cl, Y = H	18%	3%
X = H, Y = Cl	2%	<1%

Scheme 2-249. C1-C5 photochemical cyclization of 1,2-bis(tetrafluoropyridine) bnediynes **690**.

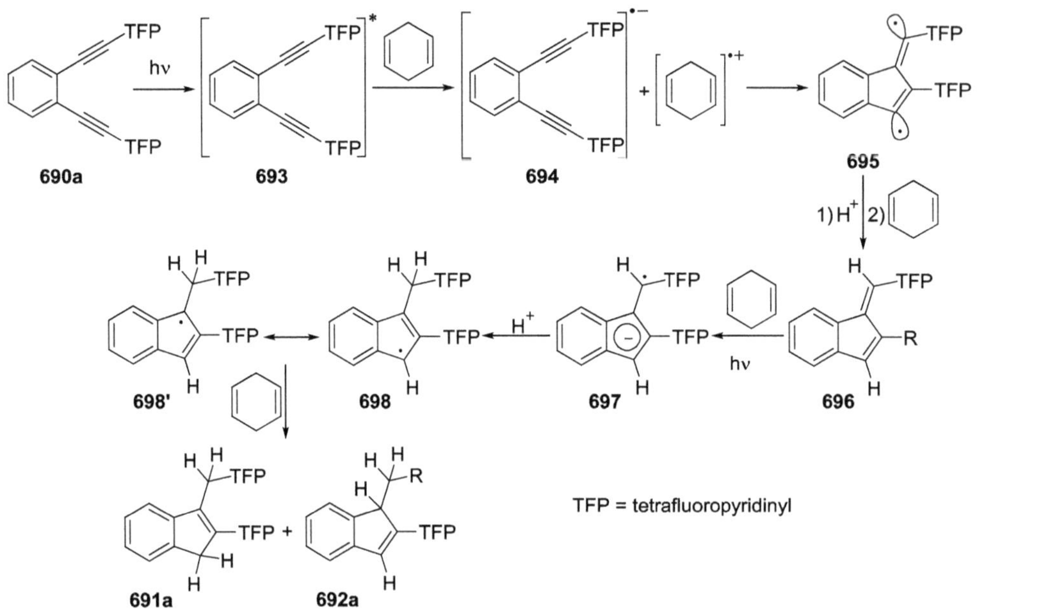

Scheme 2-250. Possible scheme for formation of the photochemical products.

Photoreaction of pentafluoropyridine with cyclohexane in the presence of benzophenone has been leaded to formation of 4-cyclohexyltetafluoropyridine and 1,2-dihydroxytetraphenylethane (Scheme 2 - 251), *via* free-radical mechanism (Scheme 2 - 252) [207].

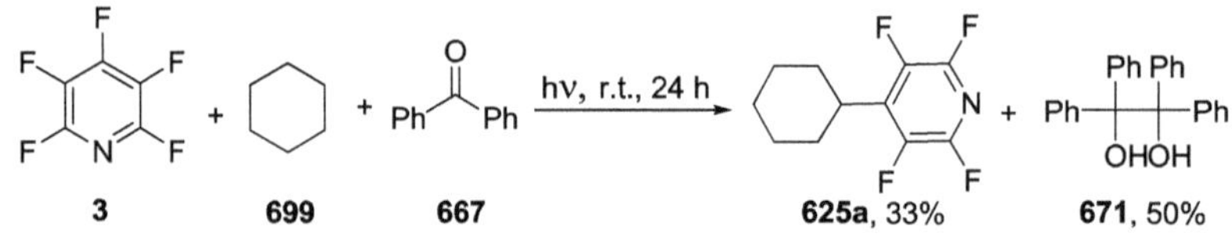

Scheme 2-251. Photoreaction of pentafluoropyridine **3** with cyclohexane **699**.

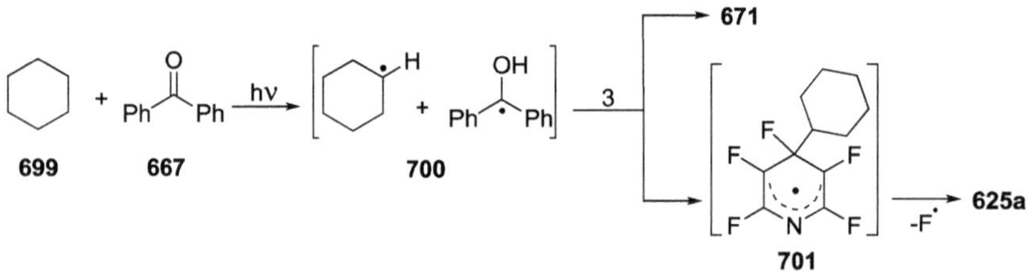

Scheme 2-252. Mechanism irradiation of pentafluoropyridine **3** in cyclohexane **699**.

8. COPOLYMERIZATION OF PENTAFLUOROPYRIDINE

A convenient method for the synthesis of novel copolymers is addition of bisfluoroxyperfluoroalkanes to perfluoro-*N*-heteroaromatics and variety of perfluoro-*N*-heterocyclic ethers [208]. The reactions of pentafluoropyridine and $CF_2(OF)_2$ at 1:1 monomer ratio give 65-75% yield of copolymers in the presence of mainly two volatile perfluoro-*N*-heterocyclic ethers-5,6-difluoromethylene-dioxyheptafluoro-1-azacyclohex-1-ene and 5,6-difluoromethylenedioxypenta-fluoro-1-azacyclohexa-1,3-diene [208]. The proposed reaction sequence is shown in scheme 2 - 253.

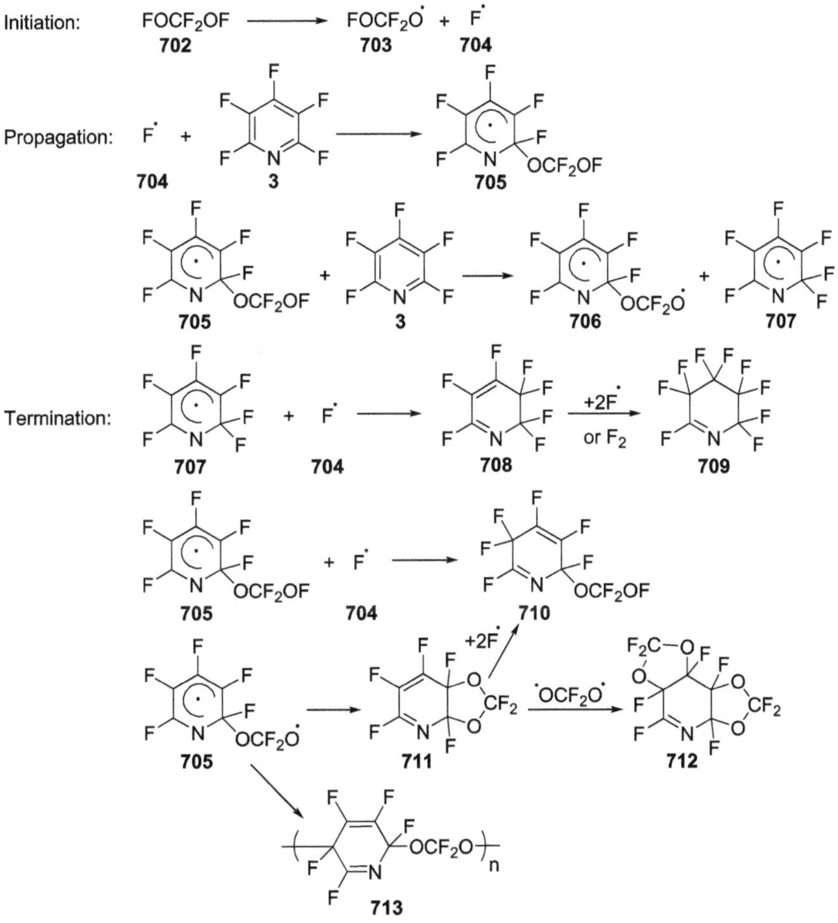

Scheme 2-253. Copolymerization of pentafluoropyridine **3**.

9. THE PENTAFLUOROPYRIDINE CATION $C_5F_5N^+$

Salts of the pentafluoropyridine cation $C_5F_5N^+$ obtained by oxidation of pentafluoropyridine with $C_5F_5N^+$ in SO_2ClF as solvent and moderator (Scheme 2 - 254) [209]. This salt decomposed at -20 °C and give a 1:1 mixture of the molecular adducts $C_5F_5N.AsF_5$ and $C_5F_7N.AsF_5$ (Scheme 2 - 255)

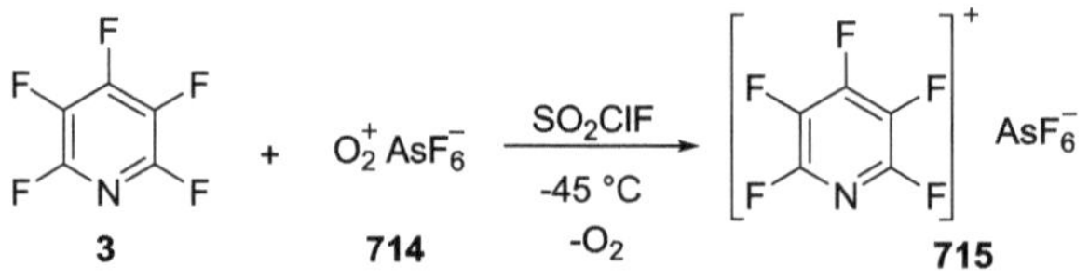

Scheme 2-254. Preparation of pentafluoropyridine salt **715**.

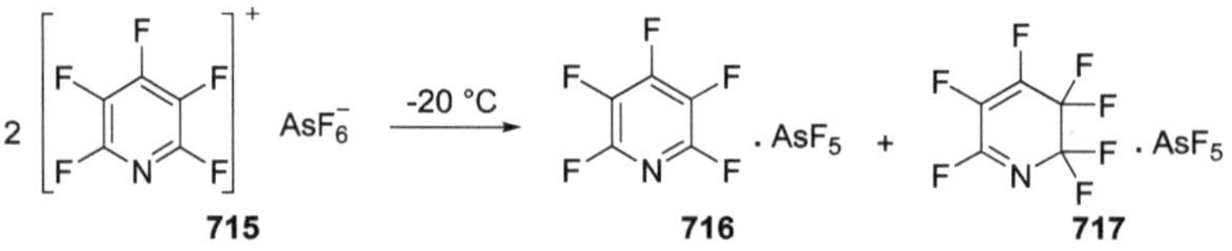

Scheme 2-255. Decomposition of salt **715**.

10. SALTS OF PERFLUOROPYRIDINE

Polyhalogenated pyridines have considerable low basicity because of the strong inductive effect of the halogen atoms and usually are resistance toward *N*-alkylation. However, methyl fluorosulphonate has been successfully reacted with 3,5 dichlorotrifluoropyridine in the absence of a solvent and give corresponding *N*-methylated pyridiniumfluorosulphonate (Scheme 2 - 256) [210]. The strong inductive effect of the positively charged nitrogen atom is activate the 2(6)-positions of ring toward nucleophilic substitution (Scheme 2 - 257).

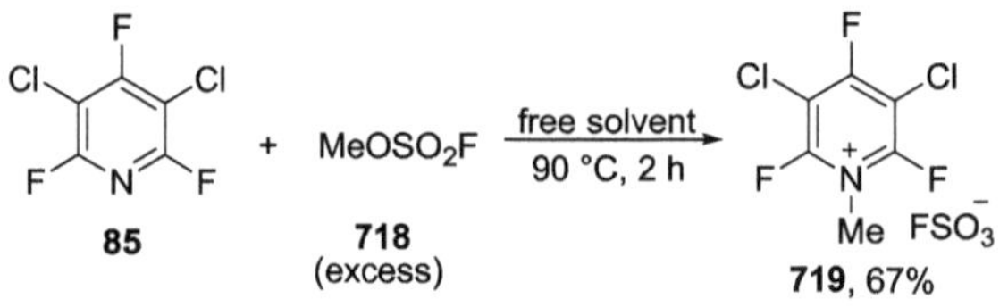

Scheme 2-256. Reaction of 3,5-dichlorotritluoropyridine **85** with methyl fluorosulphonate **718**.

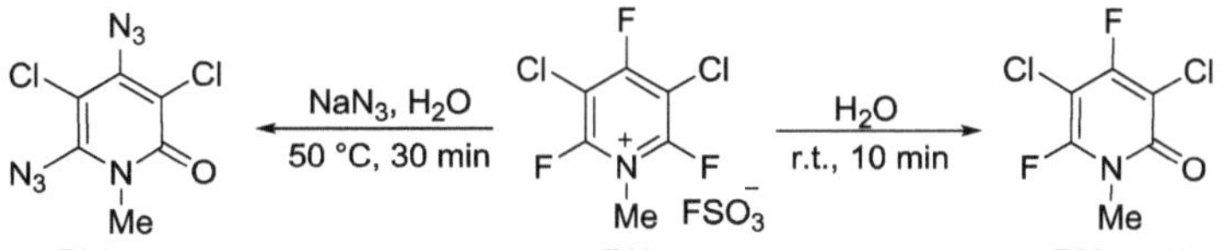

Scheme 2-257. Reactions of *N*-Methyl 3,5-dichlorotrifluoropyridinium fluorosulphonate **719** with H_2O and NaN_3.

11. SYNTHESIS OF MACROCYCLIC COMPOUNDS FROM POLYFLUOROPYRIDINES

Supramolecular chemistry has developed as an important research filed in organic chemistry [211, 212]. Macrocyclic systems have been utilized as sensors, ion analysis, imaging agents and catalysts [212]. Presence of pyridine in macrocycle ring have attracted considerable interest because of physical and biological properties of these systems [212]. Common method for synthesis of macrocyclic compounds includes nucleophilic substitution in C-sp^3 or nucleophilic addition-elimination reactions at carbonyl groups in the ring-closing step [213]. Synthesis of macrocycles by aromatic nucleophilic substitutions are less common. Pyridine derivatives with halogen atom at ortho position are useful building blocks for synthesis of macrocyclic systems, *e.g.*, from 2,6-dibromopyridine at presence of polyethylene glycol has been used for synthesis of macrocycles [214].

Formation of macrocyclic systems have been reported by aromatic nucleophilic substitution processes [215, 216]. Perhalogenated heterocycles used for synthesis of a wide range of macrocyclic derivatives. It has been found that fluorine is more active than chlorine and bromine in aromatic nucleophilic substitution reactions [217, 218]. Perfluorinated heterocycles are more appropriate starting materials than corresponding perchlorinated derivatives for synthesis of macrocycles, because of [219]:

1- In heterocyclic systems, C-F bonds are more active than C-F bonds toward nucleophilic attack.
2- Perfluoroheterocycles are more selective toward nucleophilic attack than corresponding perchlorinated derivatives.
3- The possibility of using ^{19}F NMR for identification of compound in fluoroheterocycles.

All five fluorine atoms of pentafluoropyridine can be replaced by nucleophiles that the order of replacement as shown in Scheme Fig. (**2-4**), although there are contradictions [31].

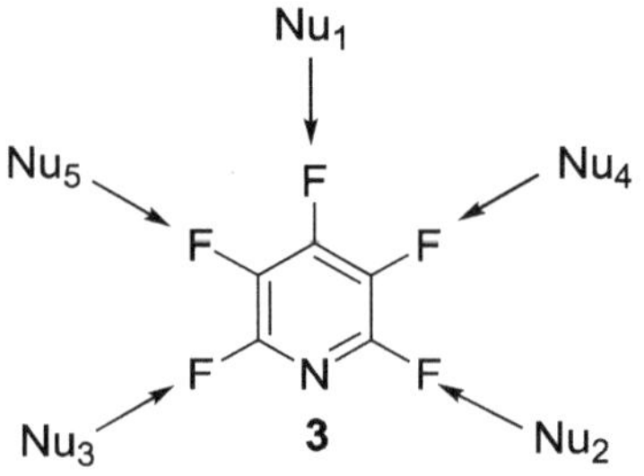

Nu_1

Nu_5 Nu_4

Nu_3 **3** Nu_2

Fig. (2-4). The order of nucleophilic addition to pentafluoropyridine **3**.

Pentafluoropyridine is a useful precursor for synthesis of macrocylic systems [220], and general route of reaction as shown in Scheme 2 - 258.

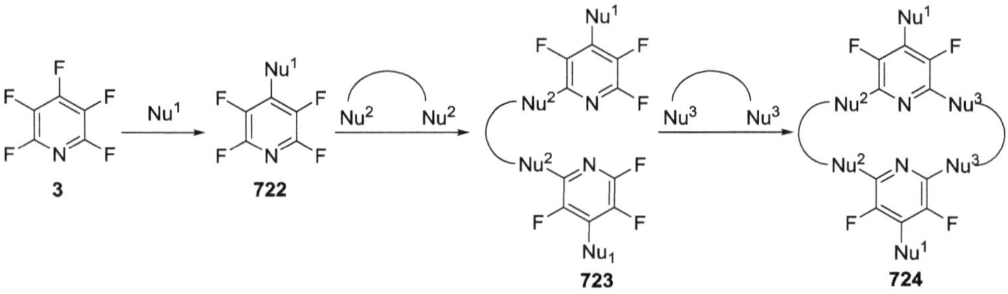

3 Nu^1 **722** Nu^2 Nu^2 **723** Nu^3 Nu^3 **724**

Scheme 2-258. General route for synthesis of macrocycle from pentafluoropyridine **3**.

Other method for synthesis of macrocycle from pentafluoropyridine has included blocking of 4-position of pyridine ring and followed by attack of bidentate nucleophile to two α-positions of ring nitrogen (Scheme 2 - 259) [221].

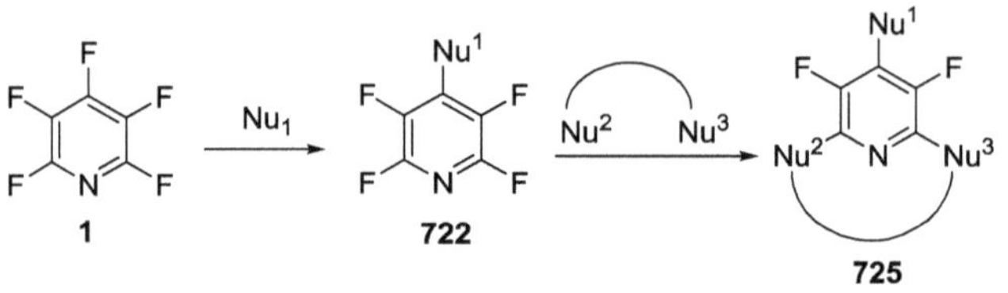

1 Nu_1 **722** Nu^2 Nu^3 **725**

Scheme 2-259. Synthesis of macrocycle from pentafluoropyridine **3**.

Perfluoro-4-isopropylpyridine used as a building block for two steps synthesis of macrocycles with pyridine unit [219, 221]. Perfluoroalkylation of pentafluoropyridine has been carried out by heating in hexafluoropropene at the presence of tetrakis(bisdimethylamino)ethane to gave compound **83**. Reaction of compound **83** with various bidentate nucleophiles produced macrocyclic systems (Table **2-7**, Schemes 2 - 260 to 2-262) [219, 221].

Table 2-7. Synthesis of macrocycle by using 4-perfluoroalkyl tetrafluoropyridine 83 and bis-silane derivatives 726.

726	727	728
726a Me₃SiO—CH₂CH₂—OSiMe₃	**727a**, 90%	**728a**, 43%
726b Me₃SiO—CH₂CH₂—O—CH₂CH₂—OSiMe₃	**727b**, 64%[a], 83%[b]	**728b**, 40%

(Table 2-7) cont.....

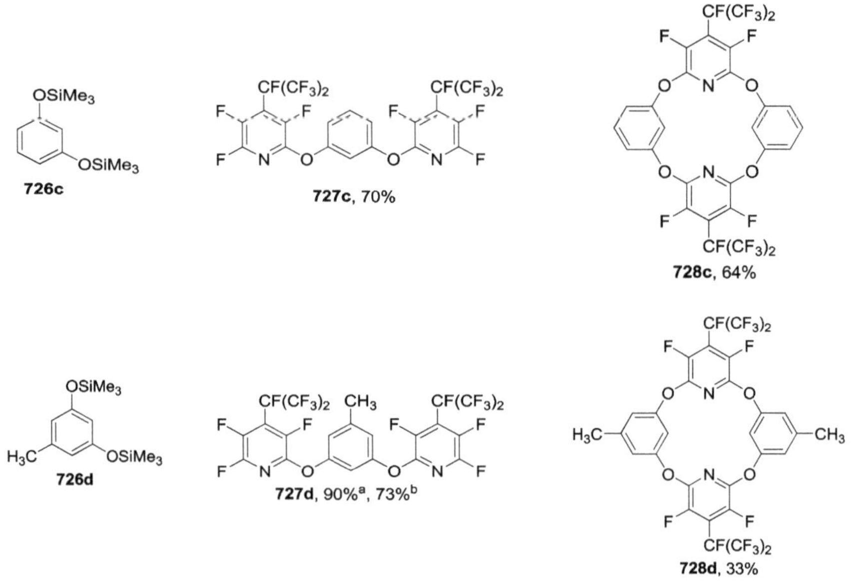

726c

727c, 70%

728c, 64%

726d

727d, 90%[a], 73%[b]

728d, 33%

[a] ref. [219], [b] ref. [221]

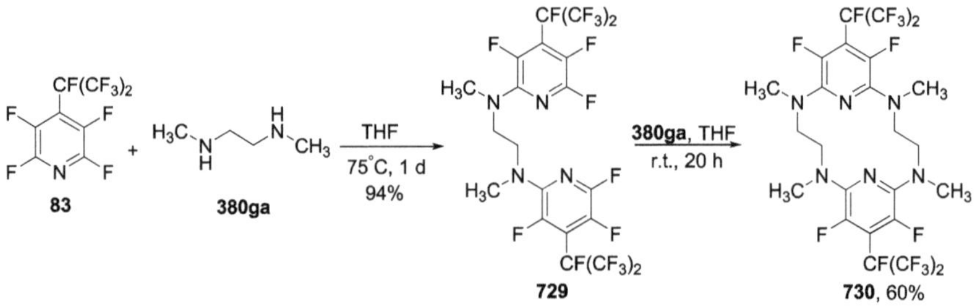

83   +   **380ga**   THF, 75°C, 1 d, 94%   **729**   380ga, THF, r.t., 20 h   **730**, 60%

Scheme 2-260. Synthesis of macrocycle **730** by reaction of **83** with diamine **380ga**.

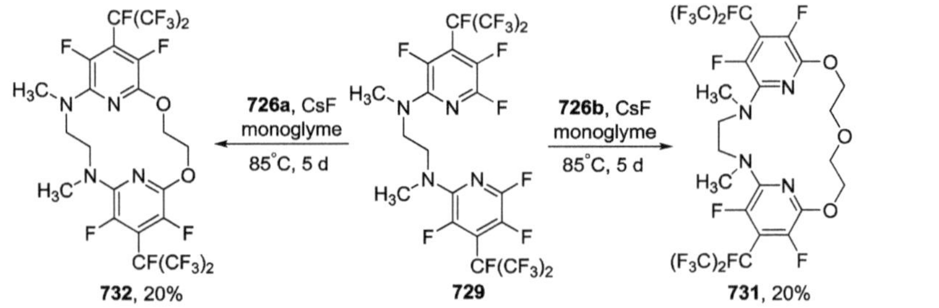

732, 20%   726a, CsF, monoglyme, 85°C, 5 d   **729**   726b, CsF, monoglyme, 85°C, 5 d   **731**, 20%

Scheme 2-261. Synthesis of macrocycles **731** and **732** by reaction of compound **729** with dilos.

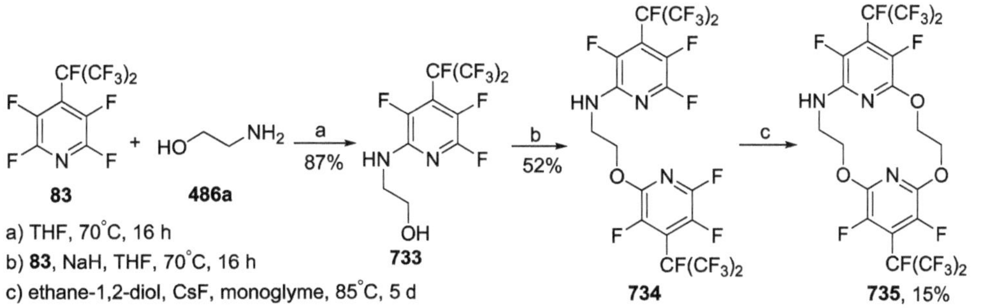
CF(CF3)2
83
486a
a
87%
733
b
52%
734
c
735, 15%
a) THF, 70°C, 16 h
b) 83, NaH, THF, 70°C, 16 h
c) ethane-1,2-diol, CsF, monoglyme, 85°C, 5 d

Scheme 2-262. Synthesis of macrocycle **735** from compound **83**.

Pentafluoropyridine reacted effectively with various *O*-centered nucleophiles and produced 4-alkoxytetrafluoropyridine derivatives, which used as starting materials for synthesis of macrocyclic systems [222]. 4-methoxytetrafluoropridine converted to macrocycles **737** and **739** on reaction with bis-silane **726a** (Scheme 2 - 263) and **726c** (Scheme 2 - 264). Similarly, macrocyclic system **742** obtained from reaction of 4-alkoxy perfluoropyridine **740** with diamine **380ga** (Scheme 2 - 265).

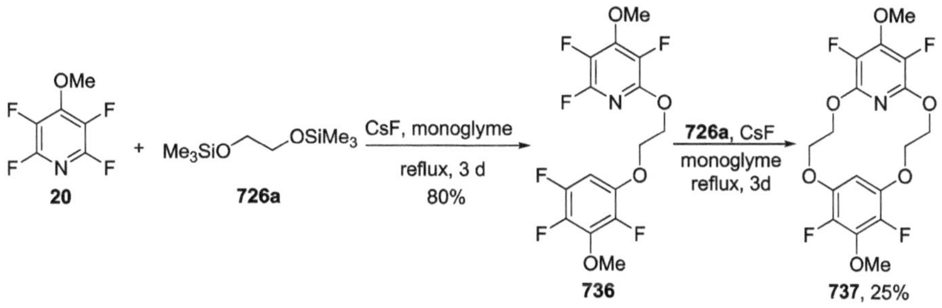
20
726a
CsF, monoglyme
reflux, 3 d
80%
736
726a, CsF
monoglyme
reflux, 3d
737, 25%

Scheme 2-263. Synthesis of macrocycle **737** by reaction of **20** with bis-silane **726a**.

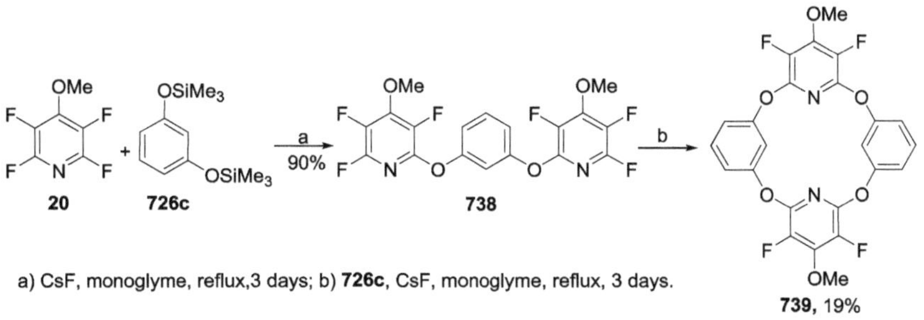
20
726c
a
90%
738
b
739, 19%
a) CsF, monoglyme, reflux,3 days; b) 726c, CsF, monoglyme, reflux, 3 days.

Scheme 2-264. Synthesis of macrocycle **739** by reaction of **20** with bis-silane **726c**.

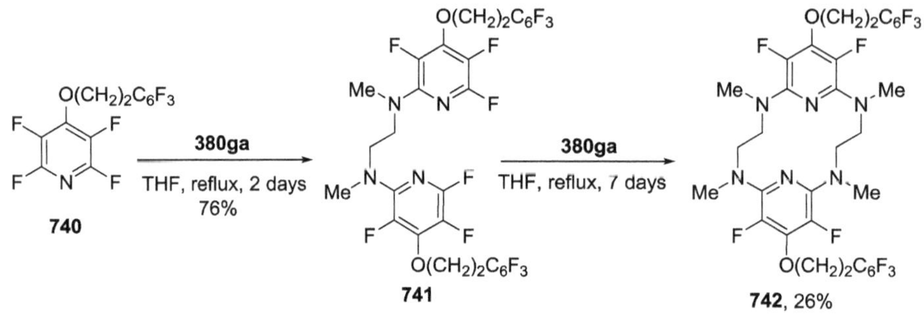

Scheme 2-265. Synthesis of macrocycle **742** by reaction of compound **740** with **380ga**.

3,5-Dichloro-2,4,6-trifluoropyridine has been obtained directly from reaction of pentachloropyridine with KF in sulfolane (Scheme 2 - 266) [3]. Other route for its synthesis is reaction of pentachloropyridine with KF in the presence of perfluoroperhydrophenanthrene in sulfolane (Scheme 2 - 266) [223]. It reacted selectively at 4-position of pyridine ring with sodium methoxy and produced 3,5-dichloro-2,6-difluoro-4-methoxypyridine **744** (Scheme 2 - 267). Reaction of compound **744** with bifunctional *O*-centered nucleophiles produced macrocyclic systems **746** and **748** (Scheme 2 - 268) [224].

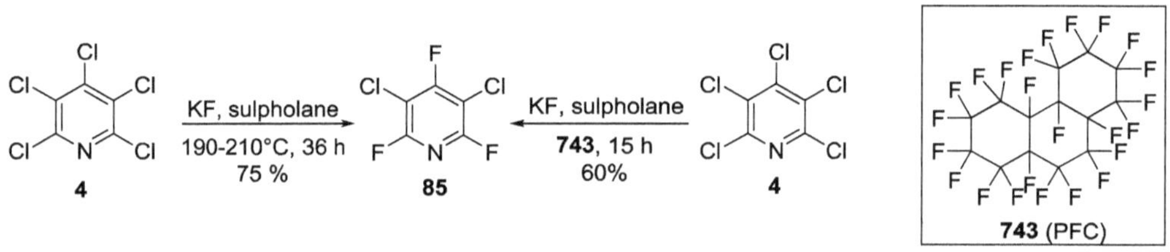

Scheme 2-266. Synthesis of 3,5-dichloro-2,4,6-trifluoropyridine **85**.

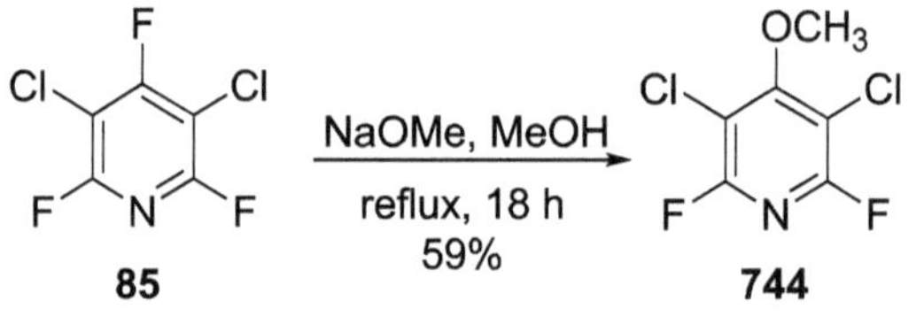

Scheme 2-267. Synthesis of 3,5-dichloro-2,6-difluoro-4-methoxypyridine **744**.

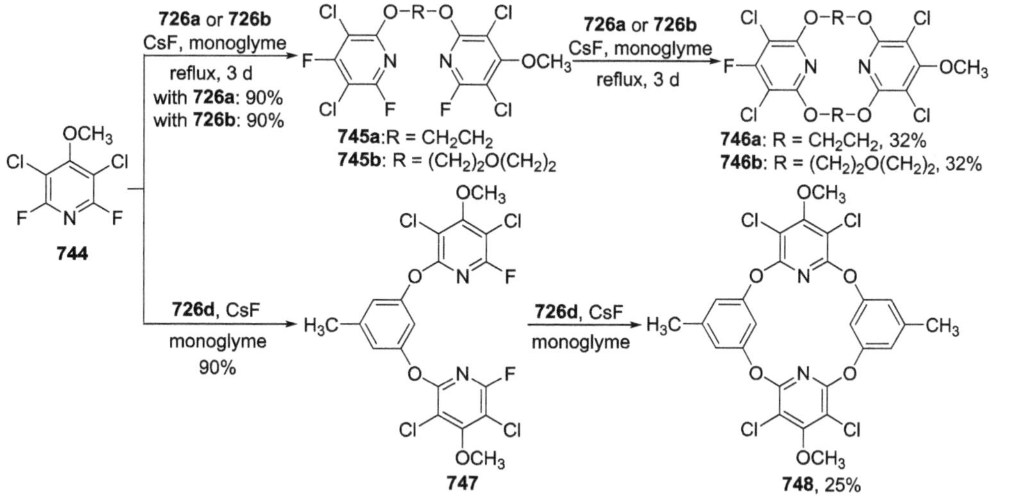

Scheme 2-268. Synthesis of macrocycls systems **746a,b** and **748** by using **744**.

12. PENTAFLUOROPYRIDINE IN MEDICINAL CHEMISTRY AND BIOCHEMISTRY

A few samples have been existed from using pentafluoropyridine as a scaffold for drug discovery. Synthesized 3,5-difluoro-4-methyl-diaryloxypyridine derivatives from 4-methyl tetrafluoropyridine have been shown medium inhibitory effect for Xa factor. A series of 3,5-difluoro-triaryloxypyridine compounds have been synthesized from pentafluoropyridine **3** for inhibition of Xa factor (Scheme 2 - 269) [225].

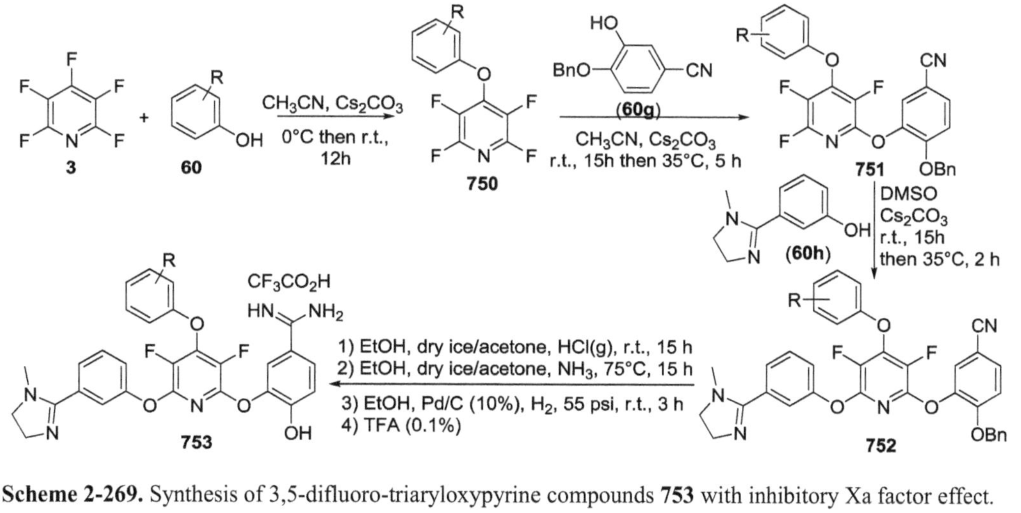

Scheme 2-269. Synthesis of 3,5-difluoro-triaryloxypyrine compounds **753** with inhibitory Xa factor effect.

Also, a series of complex VII/TF factor inhibitors have been synthesized based on pentafluoropyridine (Scheme 2 - 270) [226]. This factor played important role in blood clots formation, that inhibitory of this complex may lead to anti-clotting drugs.

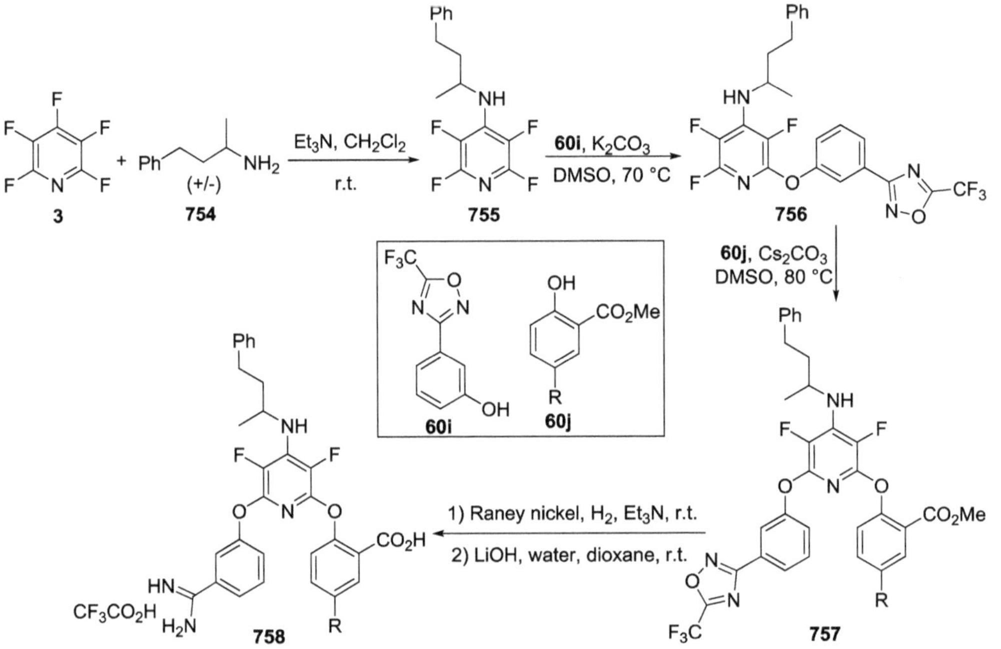

Scheme 2-270. Synthesis pf 3,5-difluoro-4-alkylamino-diaryloxypyridine derivatives **758**.

Inhibition of kinase protein p38 cause chronic inflammatory diseases. 4-substituted perfluoropyridine heterocycles with inhibitory property of p38α have been synthesized using penafluoropyridine (Schemes 2 - 271 to 2-274) [227].

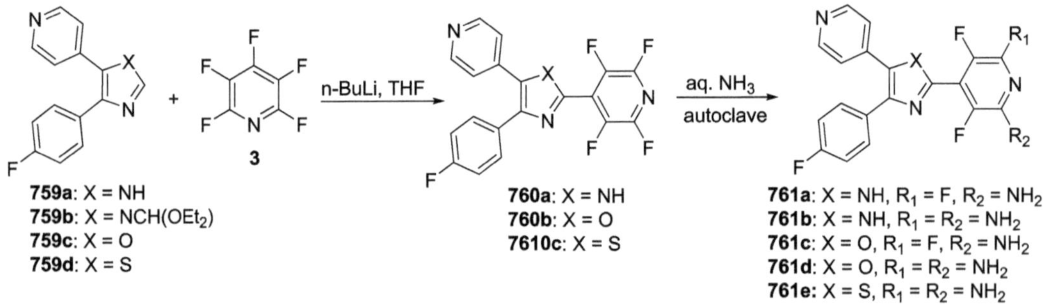

759a: X = NH
759b: X = NCH(OEt₂)
759c: X = O
759d: X = S

760a: X = NH
760b: X = O
7610c: X = S

761a: X = NH, R₁ = F, R₂ = NH₂
761b: X = NH, R₁ = R₂ = NH₂
761c: X = O, R₁ = F, R₂ = NH₂
761d: X = O, R₁ = R₂ = NH₂
761e: X = S, R₁ = R₂ = NH₂

Scheme 2-271. Synthesis of 4-substituted 2,6-diamino-3,5-difluoropyrine heterocycles **761**.

762a: $R_1 = R_2 = H$
762b: $R_1 = Br$, $R_2 = SEM$
763
764a: R = SEM
764b: R = H

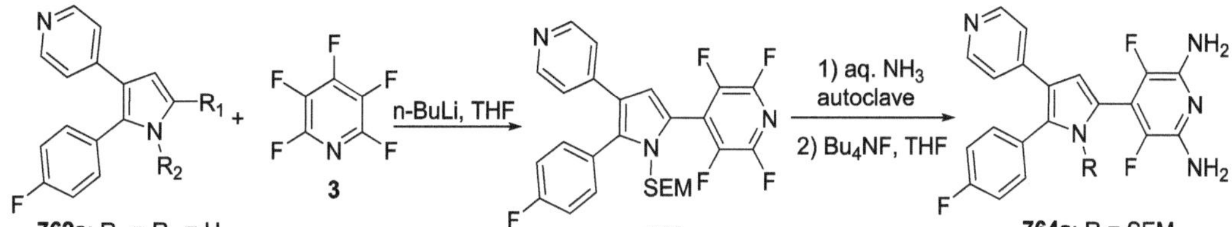

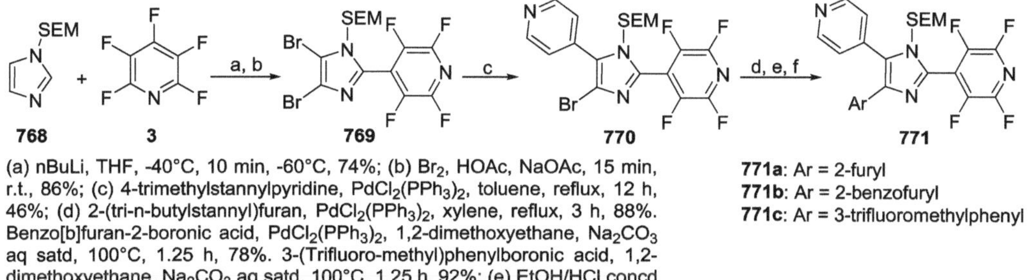

Scheme 2-272. Synthesis of 4-pyrrolo 2,6-diamino-3,5-difluoropyrines.

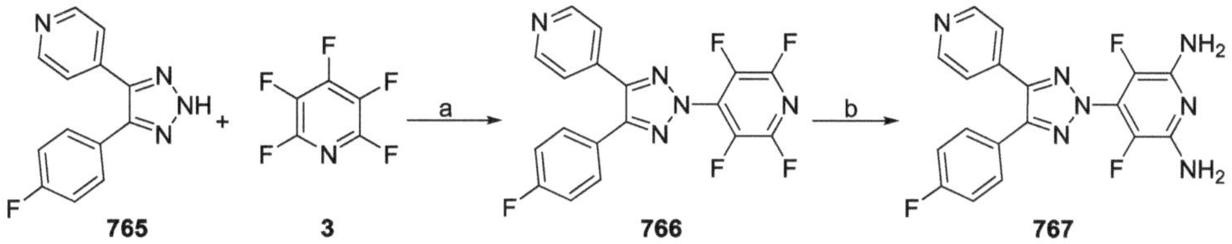

a) $KN(TMS)_2$, THF, 0°C to r.t., 20 min, 49%; b) 25% aq NH_3, 170C, autoclave, 17 h, 24%.

Scheme 2-273. Synthesis of 3,5-difluoro-4-(triazole-2-yl)pyridine-2,6-diamine **767**.

(a) nBuLi, THF, -40°C, 10 min, -60°C, 74%; (b) Br_2, HOAc, NaOAc, 15 min, r.t., 86%; (c) 4-trimethylstannylpyridine, $PdCl_2(PPh_3)_2$, toluene, reflux, 12 h, 46%; (d) 2-(tri-n-butylstannyl)furan, $PdCl_2(PPh_3)_2$, xylene, reflux, 3 h, 88%. Benzo[b]furan-2-boronic acid, $PdCl_2(PPh_3)_2$, 1,2-dimethoxyethane, Na_2CO_3 aq satd, 100°C, 1.25 h, 78%. 3-(Trifluoro-methyl)phenylboronic acid, 1,2-dimethoxyethane, Na_2CO_3 aq satd, 100°C, 1.25 h, 92%; (e) EtOH/HCl concd 1:1, r.t., 1 h,78–85%; (f) 25% aq NH_3, 170°C, autoclave, 12 h, 30–36%.

771a: Ar = 2-furyl
771b: Ar = 2-benzofuryl
771c: Ar = 3-trifluoromethylphenyl

Scheme 2-274. Synthesis of tetrafluoro-4-(imidazole-2-yl)pyridines **771**.

Among antibacterial agents, the fluoroquinolones have attracted considerable interest in both clinically and economically. Similar to bioisosters of quinolones, 2-pyridones are a valuable source of new therapeutic agents (Scheme 2 - 275) [228].

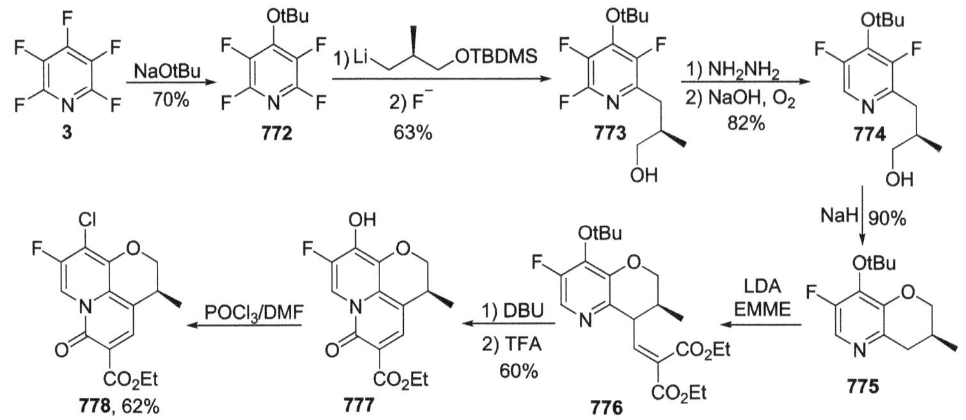

Scheme 2-275. Synthesis of pyrano[2,3,4-ij]quinazoline-6-one **778**.

Porphyrines played important role in field of catalyst, solar energy conversion, spectroscopy, cancer and alzheimer therapy [229]. Porphyrine **779a** and **779b** with potential AChE inhibitors produced in two and six steps from tetrafluoropyridine-4-carbonitrile in overall yield 3% and 5%, respectively (Scheme 2 - 276) [229].

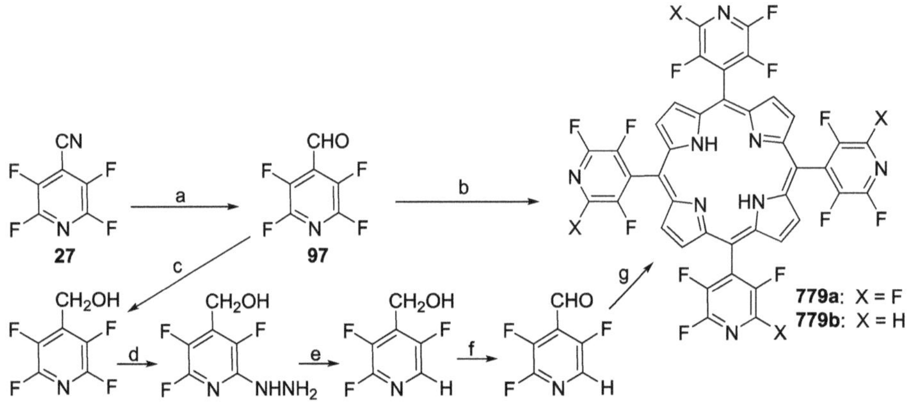

a) 1M DIBAH in hexane, Ether, 0 °C, 45%; b) Propionic acid, Pyrrole, reflux; 7%; c) MeOH, NaBH₄, 0 °C, 90%; d) THF, Hydrazine, 50 °C; e) EtOH, CuSO₄, 30 °C, NaOH, 51% yield in two steps; f) Oxalylchloride, DMSO, CH₂Cl₂, -30 °C, 78%; g) CH₂Cl₂, Pyrrole, BF₃.Et₂O then p-Chloranile,Et₃N, 45 °C, 29%.

Scheme 2-276. Synthesis of porphyrines **779** from tetrafluoropyridine-4-carbonitrile **27**.

Benzimidazoles played important role in medicinal chemistry, and used as suitable building blocks in the design and construction of bioactive compounds [230 - 232]. A series of *N*-perfluoropyridylbenzimidazole derivatives have been synthesized with inhibitory activity against K-562, MCF-7, G361 and HOS cell lines (Schemes 2 - 277 and 2 - 278) [233].

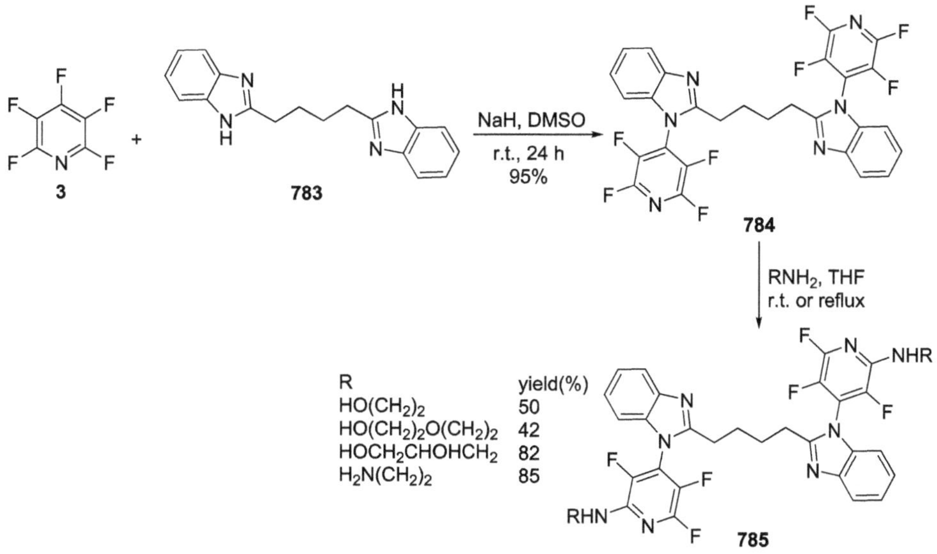

R	yield(%)
$HO(CH_2)_2$	50
$HO(CH_2)_2O(CH_2)_2$	42
$HOCH_2CHOHCH_2$	82
$H_2N(CH_2)_2$	85

Scheme 2-277. Reaction of bisimidazoles **785** with pentafluoropyridine **3**.

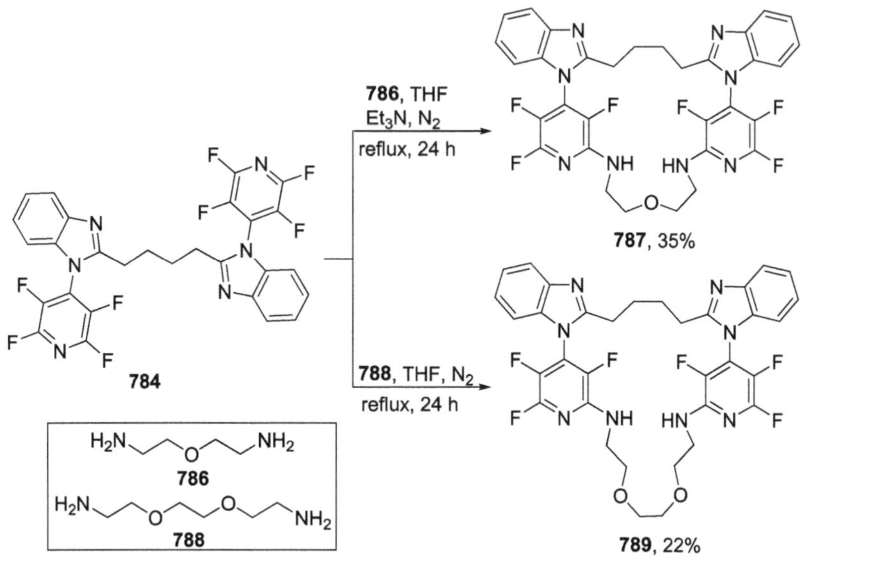

Scheme 2-278. Synthesis of macrocycle using compound **784**.

Ciprofloxacin **790** is a fluoroquinolone antibiotic with *in vitro* activity against Bacillus and Staphylococcus species and most gram-negative microorganisms, also has shown antiproliferative and apoptotic activities in several cancer cell lines [234, 235]. A new class of piperazinylquinolone with antibacterial Effects including coupling of perfluoropyridines **3** and **24** with Ciprofloxacin **790** have been reported (scheme 2 - 279) [236].

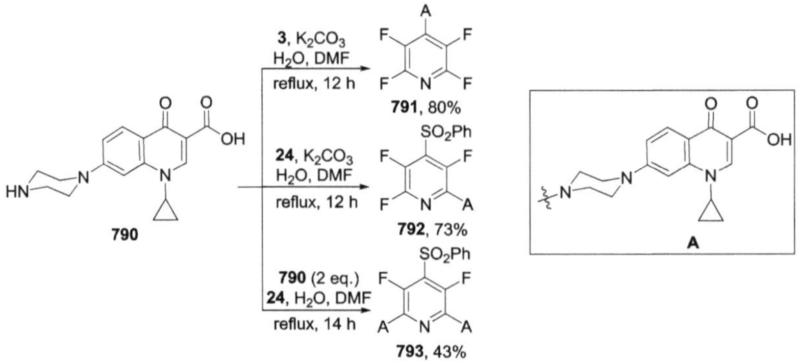

Scheme 2-279. Synthesis of *N*-perfluoropyridyl substituted piperazinylquinolone derivatives **791-793**.

Quinolines are an important class of heterocycle and the most common use of quinoline nucleus is antimalarial activity. A series of hybrid of 4-aminoquinoline and fluorinated pyridine derivatives have been synthesized by the reaction of perfluoropyridines **3** and **24** with hydroxy- and amino-functionalized quinolines (Scheme **2 - 280**), and evaluated against one Gram-positive and one Gram-negative bacteria to assess their *in vitro* antibacterial activity [237]. Compounds **795a**, **795b**, **796a** and **796b** have been showed moderate antibacterial activity against Gram-positive bacterium, Staphylococcus aureus.

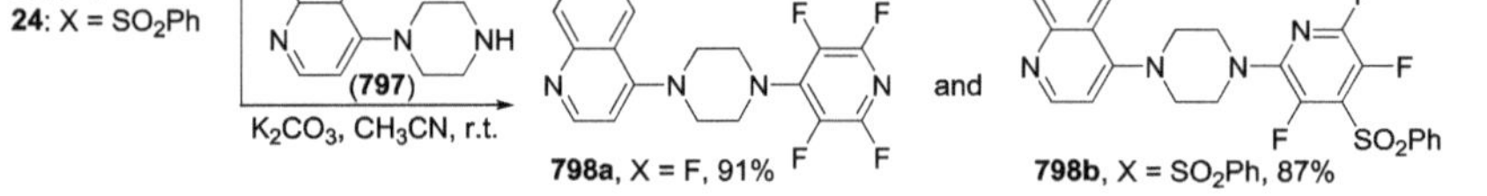

Scheme 2-280. Reaction of hydroxy- and amino-functionalized quinolines with perfluoropyridines **3** and **24**.

REFERENCES

[1]   Petrov, V.A. *Fluorinated heterocyclic compounds: synthesis, chemistry, and applications*; John Wiley & Sons, **2009**.
        [http://dx.doi.org/10.1002/9780470528952]

[2]   Banks, R. E.; Ginsberg, A. E.; Haszeldine, R. N. Heterocyclic polyfluoro-compounds. Part I. Pentafluoropyridine. *Journal of the Chemical Society (Resumed)*, **1961**, *338*(0), 1740-1743.

[3]   Chambers, R. D.; Hutchinson, J.; Musgrave, W. K. R. Polyfluoro-heterocyclic compounds. Part I. The preparation of fluoro-, chlorofluoro-, and chlorofluorohydro-pyridines. *Journal of the Chemical Society (Resumed)*, **1964**, *691*(0), 3573-3576.

[4]   Plevey, R.G.; Rendell, R.W.; Tatlow, J.C. Fluorinations with complex metal fluorides. Part 6 [1] fluorination of yridine and related compounds with caesium tetrafluorocobaltate(III). *J. Fluor. Chem.*, **1982**, *21*(2), 159-169. [2].
        [http://dx.doi.org/10.1016/S0022-1139(00)81239-7]

[5]   Terrier, F. *Modern nucleophilic aromatic substitution*; John Wiley & Sons, **2013**.
        [http://dx.doi.org/10.1002/9783527656141]

[6]   Longuet-Higgins, H.; Coulson, C.A. A theoretical investigation of the distribution of electrons in some heterocyclic molecules containing nitrogen. *Trans. Faraday Soc.*, **1947**, *43*, 87-94.
        [http://dx.doi.org/10.1039/tf9474300087]

[7]   Brooke, G.M. The preparation and properties of polyfluoro aromatic and heteroaromatic compounds. *J. Fluor. Chem.*, **1997**, *86*(1), 1-76.
        [http://dx.doi.org/10.1016/S0022-1139(97)00006-7]

[8]   Chambers, R.D.; Sargent, C.R. Polyfluoroheteroaromatic Compounds.*Adv. Heterocycl. Chem*; Katritzky, A.R.; Boulton, A.J., Eds.; Academic Press, **1981**, Vol. 28, pp. 1-71.

[9]   Bressan, G. B.; Giardi, I.; Illuminati, G.; Linda, P.; Sleiter, G. Nucleophilic heteroaromatic substitution. Part XXXIV. Fluorine *versus* chlorine mobility in reactions with methanolic methoxide ion and with piperidine in various solvents. *J. Chem. Soc. B: Phys. Org.*, **1971**, *1*(0), 225-230.

[10]   Levine, R.; Leake, W.W. Rearrangement in the reaction of 3-bromopyridine with sodium amide and sodioacetophenone. *Science*, **1955**, *121*(3152), 780-780.
        [http://dx.doi.org/10.1126/science.121.3152.780] [PMID: 17773207]

[11]   Burdon, J.; Fisher, D.; King, D.; Tatlow, J. A solvent effect in the reaction of sodium methoxide with pentafluoronitrobenzene. *Chem. Commun. (Camb.)*, **1965**, (4), 65-66.

[12]   Burdon, J.; King, D.R.; Tatlow, J.C. Aromatic polyfluoro compounds—XXXIV: Nucleophilic replacement reactions of some tetrafluorohalogenobenzenes. *Tetrahedron*, **1966**, *22*(8), 2541-2549.
        [http://dx.doi.org/10.1016/S0040-4020(01)99045-3]

[13]   De Pasquale, R.J.; Tamborski, C. Reactions of sodium pentafluorophenolate with substituted pentafluorobenzenes. *J. Org. Chem.*, **1967**, *32*(10), 3163-3168.
        [http://dx.doi.org/10.1021/jo01285a051]

[14]   Burdon, J. A rationalization of orientation and reactivity in the nucleophilic replacement reactions of aromatic polyhalo-compounds. *Tetrahedron*, **1965**, *21*(12), 3373-3380.
        [http://dx.doi.org/10.1016/S0040-4020(01)96958-3]

[15]   Flowers, W.T.; Haszeldine, R.N.; Majid, S.A. Synthesis and reactions of pentachloropyridine. *Tetrahedron Lett.*, **1967**, *8*(26), 2503-2505.
        [http://dx.doi.org/10.1016/S0040-4039(00)90842-6]

[16]   Banks, R.; Burgess, J.; Cheng, W.; Haszeldine, R. *93. Heterocyclic polyfluoro-compounds. Part IV. Nucleophilic substitution in pentafluoropyridine: the preparation and properties of some 4-substituted 2, 3, 5, 6-tetrafluoropyridines. Journal of the Chemical Society*; Resumed, **1965**, pp. 575-581.

[17]   Chambers, R. D.; Hutchinson, J.; Musgrave, W. K. R. 722. Polyfluoro-heterocyclic compounds. Part
        II. Nucleophilic substitution in pentafluoropyridine. *J. Chem. Soc. (Resumed)*, **1964**, *1*(0), 3736-3739.

[18]   Banks, R. E.; Haszeldine, R. N.; Karsa, D. R.; Rickett, F. E.; Young, I. M. Heterocyclic polyfluoro-
        compounds. Part XV. Synthesis of tetrafluoropyridine-4-sulphonic acid and related sulphur-containing
        derivatives of pentafluoropyridine. *J. Chem. Soc. C: Organ.*, **1969**, *0*(12), 1660-1662.

[19]   Efremov, I.v.; Sipyagin, A.M.; Pomytkin, I.A. Reactions of polyhalogenopyridines. 12. Reactions of
        4-pentafluoroethylthio-2,3, 5,6-tetrafluoropyridine with nucleophilic agents. *Chem. Heterocycl.
        Compd.*, **1996**, *32*(7), 796-799.
        [http://dx.doi.org/10.1007/BF01165723]

[20]   Sipyagin, A.M.; Enshov, V.S.; Lebedev, A.T.; Karakhanova, N.K. Reactions of Polyhalopyridines. 16.
        Synthesis and Reactions of 2,3,5,6-Tetrafluoro-4-perfluoroalkylthiopyridines. *Chem. Heterocycl.
        Compd.*, **2003**, *39*(8), 1022-1028.

[21]   Yin, X.; Guo, Y.; Liu, C.; Wang, Z.; Zhang, B. One-pot two-step facile synthesis of 2,3,5,6-
        tetrafluorobenzonitrile-containing dithiocarbamic acid esters. *Tetrahedron Lett.*, **2015**, *56*(36), 5135-
        5139.
        [http://dx.doi.org/10.1016/j.tetlet.2015.07.009]

[22]   Gingras, M.; Raimundo, J-M.; Chabre, Y.M. Persulfurated aromatic compounds. *Angew. Chem. Int.
        Ed. Engl.*, **2006**, *45*(11), 1686-1712.
        [http://dx.doi.org/10.1002/anie.200500032] [PMID: 16511821]

[23]   Testaferri, L.; Tiecco, M.; Tingoli, M.; Bartoli, D.; Massoli, A. The reactions of some halogenated
        pyridines with methoxide and methanethiolate ions in dimethylformamide. *Tetrahedron*, **1985**, *41*(7),
        1373-1384.
        [http://dx.doi.org/10.1016/S0040-4020(01)96539-1]

[24]   Gilmore, C.J.; MacNicol, D.D.; Murphy, A.; Russell, M.A. Discovery and x-ray crystal structure of a
        new host compound: 1,3,4-tris(phenylthio)[1]benzothieno[3,2-c]pyridine. *Tetrahedron Lett.*, **1984**,
        25(38), 4303-4306.
        [http://dx.doi.org/10.1016/S0040-4039(01)81423-4]

[25]   Tucker, H.R. J.; Gingras, M.; Brand, H.; Lehn, J.-M., Redox properties of polythiaarene derivatives. A
        novel class of electron acceptors. *J. Chem. Soc., Perkin Trans. 2*, **1997**, (7), 1303-1308.
        [http://dx.doi.org/10.1039/a608455i]

[26]   Dmowski, W.; Haas, A. Trifluoromethanethiolate ion. Part 2. Nucleophilic substitution in
        pentafluoropyridine. Synthesis and characteristics of trifluoromethylthio and trifluoromethylsulphonyl
        derivatives. *J. Chem. Soc., Perkin Trans. 1*, **1987**, (0), 2119-2124.
        [http://dx.doi.org/10.1039/p19870002119]

[27]   Smith, J.D.; Ansari, T.N.; Andersson, M.P.; Yadagiri, D.; Ibrahim, F.; Liang, S.; Hammond, G.B.;
        Gallou, F.; Handa, S. Micelle-enabled clean and selective sulfonylation of polyfluoroarenes in water
        under mild conditions. *Green Chem.*, **2018**, *20*(8), 1784-1790.
        [http://dx.doi.org/10.1039/C7GC03514D]

[28]   Vlasov, V.M.; Aksenov, V.V.; Rodionov, P.P.; Beregovaya, I.V.; Shchegoleva, L.N. *Russ. J. Org.
        Chem.*, **2002**, *38*(1), 115-125.
        [http://dx.doi.org/10.1023/A:1015371212613]

[29]   Aksenov, V.V.; Vlasov, V.M.; Yakobson, G.G. Interaction of pentafluoropyridine with 4-nitrophenol
        and pentafluorophenol in the presence of potassium fluoride and 18-crown-6-ether. *J. Fluor. Chem.*,
        1982, *20*(4), 439-458.
        [http://dx.doi.org/10.1016/S0022-1139(00)82271-X]

[30]   Cheong, C.L.; Wakefield, B.J. Polyhalogenoaromatic compounds. Part 53. Substitution in
        polyfluoroaromatic compounds by bulky nucleophiles. *J. Chem. Soc., Perkin Trans. 1*, **1988**, (12),
        3301-3305.

[http://dx.doi.org/10.1039/p19880003301]

[31]   Banks, R.E.; Jondi, W.; Tipping, A.E. SNAr displacement of fluorine from pentafluoropyridin by sodium oximates: unprecedented substitution patterns. *J. Chem. Soc. Chem. Commun.,* **1989**, (17), 1268-1269.
[http://dx.doi.org/10.1039/c39890001268]

[32]   Huchel, U.; Schmidt, C.; Schmidt, R.R. Synthesis of Hetaryl Glycosides and Their Glycosyl Donor Properties. *Eur. J. Org. Chem.,* **1998**, *1998*(7), 1353-1360.
[http://dx.doi.org/10.1002/(SICI)1099-0690(199807)1998:7<1353::AID-EJOC1353>3.0.CO;2-C]

[33]   Banks, R.E.; Falou, M.S.; Fields, R.; Olawore, N.O.; Tipping, A.E. Fluorocarbon derivatives of nitrogen. Part 14. Studies on some (CF3)2 no-substituted fluoroaromatics; thermal rearrangement of 4-[bis(trifluoromethyl)amino-oxy]tetrafluoropyridine. *J. Fluor. Chem.,* **1988**, *38*(2), 217-241.
[http://dx.doi.org/10.1016/S0022-1139(00)83031-6]

[34]   Chambers, R.D.; Nishimura, S.; Sandford, G. Reactions involving fluoride ion Part 431 Oligomerisations of hexafluoro-1,3-butadiene and -but-2-yne1Fax: +44-191-384-4737. *J. Fluor. Chem.,* **1998**, *91*(1), 63-68.
[http://dx.doi.org/10.1016/S0022-1139(98)00213-9]

[35]   Chambers, R.D.; Partington, S.; Speight, D.B. Reactions involving fluoride ion. Part XI. Syntheses from hexafluorobut-2-yne. *J. Chem. Soc., Perkin Trans. 1,* **1974**, (0), 2673-2678.
[http://dx.doi.org/10.1039/p19740002673]

[36]   Hammond, P.I.; Kern, C.; Hong, F.; Kollmeyer, T.M.; Pang, Y-P.; Brimijoin, S. Cholinesterase reactivation *in vivo* with a novel bis-oxime optimized by computer-aided design. *J. Pharmacol. Exp. Ther.,* **2003**, *307*(1), 190-196.
[http://dx.doi.org/10.1124/jpet.103.053405] [PMID: 12893843]

[37]   Timperley, C.M.; Banks, R.E.; Young, I.M.; Haszeldine, R.N. Synthesis of some fluorine-containing pyridinealdoximes of potential use for the treatment of organophosphorus nerve-agent poisoning. *J. Fluor. Chem.,* **2011**, *132*(8), 541-547.
[http://dx.doi.org/10.1016/j.jfluchem.2011.05.028]

[38]   Banks, R. E.; Haszeldine, R. N.; Young, I. M. Heterocyclic polyfluoro-compounds. Part XI. Synthesis and some reactions of 2,3,5,6-tetrafluoropyridine-4-aldehyde and -4-nitrile. *J. Chem. Soc. C: Organ,* **1967**, (0), 2089-2091.

[39]   Colgin, N.; Tatum, N.J.; Pohl, E.; Cobb, S.L.; Sandford, G. Synthesis and molecular structure of a perfluorinated pyridyl carbanion. *J. Fluor. Chem.,* **2012**, *133*, 33-37.
[http://dx.doi.org/10.1016/j.jfluchem.2011.09.013]

[40]   Chambers, R.D.; Hoskin, P.R.; Sandford, G.; Yufit, D.S.; Howard, J.A.K. Polyhalogenated heterocyclic compounds. Part 47.1 Syntheses of multi-substituted pyridine derivatives from pentafluoropyridine. *J. Chem. Soc., Perkin Trans. 1,* **2001**, (21), 2788-2795.
[http://dx.doi.org/10.1039/b105950p]

[41]   Chambers, R.D.; Hoskin, P.R.; Sandford, G. Polyhalogenated heterocyclic compounds. Part 48. Multisubstituted bis-pyridyl derivatives from pentafluoropyridine. *Collect. Czech. Chem. Commun.,* **2002**, *67*(9), 1277-1284.
[http://dx.doi.org/10.1135/cccc20021277]

[42]   Chambers, R.D.; Hassan, M.A.; Hoskin, P.R.; Kenwright, A.; Richmond, P.; Sandford, G. Polyhalogenated heterocyclic compounds: Part 45. Reactions of perfluoro-(4-isopropylpyridine) with oxygen, nitrogen and carbon nucleophiles. *J. Fluor. Chem.,* **2001**, *111*(2), 135-146. [1].

[43]   Chambers, R.D.; Hoskin, P.R.; Sandford, G. Polyhalogenated heterocyclic compounds. Part 48. Synthesis of perfluoroisopropyl-2, 2'-bipyridyl derivatives. *ARKIVOC,* **2002**, *2002*(6), 279-283.
[http://dx.doi.org/10.3998/ark.5550190.0003.624]

[44]   Yu, G.; Yin, S.; Liu, Y.; Shuai, Z.; Zhu, D. Structures, electronic states, and electroluminescent

properties of a zinc(II) 2-(2-hydroxyphenyl)benzothiazolate complex. *J. Am. Chem. Soc.,* **2003**, *125*(48), 14816-14824.
[http://dx.doi.org/10.1021/ja0371505] [PMID: 14640657]

[45] Dey, S.; Efimov, A.; Giri, C.; Rissanen, K.; Lemmetyinen, H. Electronic Structure Manipulation of (Benzothiazole)zinc Complexes: Synthesis, Optical and Electrochemical Studies of 5-Substituted Derivatives. *Eur. J. Org. Chem.,* **2011**, *2011*(31), 6226-6232.
[http://dx.doi.org/10.1002/ejoc.201100186]

[46] Suschitzky, H.; Wakefield, B.J.; Whitten, J.P. Polyhalogenoaromatic compounds. Part 44. Reactions of enamines with polyhalogenopyridines and their N-oxides. *J. Chem. Soc., Perkin Trans. 1,* **1980**, (0), 2709-2716.
[http://dx.doi.org/10.1039/p19800002709]

[47] Amii, H.; Uneyama, K.; Bond Activation, C.F. C-F bond activation in organic synthesis. *Chem. Rev.,* **2009**, *109*(5), 2119-2183.
[http://dx.doi.org/10.1021/cr800388c] [PMID: 19331346]

[48] Lindup, R.J.; Marder, T.B.; Perutz, R.N.; Whitwood, A.C. Sequential C-F activation and borylation of fluoropyridines *via* intermediate Rh(I) fluoropyridyl complexes: a multinuclear NMR investigation. *Chem. Commun. (Camb.),* **2007**, (35), 3664-3666.
[http://dx.doi.org/10.1039/b707840d] [PMID: 17728887]

[49] Nova, A.; Mas-Ballesté, R.; Ujaque, G.; González-Duarte, P.; Lledós, A. Aromatic C-F activation by complexes containing the Pt2S2 core *via* nucleophilic substitution: a combined experimental and theoretical study. *Dalton Trans.,* **2009**, (30), 5980-5988.
[http://dx.doi.org/10.1039/b901697j] [PMID: 19623398]

[50] Jana, A. Samuel, P. P.; Tavčar, G.; Roesky, H. W.; Schulzke, C., Selective Aromatic C−F and C−H Bond Activation with Silylenes of Different Coordinate Silicon. *JACS,* **2010**, *132*(29), 10164-10170.
[http://dx.doi.org/10.1021/ja103988d] [PMID: 20608652]

[51] Breyer, D.; Braun, T.; Kläring, P. Synthesis and reactivity of the fluoro complex trans-[Pd (F)(4-C5NF4)(i Pr2PCH2CH2OCH3) 2]: C−F bond formation and catalytic C–F bond activation reactions. *Organometallics,* **2012**, *31*(4), 1417-1424.
[http://dx.doi.org/10.1021/om200998d]

[52] Breyer, D.; Berger, J.; Braun, T.; Mebs, S. Nickel fluoro complexes as intermediates in catalytic cross-coupling reactions. *J. Fluor. Chem.,* **2012**, *143*, 263-271.

[53] Kuehnel, M.F.; Lentz, D.; Braun, T. Synthese fluorierter Bausteine durch Übergangsmetall-vermittelte Hydrodefluorierungsreaktionen. *Angew. Chem.,* **2013**, *125*(12), 3412-3433.
[http://dx.doi.org/10.1002/ange.201205260]

[54] Samuel, P.P.; Singh, A.P.; Sarish, S.P.; Matussek, J.; Objartel, I.; Roesky, H.W.; Stalke, D. Oxidative addition *versus* substitution reactions of group 14 dialkylamino metalylenes with pentafluoropyridine. *Inorg. Chem.,* **2013**, *52*(3), 1544-1549.
[http://dx.doi.org/10.1021/ic302344a] [PMID: 23343458]

[55] Kuhn, N.; Fahl, J.; Boese, R.; Henkel, G. Zur Reaktion von 2, 3-Dihydroimidazol-2-ylidenen mit Pentafluorpyridin: Carbene als Reaktionspartner in der nucleophilen aromatischen Substitution/On the Reaction of 2, 3-Dihydroimidazol-2-ylidenes with Pentafluoropyridine: Carbenes as Reactants in Nucleophilic Aromatic Substitution. *Z. Naturforsch. B,* **1998**, *53*(8), 881-886.
[http://dx.doi.org/10.1515/znb-1998-0818]

[56] Ung, G.; Frey, G.D.; Schoeller, W.W.; Bertrand, G. Bond activation with an apparently benign ethynyl dithiocarbamate Ar-C≡C-S-C(S)NR2. *Angew. Chem. Int. Ed. Engl.,* **2011**, *50*(42), 9923-9925.
[http://dx.doi.org/10.1002/anie.201104303] [PMID: 23210141]

[57] Styra, S.; Melaimi, M.; Moore, C.E.; Rheingold, A.L.; Augenstein, T.; Breher, F.; Bertrand, G. Crystalline Cyclic (Alkyl)(amino)carbene-tetrafluoropyridyl Radical. *Chemistry,* **2015**, *21*(23), 8441-8446.

[http://dx.doi.org/10.1002/chem.201500740] [PMID: 25925367]

[58]	Barlow, M.G.; Haszeldine, R.N.; Dingwall, J.G. Valence-bond isomer chemistry. Part IV. The valence-bond isomers of pentakis(pentafluoroethyl)pyridine. *J. Chem. Soc., Perkin Trans. 1*, **1973**, (0), 1542-1545.
[http://dx.doi.org/10.1039/p19730001542]

[59]	Igor Alabugin, W.-Y. Y. *Saumya Roy, Kemal Kaya, Qing-Xiang Sang Dipeptide acetylene conjugates and a method for photocleavage of double strand dna by dipeptide acetylene conjugates.*, **2012**.

[60]	Yang, W-Y.; Marrone, S.A.; Minors, N.; Zorio, D.A.R.; Alabugin, I.V. Fine-tuning alkyne cycloadditions: Insights into photochemistry responsible for the double-strand DNA cleavage *via* structural perturbations in diaryl alkyne conjugates. *Beilstein J. Org. Chem.*, **2011**, *7*, 813-823.
[http://dx.doi.org/10.3762/bjoc.7.93] [PMID: 21804877]

[61]	Chang, J.W.W.; Chia, E.Y.; Chai, C.L.L.; Seayad, J. Scope of direct arylation of fluorinated aromatics with aryl sulfonates. *Org. Biomol. Chem.*, **2012**, *10*(11), 2289-2299.
[http://dx.doi.org/10.1039/c2ob06840k] [PMID: 22354478]

[62]	Khaled, M.B.; El Mokadem, R.K.; Weaver, J.D., III Hydrogen Bond Directed Photocatalytic Hydrodefluorination: Overcoming Electronic Control. *J. Am. Chem. Soc.*, **2017**, *139*(37), 13092-13101.
[http://dx.doi.org/10.1021/jacs.7b06847] [PMID: 28837319]

[63]	Chambers, R.; Hutchinson, J.; Musgrave, W. *925. Polyfluoroheterocyclic compounds. Part IV. Compounds derived from 4-aminotetrafluoropyridine. Journal of the Chemical Society*; Resumed, **1965**, pp. 5040-5045.

[64]	Christopher, J.A.; Brophy, L.; Lynn, S.M.; Miller, D.D.; Sloan, L.A.; Sandford, G. Synthetic utility of 4-bromo-2,3,5,6-tetrafluoropyridine. *J. Fluor. Chem.*, **2008**, *129*(5), 447-454.
[http://dx.doi.org/10.1016/j.jfluchem.2008.01.004]

[65]	Chambers, R. D.; Hutchinson, J.; Musgrave, W. K. R. Polyfluoro-heterocyclic compounds. Part VI. Nucleophilic substitution in tetrafluoro-4-nitropyridine. *J. Chem. Soc. C: Organ*, **1966**, (0), 220-224.

[66]	Purrington, S.T.; Jones, W.A. 1-Fluoro-2-pyridone: a useful fluorinating reagent. *J. Org. Chem.*, **1983**, *48*(5), 761-762.
[http://dx.doi.org/10.1021/jo00153a037]

[67]	Satyamurthy, N.; Bida, G.T.; Phelps, M.E.; Barrio, J.R. N-Fluoro lactams: rapid, mild, and regiospecific fluorinating agents. *J. Org. Chem.*, **1990**, *55*(10), 3373-3374.
[http://dx.doi.org/10.1021/jo00297a071]

[68]	Banks, R.E.; Besheesh, M.K.; Tsiliopoulos, E. N-halogeno compounds. Part 16. Perfluoro-[N-fluoo-o-N-(4-pyridyl)acetamide] — a new site-selective electrophilic fluorinating agent. *J. Fluor. Chem.*, **1996**, *78*(1), 39-42.
[http://dx.doi.org/10.1016/0022-1139(95)03380-7]

[69]	Banks, R.E.; Khazaei, A. N-halogeno compounds. Part 11. Perfluoro-[N-fluoro-N-(4-pyridyl)-methanesulphonamide], a powerful new electrophilic fluorinating agent. *J. Fluor. Chem.*, **1990**, *46*(2), 297-305.
[http://dx.doi.org/10.1016/S0022-1139(00)80997-5]

[70]	Ronald, E. Banks, A. R. T., Haralambos S. Vellis, Azo-coupling of 2,3,5,6-tetrafluoropyridine-4-diazonium fluoride with mesitylene and anisole. *J. Fluor. Chem.*, **1983**, *22*, 499-501.
[http://dx.doi.org/10.1016/S0022-1139(00)81171-9]

[71]	Banks, R.E.; Noakes, T.J. Heterocyclic polyfluoro-compounds. Part XXII. Synthesis of octafluoro-4,4'-azopyridine and tetrafluoro-4-(pentafluorophenylazo)pyridine. *J. Chem. Soc., Perkin Trans. 1*, **1975**, (14), 1419-1420.
[http://dx.doi.org/10.1039/P19750001419]

[72]	Banks, R.E.; Farhat, I.M.; Fields, R.; Pritchard, R.G.; Saleh, M.M. N-halogeno-compounds. Part 9 [1].

Azoxy- and azo-arenes derived from 4-(dichloroamino)tetrafluoropyridine; crystal structure of trans-2,3,5,6-tetrafluoro-4-(2,4,6-trimethylphenyl-onn-azoxy)pyridine. *J. Fluor. Chem.,* **1985**, *28*(3), 325-340.
[http://dx.doi.org/10.1016/S0022-1139(00)80544-8]

[73]   Chambers, R.D.; Sandford, G.; Trmcic, J. Continuous flow glassware reactors for the laboratory: Synthesis of 2-alkoxy-4-aminotrifluoropyridine derivatives from pentafluoropyridine. *J. Fluor. Chem.,* **2007**, *128*(12), 1439-1443.
[http://dx.doi.org/10.1016/j.jfluchem.2007.07.010]

[74]   Steglich, W.; Höfle, G. N,N-Dimethyl-4-pyridinamine, a Very Effective Acylation Catalyst. *Angew. Chem. Int. Ed. Engl.,* **1969**, *8*(12), 981-981.
[http://dx.doi.org/10.1002/anie.196909811]

[75]   Höfle, G.; Steglich, W.; Vorbrüggen, H. 4-Dialkylaminopyridines as Highly Active Acylation Catalysts. *Angew. Chem. Int. Ed. Engl.,* **1978**, *17*(8), 569-583. [New synthetic method (25)].
[http://dx.doi.org/10.1002/anie.197805691]

[76]   Scriven, E.F. 4-Dialkylaminopyridines: super acylation and alkylation catalysts. *Chem. Soc. Rev.,* **1983**, *12*(2), 129-161.
[http://dx.doi.org/10.1039/cs9831200129]

[77]   Schmidt, A.; Mordhorst, T.; Habeck, T. Synthesis of new pyridines with oligocations and oxygen nucleophiles. *Org. Lett.,* **2002**, *4*(8), 1375-1377.
[http://dx.doi.org/10.1021/ol0256926] [PMID: 11950366]

[78]   Schmidt, A.; Mordhorst, T. Synthesis of Alkoxy-Substituted Pyridines from Mono- and Tricationic Pyridinium Salts. *Synthesis,* **2005**, *2005*(05), 781-786.
[http://dx.doi.org/10.1055/s-2005-861827]

[79]   Schmidt, A.; Mordhorst, T. Synthesis of pyridine-thioethers *via* mono-and tricationic pyridinium salts. *Z. Naturforsch. B,* **2005**, *60*(6), 683-687.
[http://dx.doi.org/10.1515/znb-2005-0613]

[80]   Schmidt, A.; Mordhorst, T.; Nieger, M. Heteroarenium salts in synthesis. Highly functionalized tetra- and pentasubstituted pyridines. *Tetrahedron,* **2006**, *62*(8), 1667-1674.
[http://dx.doi.org/10.1016/j.tet.2005.11.065]

[81]   Schmidt, A.; Mordhorst, T.; Namyslo, J.C.; Telle, W. Hetarenium salts from pentafluoropyridine. Syntheses, spectroscopic properties, and applications. *J. Heterocycl. Chem.,* **2007**, *44*(3), 679-684.
[http://dx.doi.org/10.1002/jhet.5570440326]

[82]   Murray, C.B.; Sandford, G.; Korn, S.R.; Yufit, D.S.; Howard, J.A.K. New fluoride ion reagent from pentafluoropyridine. *J. Fluor. Chem.,* **2005**, *126*(4), 569-574.
[http://dx.doi.org/10.1016/j.jfluchem.2004.12.013]

[83]   Banks, R.E.; Sparkes, G.R. Studies in azide chemistry. Part V. Synthesis of 4-azido-2,3,5-6-tetrafluoro-, 4-azido-3-chloro-2,5,6-trifluoro-, and 4-azido-3,5-dichloro-2,6-difluoro-pyridine, and some thermal reactions of the tetrafluoro-compound. *J. Chem. Soc., Perkin Trans. 1,* **1972**, (0), 2964-2970.
[http://dx.doi.org/10.1039/p19720002964]

[84]   Wu, J.; Fu, D.; Cao, S. Synthesis of polyfluoroaryl-containing 1,2,3-triazoles by reaction of polyfluoroarenes, sodium azide and active methylene ketones/esters. *J. Fluor. Chem.,* **2014**, *168*, 230-235.
[http://dx.doi.org/10.1016/j.jfluchem.2014.10.009]

[85]   Xie, S.; Fukumoto, R.; Ramström, O.; Yan, M. Anilide formation from thioacids and perfluoroaryl azides. *J. Org. Chem.,* **2015**, *80*(9), 4392-4397.
[http://dx.doi.org/10.1021/acs.joc.5b00240] [PMID: 25837012]

[86]   Law, K.Y.; Bailey, F.C. Squaraine chemistry. Synthesis, characterization, and optical properties of a

class of novel unsymmetrical squaraines:[4-(dimethylamino) phenyl](4'-methoxyphenyl) squaraine and its derivatives. *J. Org. Chem.,* **1992**, *57*(12), 3278-3286.
[http://dx.doi.org/10.1021/jo00038a010]

[87]   Law, K.Y. Squaraine chemistry: effects of structural changes on the absorption and multiple fluorescence emission of bis [4-(dimethylamino) phenyl] squaraine and its derivatives. *J. Phys. Chem.,* **1987**, *91*(20), 5184-5193.
[http://dx.doi.org/10.1021/j100304a012]

[88]   Beverina, L.; Drees, M.; Facchetti, A.; Salamone, M.; Ruffo, R.; Pagani, G.A. Bulk heterojunction solar cells–tuning of the HOMO and LUMO energy levels of pyrrolic squaraine dyes. *Eur. J. Org. Chem.,* **2011**, *2011*(28), 5555-5563.
[http://dx.doi.org/10.1002/ejoc.201100940]

[89]   Laot, Y.; Petit, L.; Zard, S.Z. Synthesis of fluoroazaindolines by an uncommon radical ipso substitution of a carbon-fluorine bond. *Org. Lett.,* **2010**, *12*(15), 3426-3429.
[http://dx.doi.org/10.1021/ol101240f] [PMID: 20670008]

[90]   Mérour, J-Y.; Routier, S.; Suzenet, F.; Joseph, B. Recent advances in the synthesis and properties of 4-, 5-, 6- or 7-azaindoles. *Tetrahedron,* **2013**, *69*(24), 4767-4834.
[http://dx.doi.org/10.1016/j.tet.2013.03.081]

[91]   Popowycz, F.; Routier, S.; Joseph, B.; Mérour, J-Y. Synthesis and reactivity of 7-azaindole (1H-pyrrolo[2,3-b]pyridine). *Tetrahedron,* **2007**, *63*(5), 1031-1064.
[http://dx.doi.org/10.1016/j.tet.2006.09.067]

[92]   Popowycz, F.; Mérour, J-Y.; Joseph, B. Synthesis and reactivity of 4-, 5- and 6-azaindoles. *Tetrahedron,* **2007**, *63*(36), 8689-8707.
[http://dx.doi.org/10.1016/j.tet.2007.05.078]

[93]   Song, J.J.; Reeves, J.T.; Gallou, F.; Tan, Z.; Yee, N.K.; Senanayake, C.H. Organometallic methods for the synthesis and functionalization of azaindoles. *Chem. Soc. Rev.,* **2007**, *36*(7), 1120-1132.
[http://dx.doi.org/10.1039/b607868k] [PMID: 17576479]

[94]   Schirok, H. Microwave-assisted flexible synthesis of 7-azaindoles. *J. Org. Chem.,* **2006**, *71*(15), 5538-5545.
[http://dx.doi.org/10.1021/jo060512h] [PMID: 16839132]

[95]   Humphrey, G.R.; Kuethe, J.T. Practical methodologies for the synthesis of indoles. *Chem. Rev.,* **2006**, *106*(7), 2875-2911.
[http://dx.doi.org/10.1021/cr0505270] [PMID: 16836303]

[96]   Cacchi, S.; Fabrizi, G. Synthesis and functionalization of indoles through palladium-catalyzed reactions. *Chem. Rev.,* **2005**, *105*(7), 2873-2920.
[http://dx.doi.org/10.1021/cr040639b] [PMID: 16011327]

[97]   Zhang, A.; Neumeyer, J.L.; Baldessarini, R.J. Recent progress in development of dopamine receptor subtype-selective agents: potential therapeutics for neurological and psychiatric disorders. *Chem. Rev.,* **2007**, *107*(1), 274-302.
[http://dx.doi.org/10.1021/cr050263h] [PMID: 17212477]

[98]   Liu, Z.; Qin, L.; Zard, S.Z. Radical ipso-substitution of a carbon-fluorine bond leading to fluoro--azaindolines and fluoro-7-azaindoles. *Org. Lett.,* **2014**, *16*(10), 2704-2707.
[http://dx.doi.org/10.1021/ol500985f] [PMID: 24773583]

[99]   Claridge, P. R.; W. Millar, R.; P. B. Sandall, J.; Thompson, C., Preparation of a Series of N-Aryl-S-S-diphenylsulfilimines by Nucleophilic Attack of S,S-Diphenyl-sulfilimine on Activated Halogenoaromatic Compounds. *J. Chem. Res. Synop.,* **1999**, (8), 520-520.
[http://dx.doi.org/10.1039/a901862j]

[100] Benmansour, H.; Chambers, R.D.; Hoskin, P.R.; Sandford, G. Multi-substituted heterocycles. *J. Fluor. Chem.,* **2001**, *112*(1), 133-137.

[http://dx.doi.org/10.1016/S0022-1139(01)00480-8]

[101]   Benmansour, H.; Chambers, R.D.; Sandford, G.; McGowan, G.; Dahaoui, S.; Yufit, D.S.; Howard, J.A. Polyhalogenated heterocyclic compounds: Part 46. Multifunctional heterocycles from bromofluoropyridine derivatives. *J. Fluor. Chem.,* **2001**, *112*(2), 349-354.
[http://dx.doi.org/10.1016/S0022-1139(01)00534-6]

[102]   Banks, R.; Haszeldine, R.; Phillips, E.; Young, I. Heterocyclic polyfluoro-compounds. Part XII. Synthesis and some reactions of 2, 3, 5, 6-tetrafluoro-4-iodopyridine. *J. Chem. Soc. C: Organ,* **1967**, 2091-2095.

[103]   Senaweera, S.; Weaver, J.D. S_NAr catalysis enhanced by an aromatic donor-acceptor interaction; facile access to chlorinated polyfluoroarenes. *Chem. Commun. (Camb.),* **2017**, *53*(54), 7545-7548.
[http://dx.doi.org/10.1039/C7CC03996D] [PMID: 28634609]

[104]   Chambers, D. R.; W. Hall, C.; Hutchinson, J.; W. Millar, R., Polyhalogenated heterocyclic compounds. Part 42.1 Fluorinated nitrogen heterocycles with unusual substitution patterns. *J. Chem. Soc., Perkin Trans. 1,* **1998**, (10), 1705-1714.
[http://dx.doi.org/10.1039/a709291a]

[105]   Arévalo, A.; Tlahuext-Aca, A.; Flores-Alamo, M.; García, J.J. On the catalytic hydrodefluorination of fluoroaromatics using nickel complexes: the true role of the phosphine. *J. Am. Chem. Soc.,* **2014**, *136*(12), 4634-4639.
[http://dx.doi.org/10.1021/ja412268y] [PMID: 24432839]

[106]   Coe, P.L.; Rees, A.J. Preparation and reactions of 2, 3, 4, 6-tetrafluoropyridine and its derivatives. *J. Fluor. Chem.,* **2000**, *101*(1), 45-60.
[http://dx.doi.org/10.1016/S0022-1139(99)00189-X]

[107]   Bobbio, C.; Rausis, T.; Schlosser, M. Removal of fluorine from and introduction of fluorine into polyhalopyridines: an exercise in nucleophilic hetarenic substitution. *Chemistry,* **2005**, *11*(6), 1903-1910.
[http://dx.doi.org/10.1002/chem.200400837] [PMID: 15685584]

[108]   Ranjbar-Karimi, R.; Heidari, E. Survey of reactivity of some enolates with pentafluoropyridine and 4-phenylsulfonyl-2, 3, 5, 6-tetrafluoropyridine. *J. Fluor. Chem.,* **2013**, *154*, 47-52.
[http://dx.doi.org/10.1016/j.jfluchem.2013.06.008]

[109]   Cartwright, M.W.; Parks, E.L.; Pattison, G.; Slater, R.; Sandford, G.; Wilson, I.; Yufit, D.S.; Howard, J.A.; Christopher, J.A.; Miller, D.D. Annelation of perfluorinated heteroaromatic systems by 1, 3-dicarbonyl derivatives. *Tetrahedron,* **2010**, *66*(17), 3222-3227.
[http://dx.doi.org/10.1016/j.tet.2010.02.083]

[110]   Teegardin, K.A.; Weaver, J.D. Polyfluoroarylation of oxazolones: access to non-natural fluorinated amino acids. *Chem. Commun. (Camb.),* **2017**, *53*(35), 4771-4774.
[http://dx.doi.org/10.1039/C7CC01606A] [PMID: 28357423]

[111]   Senaweera, S.M.; Weaver, J.D. Selective perfluoro- and polyfluoroarylation of Meldrum's acid. *J. Org. Chem.,* **2014**, *79*(21), 10466-10476.
[http://dx.doi.org/10.1021/jo502075p] [PMID: 25271542]

[112]   Ranjbar-Karimi, R.; Karbakhsh-Ravari, A.; Poorfreidoni, A. Reactions of pentafluoropyridine with amidoximes. *J. Iran. Chem. Soc.,* **2017**, *14*(11), 2397-2405.
[http://dx.doi.org/10.1007/s13738-017-1174-1]

[113]   Ranjbar-Karimi, R.; Poorfreidoni, A.; Masoodi, H.R. Survey reactivity of some N-aryl formamides with pentafluoropyridine. *J. Fluor. Chem.,* **2015**, *180*, 222-226.
[http://dx.doi.org/10.1016/j.jfluchem.2015.10.008]

[114]   Olah, G.A. *Friedel-Crafts and Related Reactions*; Interscience Publishers: London, **1964**, Vol. 3, .

[115]   Favero, P.; Mirri, A. M.; Baker, J. G. Centrifugal effects in millimetre wave spectra: formyl fluoride. *Il Nuovo Cimento (1955-1965),* **1960**, *17*(5), 740-748.

[116] Poorfreidoni, A.; Ranjbar-Karimi, R. Synthesis of substituted imidazopyridines from perfluorinated pyridine derivatives. *Tetrahedron Lett.,* **2016**, *57*(51), 5781-5783.
[http://dx.doi.org/10.1016/j.tetlet.2016.11.045]

[117] Schenker, S.; Zamfir, A.; Freund, M.; Tsogoeva, S.B. Developments in Chiral Binaphthyl-Derived Brønsted/Lewis Acids and Hydrogen-Bond-Donor Organocatalysis. *Eur. J. Org. Chem.,* **2011**, *2011*(12), 2209-2222.
[http://dx.doi.org/10.1002/ejoc.201001538]

[118] Dabbagh, H.A.; Najafi-Chermahini, A.; Banibairami, S. A new family of bis-tetrazole (BIZOL) BINOL-type ligands. *Tetrahedron Lett.,* **2006**, *47*(23), 3929-3932.
[http://dx.doi.org/10.1016/j.tetlet.2006.03.160]

[119] Chen, Y.; Yekta, S.; Yudin, A.K. Modified BINOL ligands in asymmetric catalysis. *Chem. Rev.,* **2003**, *103*(8), 3155-3212.
[http://dx.doi.org/10.1021/cr020025b] [PMID: 12914495]

[120] Koltunov, K.Y.; Chernov, A.N. BINOL modification *via* SNAr reactions with pentafluoropyridine. *Mendeleev Commun.,* **2015**, *1*(25), 39-40.
[http://dx.doi.org/10.1016/j.mencom.2015.01.014]

[121] Ranjbar-Karimi, R.; Khaje-Khezri, A. Environmental Friendly Synthesis of Bis-Perfluoropyridine and Pyrimidine in Water. *Heterocycles: an international journal for reviews and communications in heterocyclic chemistry,* **2015**, *91*(4), 738-746.

[122] Ranjbar-Karimi, R.; Mashak-Shoshtari, M.; Darehkordi, A. Ultrasound promoted facile synthesis of some pentafluoropyridine derivatives at ambient conditions. *Ultrason. Sonochem.,* **2011**, *18*(1), 258-263.
[http://dx.doi.org/10.1016/j.ultsonch.2010.05.017] [PMID: 20630789]

[123] Ranjbar-Karimi, R.; Davodian, T.; Mehrabi, H. Reactions of pyridin-2-ol, pyridin-3-ol, and pyridin--ol with pentafluoro- and pentachloropyridine. *Chem. Heterocycl. Compd.,* **2017**, *53*(12), 1330-1334.
[http://dx.doi.org/10.1007/s10593-018-2213-2]

[124] Davodian, T.; Ranjbar-Karimi, R.; Mehrabi, H. Synthesis of diheteroaryl sulfides *via* chemoselective reaction of 4, 6-diaminopyrimidine-2 (1H)-thione with haloheteroaryl compounds. *Chem. Heterocycl. Compd.,* **2017**, *53*(10), 1120-1123.
[http://dx.doi.org/10.1007/s10593-017-2181-y]

[125] Coe, P.L.; Rees, A.J.; Whittaker, J. Reactions of polyfluoropyridines with bidentate nucleophiles: attempts to prepare deazapurine analogues. *J. Fluor. Chem.,* **2001**, *107*(1), 13-22.
[http://dx.doi.org/10.1016/S0022-1139(00)00335-3]

[126] Trawny, D.; Kunz, V.; Reissig, H.U. Modular Syntheses of Star-Shaped Pyridine, Bipyridine, and Terpyridine Derivatives by Employing Sonogashira Reactions. *Eur. J. Org. Chem.,* **2014**, *2014*(28), 6295-6302.
[http://dx.doi.org/10.1002/ejoc.201402778]

[127] Takimiya, K.; Kunugi, Y.; Konda, Y.; Niihara, N.; Otsubo, T. 2,6-Diphenylbenzo[1,2-b:4-5-b′]dichalcogenophenes: a new class of high-performance semiconductors for organic field-effect transistors. *J. Am. Chem. Soc.,* **2004**, *126*(16), 5084-5085.
[http://dx.doi.org/10.1021/ja0496930] [PMID: 15099088]

[128] Takimiya, K.; Kunugi, Y.; Ebata, H.; Otsubo, T. Molecular Modification of 2, 6-Diphenylbenzo [1, 2-b: 4, 5-b′] dichalcogenophenes by Introduction of Strong Electron-withdrawing Groups: Conversion from p-to n-Channel OFET Materials. *Chem. Lett.,* **2006**, *35*(10), 1200-1201.
[http://dx.doi.org/10.1246/cl.2006.1200]

[129] Pan, H.; Li, Y.; Wu, Y.; Liu, P.; Ong, B.S.; Zhu, S.; Xu, G. Low-temperature, solution-processed, high-mobility polymer semiconductors for thin-film transistors. *J. Am. Chem. Soc.,* **2007**, *129*(14), 4112-4113.

[http://dx.doi.org/10.1021/ja067879o] [PMID: 17362006]

[130]   Hou, J.; Park, M-H.; Zhang, S.; Yao, Y.; Chen, L-M.; Li, J-H.; Yang, Y. Bandgap and molecular energy level control of conjugated polymer photovoltaic materials based on benzo [1, 2-b: 4, 5-b'] dithiophene. *Macromolecules,* **2008**, *41*(16), 6012-6018.
[http://dx.doi.org/10.1021/ma800820r]

[131]   Wang, Y.; Parkin, S.R.; Watson, M.D. Benzodichalcogenophenes with perfluoroarene termini. *Org. Lett.,* **2008**, *10*(20), 4421-4424.
[http://dx.doi.org/10.1021/ol801569m] [PMID: 18800845]

[132]   Gimenez, D.; Mooney, C.A.; Dose, A.; Sandford, G.; Coxon, C.R.; Cobb, S.L. The application of perfluoroheteroaromatic reagents in the preparation of modified peptide systems. *Org. Biomol. Chem.,* **2017**, *15*(19), 4086-4095.
[http://dx.doi.org/10.1039/C7OB00283A] [PMID: 28470238]

[133]   Hudson, A.S.; Hoose, A.; Coxon, C.R.; Sandford, G.; Cobb, S.L. Synthesis of a novel tetrafluoropyridine-containing amino acid and tripeptide. *Tetrahedron Lett.,* **2013**, *54*(36), 4865-4867.
[http://dx.doi.org/10.1016/j.tetlet.2013.06.124]

[134]   Webster, A.M.; Coxon, C.R.; Kenwright, A.M.; Sandford, G.; Cobb, S.L. A mild method for the synthesis of a novel dehydrobutyrine-containing amino acid. *Tetrahedron,* **2014**, *70*(31), 4661-4667.
[http://dx.doi.org/10.1016/j.tet.2014.05.031]

[135]   Antsypovich, I. S.; S. Oretskaya, T. y., Double-helical nucleic acids with cross-linked strands: synthesis and applications in molecular biology. *Russ. Chem. Rev.,* **1998**, *67*(3), 245-262.
[http://dx.doi.org/10.1070/RC1998v067n03ABEH000345]

[136]   Mathé, C.; Gosselin, G. Synthesis and antiviral evaluation of the β-L-enantiomers of some thymine 3'-deoxypentofuranonucleoside derivatives. *Nucleosides Nucleotides Nucleic Acids,* **2000**, *19*(10-12), 1517-1530.
[http://dx.doi.org/10.1080/15257770008045443] [PMID: 11200256]

[137]   Ermolinsky, B.; Fomitcheva, M.; Efimtseva, E.; Mikhailov, S.N.; Esipov, D.; Boldyreva, E.; Korobko, V.; Van Aerschot, A.; Herdewijn, P. Modified oligonucleotides containing 1-β-D-galactopyr-anosylthymine: Synthesis and substrate properties. *uss. J. Bioorg. Chem.,* **2002**, *28*(1), 50-57.
[http://dx.doi.org/10.1023/A:1013906303698]

[138]   Litvak, V.; Mainagashev, I.Y.; Bukhanets, O. Polynucleotides and their components in the processes of aromatic nucleophilic substitution: i. Chemistry and dynamics of nucleotide arylation with pentafluoropyridine; obtaining of synthons for molecular design of nucleic acid analogues. *uss. J. Bioorg. Chem.,* **2004**, *30*(1), 47-52.
[http://dx.doi.org/10.1023/B:RUBI.0000015773.37915.3b]

[139]   Jarman, M.; McCague, R. Heptafluoro-p-tolyl and tetrafluoro-4-pyridyl as novel and selective protecting groups for phenolic and alcoholic functions: synthesis and cleavage of perfluoroaryl ethers of steroids. *J. Chem. Soc. Chem. Commun.,* **1984**, (2), 125-127.
[http://dx.doi.org/10.1039/c39840000125]

[140]   Ranjbar-Karimi, R.; Mashak-Shoshtari, M.; Hashemi-Uderji, S.; Kia, R. Synthesis and structural study of bis-perfluoropyridyl bridged by 1, 4 and 1, 2 dihydropyridine. *J. Fluor. Chem.,* **2011**, *132*(4), 285-290.
[http://dx.doi.org/10.1016/j.jfluchem.2011.02.007]

[141]   Sandford, G.; Slater, R.; Yufit, D.S.; Howard, J.A.; Vong, A. Tetrahydropyrido[3,4-b]pyrazine scaffolds from pentafluoropyridine. *J. Org. Chem.,* **2005**, *70*(18), 7208-7216.
[http://dx.doi.org/10.1021/jo0508696] [PMID: 16122239]

[142]   Baron, A.; Sandford, G.; Slater, R.; Yufit, D.S.; Howard, J.A.; Vong, A. Polyfunctional tetrahydropyrido[2,3-b]pyrazine scaffolds from 4-phenylsulfonyl tetrafluoropyridine. *J. Org. Chem.,* **2005**, *70*(23), 9377-9381.
[http://dx.doi.org/10.1021/jo051453v] [PMID: 16268611]

[143] Cartwright, M.W.; Convery, L.; Kraynck, T.; Sandford, G.; Yufit, D.S.; Howard, J.A.; Christopher, J.A.; Miller, D.D. Dipyrido [1, 2-a; 3', 4'-d] imidazole systems. *Tetrahedron*, **2010**, *66*(2), 519-529.
[http://dx.doi.org/10.1016/j.tet.2009.11.036]

[144] Ranjbar-Karimi, R.; Hashemi-Uderji, S.; Danesteh, R. Synthesis of some di-and trifluoro quinoxaline and dioxine derivatives from pentafluoropyridine. *J. Iran. Chem. Soc.*, **2012**, *9*(5), 747-755.
[http://dx.doi.org/10.1007/s13738-012-0091-6]

[145] Hargreaves, C.A.; Sandford, G.; Slater, R.; Yufit, D.S.; Howard, J.A.; Vong, A. Synthesis of tetrahydropyrido [2, 3-b] pyrazine scaffolds from 2, 3, 5, 6-tetrafluoropyridine derivatives. *Tetrahedron*, **2007**, *63*(24), 5204-5211.
[http://dx.doi.org/10.1016/j.tet.2007.03.164]

[146] Sandford, G.; Slater, R.; Yufit, D.S.; Howard, J.A.; Vong, A. Pyrido [3, 2-b][1, 4] oxazine and pyrido [2, 3-b][1, 4] benzoxazine systems from tetrafluoropyridine derivatives. *J. Fluor. Chem.*, **2014**, *167*, 91-95.
[http://dx.doi.org/10.1016/j.jfluchem.2014.05.003]

[147] Ranjbar-Karimi, R.; Mousavi, M. Regiochemistry of nucleophilic substitution of 4-phenylsulfonyl tetrafluoropyridine with unequal bidentate nucleophiles. *J. Fluor. Chem.*, **2010**, *131*(5), 587-591.
[http://dx.doi.org/10.1016/j.jfluchem.2010.01.006]

[148] Cartwright, M.W.; Sandford, G.; Bousbaa, J.; Yufit, D.S.; Howard, J.A.; Christopher, J.A.; Miller, D.D. Imidazopyridine and pyrimidinopyridine systems from perfluorinated pyridine derivatives. *Tetrahedron*, **2007**, *63*(30), 7027-7035.
[http://dx.doi.org/10.1016/j.tet.2007.05.016]

[149] Ranjbar-Karimi, R.; Danesteh, R.; Beiki-Shoraki, K. Synthesis of some fluorinated thiazolopyridine from pentafluoropyridine and 4-phenylsulfonyl tetrafluoropyridine. *Arab. J. Chem.*, **2015**.

[150] Ranjbar-Karimi, R.; Darehkordi, A.; Bahadornia, F.; Poorfreidoni, A. Dipyrido [1, 2-b: 3', 4'-e][1, 2, 4] triazine Scaffolds from Pentafluoropyridine. *J. Heterocycl. Chem.*, **2018**, *55*(11), 2516-2521.
[http://dx.doi.org/10.1002/jhet.3283]

[151] White, W. L.; Filler, R. New reactions of polyfluoroaromatic compounds. Part II. Polyfluoroaralkyl amines. *J. Chem. Soc. C: Organ*, **1971**, 2062-2068.

[152] Haas, A.; Koehler, J. Darstellung von polyfluororganotrichlorsilanen. *J. Fluor. Chem.*, **1981**, *17*(6), 531-537.
[http://dx.doi.org/10.1016/S0022-1139(00)82259-9]

[153] Miller, A.O.; Krasnov, V.I.; Peters, D.; Platonov, V.E.; Miethchen, R. Perfluorozinc aromatics by direct insertion of zinc into C–F or C–Cl bonds. *Tetrahedron Lett.*, **2000**, *41*(20), 3817-3819.
[http://dx.doi.org/10.1016/S0040-4039(00)00527-X]

[154] Krasnov, B.; Platonov, V. Reductive transformations of organofluorine compounds: III. Hydrodefluorination of perfluoroalkylbenzenes effected by Zn (Cu). The unusual behavior of compounds containing perfluorinated tert-butyl group. *Russ. J. Org. Chem.*, **2001**, *37*(4), 517-522.
[http://dx.doi.org/10.1023/A:1012429802321]

[155] Vinogradov, A.; Krasnov, V.; Platonov, V. Organozinc reagents from polyfluoroarenes: Preparation and reactions with allyl halides. Synthesis of allylpolyfluoroarenes. *Russ. J. Org. Chem.*, **2008**, *44*(1), 95-102.
[http://dx.doi.org/10.1134/S1070428008010119]

[156] Tamborski, C.; Soloski, E.J.; De Pasquale, R.J. Novel synthesis of perhalostyrene compounds. *J. Organomet. Chem.*, **1968**, *15*(2), 494-496.
[http://dx.doi.org/10.1016/S0022-328X(00)91328-7]

[157] Jukes, A.E.; Dua, S.S.; Gilman, H. Polyhalo-organometallic and -organometalloidal compounds XVIII. bis(polyhaloaryl)acetylenes *via* organocopper compounds. *J. Organomet. Chem.*, **1968**, *12*(3), 44-P46.

[http://dx.doi.org/10.1016/S0022-328X(00)88692-1]

[158]   DePasquale, R.J.; Tamborski, C. Reactions of pentafluorophenylcopper reagent. *J. Org. Chem.,* **1969**, *34*(6), 1736-1740.
[http://dx.doi.org/10.1021/jo01258a046]

[159]   Soloski, E.; Ward, W.; Tamborski, C. Synthesis of trifluorovinylpolyhaloaryl compounds *via* polyhaloarylcopper complexes. *J. Fluor. Chem.,* **1973**, *2*(4), 361-371.
[http://dx.doi.org/10.1016/S0022-1139(00)83193-0]

[160]   Sartori, P.; Adelt, H. Darstellung und eigenschaften von tetrafluorisonicotinsäure-derivaten der nebengruppe II. *J. Fluor. Chem.,* **1974**, *3*(3-4), 275-283.
[http://dx.doi.org/10.1016/S0022-1139(00)82627-5]

[161]   Nguyen, B.V.; Burton, D.J. Preparation and reactions of the 2, 3, 5, 6-tetrafluoropyridylcopper reagent. *J. Fluor. Chem.,* **1994**, *67*(3), 205-206.
[http://dx.doi.org/10.1016/0022-1139(93)03058-T]

[162]   Schaub, T.; Backes, M.; Radius, U.; Catalytic, C. Catalytic C-C bond formation accomplished by selective C-F activation of perfluorinated arenes. *J. Am. Chem. Soc.,* **2006**, *128*(50), 15964-15965.
[http://dx.doi.org/10.1021/ja064068b] [PMID: 17165711]

[163]   Nakamura, Y.; Yoshikai, N.; Ilies, L.; Nakamura, E. Nickel-catalyzed monosubstitution of polyfluoroarenes with organozinc reagents using alkoxydiphosphine ligand. *Org. Lett.,* **2012**, *14*(13), 3316-3319.
[http://dx.doi.org/10.1021/ol301195x] [PMID: 22691135]

[164]   Böhm, V.P.; Gstöttmayr, C.W.; Weskamp, T.; Herrmann, W.A. Katalytische C-C-Bindungsknüpfung durch selektive Aktivierung von C-F-Bindungen. *Angew. Chem.,* **2001**, *113*(18), 3500-3503.
[http://dx.doi.org/10.1002/1521-3757(20010917)113:18<3500::AID-ANGE3500>3.0.CO;2-B]

[165]   Tobisu, M.; Xu, T.; Shimasaki, T.; Chatani, N. Nickel-catalyzed Suzuki-Miyaura reaction of aryl fluorides. *J. Am. Chem. Soc.,* **2011**, *133*(48), 19505-19511.
[http://dx.doi.org/10.1021/ja207759e] [PMID: 22023167]

[166]   Steffen, A.; Sladek, M.I.; Braun, T.; Neumann, B.; Stammler, H-G.; Catalytic, C. C coupling reactions at nickel by C− F activation of a pyrimidine in the presence of a C− Cl bond: the crucial role of highly reactive fluoro complexes. *Organometallics,* **2005**, *24*(16), 4057-4064.
[http://dx.doi.org/10.1021/om050080l]

[167]   Cargill, M.R.; Sandford, G.; Tadeusiak, A.J.; Yufit, D.S.; Howard, J.A.; Kilickiran, P.; Nelles, G. Palladium-catalyzed C-F activation of polyfluoronitrobenzene derivatives in Suzuki-Miyaura coupling reactions. *J. Org. Chem.,* **2010**, *75*(17), 5860-5866.
[http://dx.doi.org/10.1021/jo100877j] [PMID: 20704342]

[168]   Ohashi, M.; Doi, R.; Ogoshi, S. Palladium-catalyzed coupling reaction of perfluoroarenes with diarylzinc compounds. *Chemistry,* **2014**, *20*(7), 2040-2048.
[http://dx.doi.org/10.1002/chem.201303451] [PMID: 24431191]

[169]   Tyrra, W.; Aboulkacem, S.; Pantenburg, I. Silver compounds in synthetic chemistry. Part 3. 4-Tetrafluoropyridyl silver (I), AgC 5 F 4 N–A reagent for redox transmetallations with group 12–14 elements. *J. Organomet. Chem.,* **2006**, *691*(3), 514-522.
[http://dx.doi.org/10.1016/j.jorganchem.2005.09.017]

[170]   Tyrra, W.; Aboulkacem, S.; Hoge, B.; Wiebe, W.; Pantenburg, I. Silver compounds in synthetic chemistry: Part 4. 4-Tetrafluoropyridyl silver (I), AgC5F4N in redox transmetallations—possibilities and limitations in reactions with group 15 elements. *J. Fluor. Chem.,* **2006**, *127*(2), 213-217.
[http://dx.doi.org/10.1016/j.jfluchem.2005.10.009]

[171]   Aboulkacem, S.; Naumann, D.; Tyrra, W.; Pantenburg, I. 4-Tetrafluoropyridyl Silver (I), AgC5F4N, in Redox Transmetalations with Selenium and Tellurium. *Organometallics,* **2012**, *31*(4), 1559-1565.
[http://dx.doi.org/10.1021/om201195j]

[172] Kiplinger, J.L.; Richmond, T.G.; Osterberg, C.E. Activation of carbon-fluorine bonds by metal complexes. *Chem. Rev.,* **1994**, *94*(2), 373-431.
[http://dx.doi.org/10.1021/cr00026a005]

[173] Murphy, E.F.; Murugavel, R.; Roesky, H.W. Organometallic Fluorides: Compounds Containing Carbon− Metal− Fluorine Fragments of d-Block Metals. *Chem. Rev.,* **1997**, *97*(8), 3425-3468.
[http://dx.doi.org/10.1021/cr960365v] [PMID: 11851496]

[174] Richmond, T.G. *Activation of unreactive bonds and organic synthesis*; Springer Science & Business Media, **1999**, Vol. 3, .
[http://dx.doi.org/10.1007/3-540-68525-1_10]

[175] Braun, T.; Perutz, R.N. Routes to fluorinated organic derivatives by nickel mediated C-F activation of heteroaromatics. *Chem. Commun. (Camb.),* **2002**, (23), 2749-2757.
[http://dx.doi.org/10.1039/B206154F] [PMID: 12478732]

[176] Braun, T.; Perutz, R.N.; Sladek, M.I. Catalytic C-F activation of polyfluorinated pyridines by nickel-mediated cross-coupling reactions. *Chem. Commun. (Camb.),* **2001**, (21), 2254-2255.
[http://dx.doi.org/10.1039/b106646c] [PMID: 12240137]

[177] Hughes, R.P.; Laritchev, R.B.; Williamson, A.; Incarvito, C.D.; Zakharov, L.N.; Rheingold, A.L. Reactions of Iridium and Rhodium Complexes Containing η2-Benzyne, η2-Tetrafluorobenzyne, and η2-Trifluorobenzyne Ligands. Differential Rates of Arene Elimination by Protonation of Isomeric Fluoroaryl Complexes and Restricted Rotation of PMe3 Ligands in o rtho-Iodo and o rtho-Bromoaryl Complexes. *Organometallics,* **2003**, *22*(10), 2134-2141.
[http://dx.doi.org/10.1021/om030048w]

[178] Huheey, J.E. *E. A. K., R. L. Keiter, Inorganic chemistry: principles of structure and reactivity*; HarperCollins College Publishers: New York, **1993**.

[179] Breyer, D.; Braun, T.; Penner, A. Isolation and reactivity of palladium hydrido complexes: intermediates in the hydrodefluorination of pentafluoropyridine. *Dalton Trans.,* **2010**, *39*(32), 7513-7520.
[http://dx.doi.org/10.1039/c0dt00086h] [PMID: 20552114]

[180] Matsunami, A.; Kuwata, S.; Kayaki, Y. Hydrodefluorination of fluoroarenes using hydrogen transfer catalysts with a bifunctional iridium/NH moiety. *ACS Catal.,* **2016**, *6*(8), 5181-5185.
[http://dx.doi.org/10.1021/acscatal.6b01590]

[181] Li, J.; Zheng, T.; Sun, H.; Li, X. Selectively catalytic hydrodefluorination of perfluoroarenes by Co(PMe3)4 with sodium formate as reducing agent and mechanism study. *Dalton Trans.,* **2013**, *42*(36), 13048-13053.
[http://dx.doi.org/10.1039/c3dt50409c] [PMID: 23873379]

[182] Procacci, B.; Jiao, Y.; Evans, M.E.; Jones, W.D.; Perutz, R.N.; Whitwood, A.C. Activation of B-H, Si-H, and C-F bonds with Tp'Rh(PMe3) complexes: kinetics, mechanism, and selectivity. *J. Am. Chem. Soc.,* **2015**, *137*(3), 1258-1272.
[http://dx.doi.org/10.1021/ja5113172] [PMID: 25547430]

[183] Jana, A.; Sarish, S.P.; Roesky, H.W.; Leusser, D.; Objartel, I.; Stalke, D. Pentafluoropyridine as a fluorinating reagent for preparing a hydrocarbon soluble β-diketiminatolead(II) monofluoride. *Chem. Commun. (Camb.),* **2011**, *47*(19), 5434-5436.
[http://dx.doi.org/10.1039/c1cc11310k] [PMID: 21483924]

[184] Bellabarba, R.M.; Nieuwenhuyzen, M.; Saunders, G.C. Intramolecular dehydrofluorinative coupling of the asymmetric diphosphine Ph2PCH2CH2PPh (C5F4N-4) and pentamethylcyclopentadienyl ligands in a rhodium complex. *Organometallics,* **2003**, *22*(9), 1802-1810.
[http://dx.doi.org/10.1021/om020874p]

[185] Teltewskoi, M.; Panetier, J.A.; Macgregor, S.A.; Braun, T. A highly reactive rhodium(I)-boryl complex as a useful tool for C-H bond activation and catalytic C-F bond borylation. *Angew. Chem. Int.*

Ed. Engl., **2010**, *49*(23), 3947-3951.
[http://dx.doi.org/10.1002/anie.201001070] [PMID: 20419724]

[186]   Kohlmann, J.; Braun, T.; Laubenstein, R.; Herrmann, R. Suzuki-miyaura cross-coupling reactions of highly fluorinated arylboronic esters: catalytic studies and stoichiometric model reactions on the transmetallation step. *Chemistry,* **2017**, *23*(50), 12218-12232.
[http://dx.doi.org/10.1002/chem.201700549] [PMID: 28295723]

[187]   Cronin, L.; Higgitt, C.L.; Karch, R.; Perutz, R.N. Rapid intermolecular carbon−fluorine bond activation of pentafluoropyridine at nickel(0): comparative reactivity of fluorinated arene and fluorinated pyridine derivatives. *Organometallics,* **1997**, *16*(22), 4920-4928.
[http://dx.doi.org/10.1021/om9705160]

[188]   Braun, T.; Parsons, S.; Perutz, R.N.; Voith, M. Reactivity of a nickel fluoride complex: Preparation of new tetrafluoropyridyl derivatives. *Organometallics,* **1999**, *18*(9), 1710-1716.
[http://dx.doi.org/10.1021/om980935c]

[189]   Singh, A.; Kubik, J.J.; Weaver, J.D. Photocatalytic C-F alkylation; facile access to multifluorinated arenes. *Chem. Sci. (Camb.),* **2015**, *6*(12), 7206-7212.
[http://dx.doi.org/10.1039/C5SC03013G] [PMID: 29861956]

[190]   Selby, T.P.; Bereznak, J.F.; Bisaha, J.J.; Ding, A.X.; Hanagan, M.A.; Long, J.K.; Taggi, A.E.; Gopalsamuthiram, V. *Fungicidal substituted azoles*; Google Patents, **2011**.

[191]   Weck, M.; Dunn, A.R.; Matsumoto, K.; Coates, G.W.; Lobkovsky, E.B.; Grubbs, R.H. Influence of perfluoroarene–arene interactions on the phase behavior of liquid crystalline and polymeric materials. *Angew. Chem. Int. Ed. Engl.,* **1999**, *38*(18), 2741-2745.
[http://dx.doi.org/10.1002/(SICI)1521-3773(19990917)38:18<2741::AID-ANIE2741>3.0.CO;2-1]
[PMID: 10508367]

[192]   Hwang, D-H.; Song, S.Y.; Ahn, T.; Chu, H.Y.; Do, L-M.; Kim, S.H.; Shim, H-K.; Zyung, T. Synthesis and properties of new light-emitting polymers containing fluorinated tetraphenyl units. *Synth. Met.,* **2000**, *111-112*, 485-487.
[http://dx.doi.org/10.1016/S0379-6779(99)00424-5]

[193]   Kitamura, T.; Wada, Y.; Yanagida, S. Fluorinated aromatics as sensitizers for photo-splitting of water. *J. Fluor. Chem.,* **2000**, *105*(2), 305-311.
[http://dx.doi.org/10.1016/S0022-1139(00)00209-8]

[194]   Babudri, F.; Farinola, G.M.; Naso, F.; Ragni, R. Fluorinated organic materials for electronic and optoelectronic applications: the role of the fluorine atom. *Chem. Commun. (Camb.),* **2007**, (10), 1003-1022.
[http://dx.doi.org/10.1039/B611336B] [PMID: 17325792]

[195]   Zahn, A.; Brotschi, C.; Leumann, C.J. pentafluorophenyl-phenyl interactions in biphenyl-DNA. *Chemistry,* **2005**, *11*(7), 2125-2129.
[http://dx.doi.org/10.1002/chem.200401128] [PMID: 15714531]

[196]   Purser, S.; Moore, P.R.; Swallow, S.; Gouverneur, V. Fluorine in medicinal chemistry. *Chem. Soc. Rev.,* **2008**, *37*(2), 320-330.
[http://dx.doi.org/10.1039/B610213C] [PMID: 18197348]

[197]   Senaweera, S.; Weaver, J.D.; Dual, C-F. Dual C-F, C-H Functionalization *via* Photocatalysis: Access to Multifluorinated Biaryls. *J. Am. Chem. Soc.,* **2016**, *138*(8), 2520-2523.
[http://dx.doi.org/10.1021/jacs.5b13450] [PMID: 26890498]

[198]   Singh, A.; Fennell, C.J.; Weaver, J.D. Photocatalyst size controls electron and energy transfer: selectable *E/Z* isomer synthesis *via* C-F alkenylation. *Chem. Sci. (Camb.),* **2016**, *7*(11), 6796-6802.
[http://dx.doi.org/10.1039/C6SC02422J] [PMID: 28042465]

[199]   Sket, B.; Zupancic, N.; Zupan, M. Regio-and stereospecific [2+ 2] photoaddition of cycloalkenes to pentafluoropyridine. *J. Org. Chem.,* **1982**, *47*(23), 4462-4464.

[http://dx.doi.org/10.1021/jo00144a012]

[200] Barlow, M.G.; Brown, D.E.; Haszeldine, R.N.; Langridge, J.R. Heterocyclic polyfluoro-compounds. Part 29. 2: 1 Adducts by photochemical addition of cycloalkenes to pentafluoropyridine. *J. Chem. Soc., Perkin Trans. 1,* **1980**, 129-131.
[http://dx.doi.org/10.1039/p19800000129]

[201] Barlow, M.G.; Brown, D.E.; Haszeldine, R.N. Heterocyclic polyfluoro-compounds. Part 25. The photochemical addition of ethylene to pentafluoropyridine: formation of 1: 1- and 2: 1-adducts. *J. Chem. Soc., Perkin Trans. 1,* **1978**, (4), 363-365.
[http://dx.doi.org/10.1039/p19780000363]

[202] Barlow, M.; Brown, D.; Haszeldine, R. Heterocyclic polyfluoro-compounds. Part 38 [1]. Photochemical addition of but-2-yne to pentafluoropyridine to give 1: 1 and 2: 1 adducts. *J. Fluor. Chem.,* **1982**, *20*(6), 745-750.
[http://dx.doi.org/10.1016/S0022-1139(00)81441-4]

[203] Šket, B.; Zupan, M. Regiospecific 2+ 2 photoaddition of phenyl substituted acetylenes to pentafluoropyridine. *Tetrahedron,* **1989**, *45*(6), 1755-1758.
[http://dx.doi.org/10.1016/S0040-4020(01)80039-9]

[204] Procacci, B.; Blagg, R.J.; Perutz, R.N.; Rendón, N.; Whitwood, A.C. Photochemical reactions of fluorinated pyridines at half-sandwich rhodium complexes: Competing pathways of reaction. *Organometallics,* **2014**, *33*(1), 45-52.
[http://dx.doi.org/10.1021/om400552r] [PMID: 24563575]

[205] Sket, B.; Zupan, M. Regiospecific photohydroxyalkylation of pentafluoropyridine. *J. Heterocycl. Chem.,* **1978**, *15*(3), 527-527.
[http://dx.doi.org/10.1002/jhet.5570150336]

[206] Alabugin, I.V.; Kovalenko, S.V. C1-c5 photochemical cyclization of enediynes. *J. Am. Chem. Soc.,* **2002**, *124*(31), 9052-9053.
[http://dx.doi.org/10.1021/ja026630d] [PMID: 12149000]

[207] Boris, Š. ZUPAN, M., Photoreaction of Pentafluoropyridine with Cyclohexane. Evidence for Regiospecific Substitution. *Synthesis,* **1978**, *1978*(10), 760-760.
[http://dx.doi.org/10.1055/s-1978-24882]

[208] Toy, M.S.; Stringham, R.S. Copolymerization of pentafluoropyridine. *J. Polym. Sci. Polym. Lett. Ed.,* **1979**, *17*(9), 561-565.
[http://dx.doi.org/10.1002/pol.1979.130170903]

[209] Züchner, K.; Richardson, T.J.; Glemser, O.; Bartlett, N. The Pentafluoropyridine Cation C5F5N+. *Angew. Chem. Int. Ed. Engl.,* **1980**, *19*(11), 944-945.
[http://dx.doi.org/10.1002/anie.198009441]

[210] Ager, E.; Suschitzky, H. Reactions of polyhalogenopyridines with methyl fluorosulphonate. *J. Fluor. Chem.,* **1973**, *3*(2), 230-232.
[http://dx.doi.org/10.1016/S0022-1139(00)84167-6]

[211] Bernard Dietrich, P.V. *Jean-Marie Lehn, Macrocyclic chemistry: aspects of organic and inorganic supramolecular chemistry*; VCH: Weinheim, **1993**.

[212] Lehn, J.M. *J. L. A., J. E. D. Davies, D. D. MacNicol, F. Vogtle, Comprehensive supramolecular chemistry*; OUP: Oxford, **1996**.

[213] Parker, D. *Macrocycle synthesis: a practical approach*; Oxford University Press, **1996**, Vol. 2, .

[214] Newkome, G.R.; McClure, G.; Simpson, J.B.; Danesh-Khoshboo, F. Chemistry of heterocyclic compounds. 20. Multidentate chelating agents. Pyridine macrocyclic ether synthesis. *JACS,* **1975**, *97*(11), 3232-3234.
[http://dx.doi.org/10.1021/ja00844a060]

[215]   Tanaka, R.; Yano, T.; Nishioka, T.; Nakajo, K.; Breedlove, B.K.; Kimura, K.; Kinoshita, I.; Isobe, K. Thia-calix[n]pyridines, synthesis and coordination to Cu(I,II) ions with both N and S donor atoms. *Chem. Commun. (Camb.)*, **2002**, (16), 1686-1687. [http://dx.doi.org/10.1039/b203540e] [PMID: 12196950]

[216]   Banks, R.E. *J. C. T., B. E. Smart, Organofluorine chemistry: principles and commercial applications*; Plenum Press: New York, **1994**. [http://dx.doi.org/10.1007/978-1-4899-1202-2]

[217]   Miller, J. *Aromatic nucleophilic substitution*; Elsevier: Amsterdam, **1968**.

[218]   Chambers, R.D. *Fluorine in organic chemistry*; CRC Press Boca Raton, **2004**. [http://dx.doi.org/10.1002/9781444305371]

[219]   Sandford, G. Macrocycles from perhalogenated heterocycles. *Chemistry,* **2003**, *9*(7), 1464-1469. [http://dx.doi.org/10.1002/chem.200390165] [PMID: 12658642]

[220]   Chambers, R.D.; Hoskin, P.R.; Khalil, A.; Richmond, P.; Sandford, G.; Yufit, D.S.; Howard, J.A. Macrocycles from polyfluoro-pyridine derivatives. *J. Fluor. Chem.,* **2002**, *116*(1), 19-22. [http://dx.doi.org/10.1016/S0022-1139(02)00071-4]

[221]   Chambers, R.D.; Hoskin, P.R.; Kenwright, A.R.; Khalil, A.; Richmond, P.; Sandford, G.; Yufit, D.S.; Howard, J.A. Polyhalogenated heterocyclic compounds. Macrocycles from perfluoro--isopropylpyridine. *Org. Biomol. Chem.,* **2003**, *1*(12), 2137-2147. [http://dx.doi.org/10.1039/b303443g] [PMID: 12945904]

[222]   Chambers, R.D.; Khalil, A.; Richmond, P.; Sandford, G.; Yufit, D.S.; Howard, J.A. Polyhalogenoheterocyclic compounds: Part 51.[1] Macrocycles from 4-alkoxy-tetrafluoropyridine derivatives. *J. Fluor. Chem.,* **2004**, *125*(5), 715-720. [http://dx.doi.org/10.1016/j.jfluchem.2003.12.007]

[223]   Chambers, D. R.; R. Edwards, A., Perfluorocarbon fluids as solvent replacements. *J. Chem. Soc., Perkin Trans. 1,* **1997**, (24), 3623-3628. [http://dx.doi.org/10.1039/a704823h]

[224]   Chambers, R.D.; Khalil, A.; Murray, C.B.; Sandford, G.; Batsanov, A.S.; Howard, J.A. Polyhalogenated heterocyclic compounds: Part 52.[1] Macrocycles from 3, 5-dichloro-2, 4, 6-trifluoropyridine. *J. Fluor. Chem.,* **2005**, *126*(7), 1002-1008. [http://dx.doi.org/10.1016/j.jfluchem.2005.01.018]

[225]   Ng, H.P.; Buckman, B.O.; Eagen, K.A.; Guilford, W.J.; Kochanny, M.J.; Mohan, R.; Shaw, K.J.; Wu, S.C.; Lentz, D.; Liang, A.; Trinh, L.; Ho, E.; Smith, D.; Subramanyam, B.; Vergona, R.; Walters, J.; White, K.A.; Sullivan, M.E.; Morrissey, M.M.; Phillips, G.B. Design, synthesis, and biological activity of novel factor Xa inhibitors: 4-aryloxy substituents of 2,6-diphenoxypyridines. *Bioorg. Med. Chem.,* **2002**, *10*(3), 657-666. [http://dx.doi.org/10.1016/S0968-0896(01)00338-8] [PMID: 11814853]

[226]   Kohrt, J.T.; Filipski, K.J.; Cody, W.L.; Cai, C.; Dudley, D.A.; Van Huis, C.A.; Willardsen, J.A.; Rapundalo, S.T.; Saiya-Cork, K.; Leadley, R.J.; Narasimhan, L.; Zhang, E.; Whitlow, M.; Adler, M.; McLean, K.; Chou, Y.L.; McKnight, C.; Arnaiz, D.O.; Shaw, K.J.; Light, D.R.; Edmunds, J.J. The discovery of fluoropyridine-based inhibitors of the Factor VIIa/TF complex. *Bioorg. Med. Chem. Lett.,* **2005**, *15*(21), 4752-4756. [http://dx.doi.org/10.1016/j.bmcl.2005.07.059] [PMID: 16125385]

[227]   Revesz, L.; Di Padova, F.E.; Buhl, T.; Feifel, R.; Gram, H.; Hiestand, P.; Manning, U.; Wolf, R.; Zimmerlin, A.G. SAR of 2,6-diamino-3,5-difluoropyridinyl substituted heterocycles as novel p38MAP kinase inhibitors. *Bioorg. Med. Chem. Lett.,* **2002**, *12*(16), 2109-2112. [http://dx.doi.org/10.1016/S0960-894X(02)00336-0] [PMID: 12127515]

[228]   Li, Q.; Mitscher, L.A.; Shen, L.L. The 2-pyridone antibacterial agents: bacterial topoisomerase inhibitors. *Med. Res. Rev.,* **2000**, *20*(4), 231-293.

[http://dx.doi.org/10.1002/1098-1128(200007)20:4<231::AID-MED1>3.0.CO;2-N]   [PMID: 10861727]

[229]   S. G.; Lee, J. S.; Sin, J. H.; Mun, S. C.; Jeong, B. H.; Kim, H. S.; Yu, M. S., Synthesis of new tetrakis (multifluoro-4-pyridyl) porphyrin derivatives as the electric eel acetylcholinesterase inhibitors. *Bull. Korean Chem. Soc.,* **2000**, *21*(2), 264-266.

[230]   Gaba, M.; Singh, S.; Mohan, C. Benzimidazole: an emerging scaffold for analgesic and anti-inflammatory agents. *Eur. J. Med. Chem.,* **2014**, *76*, 494-505.
        [http://dx.doi.org/10.1016/j.ejmech.2014.01.030] [PMID: 24602792]

[231]   Welsch, M.E.; Snyder, S.A.; Stockwell, B.R. Privileged scaffolds for library design and drug discovery. *Curr. Opin. Chem. Biol.,* **2010**, *14*(3), 347-361.
        [http://dx.doi.org/10.1016/j.cbpa.2010.02.018] [PMID: 20303320]

[232]   Kaur, G.; Kaur, M.; Silakari, O. Benzimidazoles: an ideal privileged drug scaffold for the design of multitargeted anti-inflammatory ligands. *Mini Rev. Med. Chem.,* **2014**, *14*(9), 747-767.
        [http://dx.doi.org/10.2174/1389557514666140820120518] [PMID: 25138088]

[233]   Bhambra, A.S.; Edgar, M.; Elsegood, M.R.J.; Horsburgh, L.; Kryštof, V.; Lucas, P.D.; Mojally, M.; Teat, S.J.; Warwick, T.G.; Weaver, G.W.; Zeinali, F. Novel fluorinated benzimidazole-based scaffolds and their anticancer activity *in vitro. J. Fluor. Chem.,* **2016**, *188*, 99-109.
        [http://dx.doi.org/10.1016/j.jfluchem.2016.06.009]

[234]   Azéma, J.; Guidetti, B.; Dewelle, J.; Le Calve, B.; Mijatovic, T.; Korolyov, A.; Vaysse, J.; Malet-Martino, M.; Martino, R.; Kiss, R. 7-((4-Substituted)piperazin-1-yl) derivatives of ciprofloxacin: synthesis and *in vitro* biological evaluation as potential antitumor agents. *Bioorg. Med. Chem.,* **2009**, *17*(15), 5396-5407.
        [http://dx.doi.org/10.1016/j.bmc.2009.06.053] [PMID: 19595598]

[235]   Seay, T.M.; Peretsman, S.J.; Dixon, P.S. Inhibition of human transitional cell carcinoma *in vitro* proliferation by fluoroquinolone antibiotics. *J. Urol.,* **1996**, *155*(2), 757-762.
        [http://dx.doi.org/10.1016/S0022-5347(01)66516-9] [PMID: 8558720]

[236]   Darehkordi, A.; Ramezani, M.; Rahmani, F.; Ramezani, M. Design, Synthesis and Evaluation of Antibacterial Effects of a New Class of Piperazinylquinolone Derivatives. *J. Heterocycl. Chem.,* **2016**, *53*(1), 89-94.
        [http://dx.doi.org/10.1002/jhet.2391]

[237]   Ranjbar-Karimi, R.; Poorfreidoni, A. Incorporation of Fluorinated Pyridine in the Side Chain of 4-Aminoquinolines: Synthesis, Characterization and Antibacterial Activity. *Drug Res. (Stuttg.),* **2018**, *68*(1), 17-22.
        [http://dx.doi.org/10.1055/s-0043-116674] [PMID: 28847024]

CHAPTER 3

Perchloropyridines

Abstract: Preparation of pentachloropyridine is carried out by chlorination of pyridine ring or it is obtained from perchlorocyclopentene-3-one *via* several steps. Perchloropyridines are mainly involved in nucleophilic reactions and produce various substituted perchloropyridines, whereas the nature of solvent and nucleophile hindrance affect the regiochemistry of the reactions. Furthermore, these compounds participated in cross-coupling reactions and produced arylated and alkenylpyridines pyridines. Additionally, they are involved in photochemical reactions and produce ring-fused systems. Oxidation of pentachloropyridine gave pentachloropyridine-*N*-oxide, which is active toward nucleophiles at *ortho* positions. The reaction of perchloropyridines with methyl fluorosulphonate produced corresponding *N*-methylated compounds, which are active toward nucleophilic attack. Organometallic compounds obtained from pentachloropyridined in reaction with various electrophiles produced corresponding substituted products.

Keywords: Biological Activities, Heteronium Salts, *N*-ethylpentachloropyri-dinium Fluoroborate, Nucleophilic Substitution Reactions, Pentaalkynylpyridines, Pentachloropyridine, Pentachloropyridine-*N*-oxide, Sonogashira Cross-Coupling, Steric Hindrance, Suzuki–Miyaura Cross-Coupling, Tetraalkenylpyridines, Tetraalkynylpyridines, Tetrachloro-4-pyridyl Copper, Tetrachloro-4-pyridyl-lithium, Tetrachloro-4-pyridylmagnesium Chloride, Tetrachloropyridines, Tetrahydro-5H-pyrido[3,2-*b*]indoles, Tetrahydro-9H-pyridi[2,3-*b*]indoles, Thiazolo[2,3-*b*] quinazolines, Trichloro-thiazolo[3,2-*a*]pyrimidines.

1. INTRODUCTION

Pentachloropyridine is commercially available and its chemistry has been investigated in some detail. The first synthesized compound is attributed to Sell and Dooston [1], but there is a possibility that the first time was synthesized by Kekule [2]. The base strength of polychloropyridines decreased by increasing the chlorine atoms. Therefore, pyridines with high chlorine substituents are resistant toward the formation of their salts. Nevertheless, pentachloropyridine, tetrachloro-2-fluoropyridine and 3,5-dichlorotrifluoropyridine have been methylated by methyl fluorosulfonate [3, 4]. Pentachloropyridine on treatment

Reza Ranjbar-Karimi & Alireza Poorfreidoni

with a mixture of acetic acid and concerted sulfuric acid converted to tetrachloro-2-hydroxypyridine *via* protonation of pyridine nitrogen [5].

Polychloroheteroaromatic compounds have a great interest in the industry and showed a wide range of biological activities such as herbicides and pesticides [6]. Tetrachloro-4-sulfanylpyridine, 2,3,5-trichloro-4,6-bis-sulfanylpyridines and 3,5-dichloro-2,4,6-tris-sulfanylpyridines have found interest as bactericides, as pesticides for controlling bacteria, insects, crustaceans, nematodes, fungi and weeds, and as host compounds [7, 8]. Also, 2,6-dichloro-4-phenylpyridine-3,5-dicarbonitrile, 3,4,5-trichioro-2,6-dicyanopyridine and 4-pyridine-2,3,5-6-tetrachlorosulfonylacetic acid ethyl ester have been found as a fungicide for treatment against Peronosporu fungi, against soil fungi in cereals and cotton, and for seed treatment, respectively [9].

Polychlorinated heterocycles played an important role in the synthesis of the corresponding perfluoro compounds [10]. For example, pentachloropyridine is used as intermediates for the synthesis of other useful material such as pentafluoropyridine [11].

2. SYNTHESIS OF PENTACHLOROPYRIDINE

2.1. By Straight Chlorination

Vapor phase chlorination of pyridine by chlorine at 250°C produced a small amount of pentachloropyridine [12]. In a similar method, 2-chloropyridine and α-picoline produced pentachloropyridine [6]. Chlorination of pyridine in excess phosphorus pentachloride at 210-220°C for 15-20 h produced a mixture of products [1, 2]. Higher yield of pentachloropyridine is obtained at higher temperatures and reaction time and using nickel-lined autoclave [11, 13]. When a mixture of pyridine and phosphorus pentachloride in mole ratio 1:12 heated at 350°C for 14 h, pentachloropyridine obtained in 97% yield (Scheme **3-1**) [13]. A laboratorial method for synthesis of pentachloropyridine is included reaction of 2,6-diaminopyridine with chlorine at the presence of HCl and the subsequent reaction with phosphorus pentachloride and phosphoryl chloride (Scheme **3-2**) [14]. In addition, chlorination of piperidine with chlorine at the presence of carbon tetrachloride has been produced pentachloropyridine along with other products [6]. An unusual method for preparation of pentachloropyridine included self-condensing photochemical reaction of acrylonitrile and the subsequent reaction with chlorine. Pentachloropyridine produced mainly if valeronitrile to be used [6].

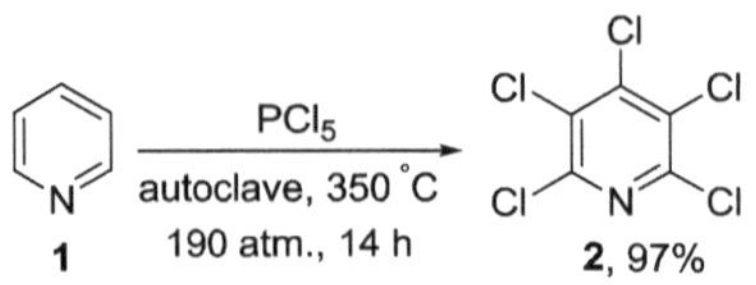

Scheme 3-1. Preparation of pentachloropyridine **2** from pyridine **1**.

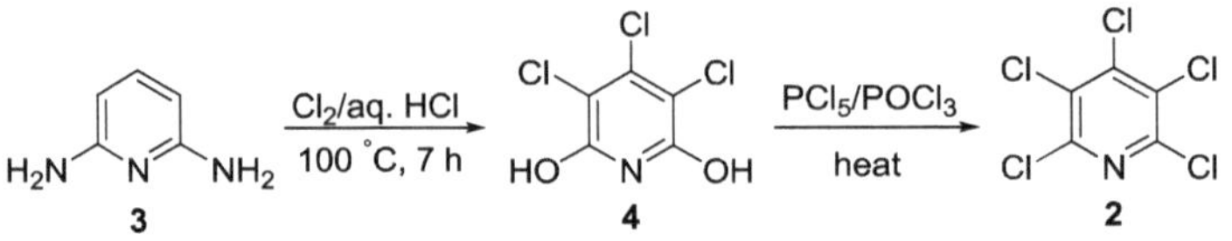

Scheme 3-2. Preparation of pentachloropyridine **2** from 2,6-diaminopyridine **3**.

2.2. By Ring-closing Method

Reaction of perchlorocyclopentene-3-one with ammonia and the subsequent reaction with phosphorus pentachloride produced pentachloropyridine as major product (Scheme **3-3**) [15]. Also, tetrachloro-*N*-methyl-2-pyridone on reaction with a mixture of phosphorus pentachloride and phosphoryl chloride converted to pentachloropyridine [16].

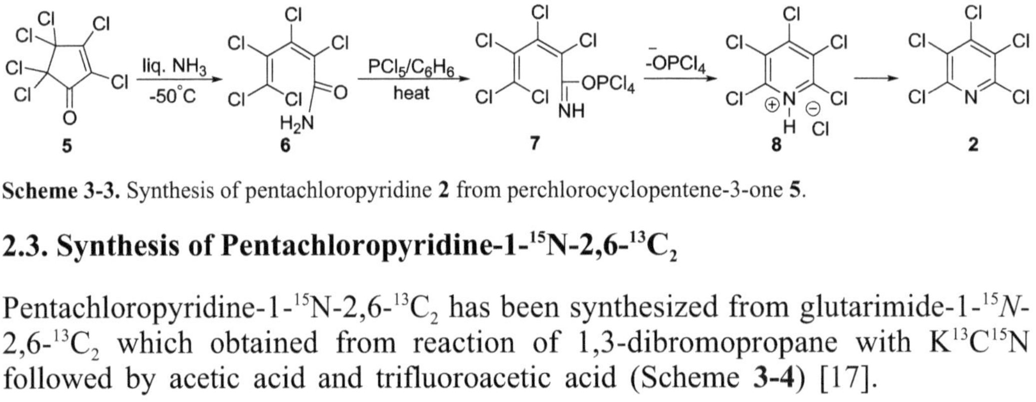

Scheme 3-3. Synthesis of pentachloropyridine **2** from perchlorocyclopentene-3-one **5**.

2.3. Synthesis of Pentachloropyridine-1-^{15}N-2,6-^{13}C$_2$

Pentachloropyridine-1-^{15}N-2,6-^{13}C$_2$ has been synthesized from glutarimide-1-^{15}N-2,6-^{13}C$_2$ which obtained from reaction of 1,3-dibromopropane with K^{13}C^{15}N followed by acetic acid and trifluoroacetic acid (Scheme **3-4**) [17].

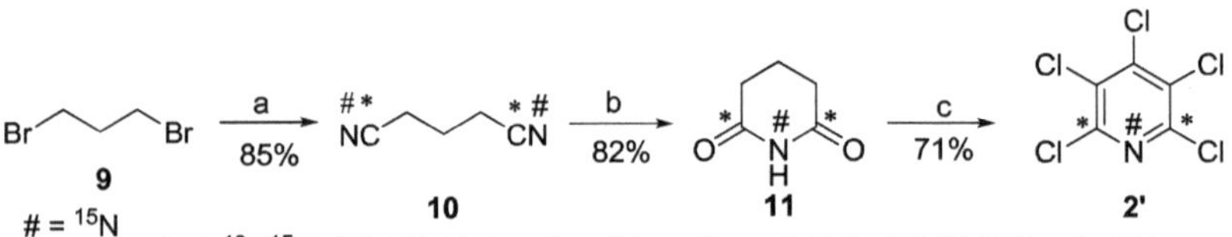

$\# = {}^{15}$N
$* = {}^{13}$C

(a) K^{13}C^{15}N, CH$_3$CN, H$_2$O, reflux; (b) acetic acid, TFA, 230°C (300 psi), 48 h; (c) PCl$_5$, Cl$_2$, FeCl$_3$ cat., I$_2$ cat., 250°C (950 psi), 28 h.

Scheme 3-4. Synthesis of pentachloropyridine-1-^{15}N-2,6-^{13}C$_2$**2′**.

3. NUCLEOPHILIC REACTIONS OF PERCHLOROPYRIDINES

3.1. Reaction of Pentachloropyridine with Various Mono Dentate Nucleophiles

Nucleophilic reactions of pentachloropyridine have been studied with various nucleophiles (Table **3-1**). Pentachloropyridine react preferentially in the less-hindered 2-position of ring on reaction with large nucleophile and at 4-position with small nucleophiles [6]. Nevertheless, nucleophilic substitution reactions of pentachloropyridine are not well-defined [6]. Substitution reactions are often solvent dependence. There is a hydrogen bonding competition between solvent and nucleophile with ring nitrogen in protic solvents, *e.g*, dimethylamine, pyrrolidine, or piperidine sited at 2-position of pentachloropyridine reacted in benzene, whereas sited at both the 2- and the 4- position of pyridine ring in ethanol [18, 19].

Table 3-1. Reaction of various nucleophiles with pentachloropyridine 2.

Reagent	Solvent	Ratio of 4:2-substitution	Ref.
NaBr	DMF	100:0	[6]
NH_3	EtOH	70:30	[14, 15, 20 - 22]
N_2H_4	EtOH	80:20	[15, 23]
$MeNH_2$	dioxane	68:32	[24]
$EtNH_2$	dioxane	68:32	[24]
$BuNH_2$	EtOH	25:75[a]	[14]
$PhCH_2NH_2$	EtOH dioxane	71:29 73:27	[24]
$ArNH_2$	EtOH DMF	100:0 100:0	[6]
Me_2NH	EtOH C_6H_6	20:80 0:100	[14, 18, 25]
Et_2NH	EtOH	1:99	[14]
Pyrrolidine	EtOH C_6H_6	20:80 0:100	[18, 25]
Piperidine	EtOH C_6H_6	37:63 4:96	[18, 25]
Morpholine	EtOH C_6H_6	0:100 0:100	[15, 18, 25]
NaOH	EtOH/H_2O	100:0	[21]
NaOMe	MeOH	85:15	[14, 26]

(Table 3-1) cont.....

Reagent	Solvent	Ratio of 4:2-substitution	Ref.
NaOEt	EtOH	65:35	[14]
NaOBu	BuOH	57:43	[14]
NaSH	various	100:0	[27, 28]
NaSR	various	100:0	[6]
various xanthates	DMF	100:0	[6]
$P(OR)_3$		100:0	[6]

[a] This is probably an error

Chlorine atoms in most of monosubstituted tetrachloropyridines replaced simply by nucleophiles. 4-substituted tetrachloropyridines give 2,4-disubstituted products and 2-substituted tetrachloropyridines give mixture of 2,4- and 2,6-disubstituted products, while the ratio of 2,4-disubstituted product to 2,6-disubstituted product is solvent dependent (Table **3-2**) [14].

Table 3-2. Reaction of monosubstituted tetrachloropyridines with nucleophiles.

Reagent	Solvent	Ratio of 2,4:2,6-disubstitution
NH_3	EtOH	100:0
Me_2NH	EtOH	30:70
NaOMe	MeOH	100:0
NaOEt	EtOH	99:1

3.1.1. Reaction of N-centered Nucleophile with Pentachloropyridine

Reaction of pentachloropyridine with aliphatic amines in boiling ethanol produced 4-alkylaminotetrachloropyridines (Scheme **3-5**) [25]. Its reaction with aromatic amines leaded to formation of 4-arylaminotetrachloropyridines (Scheme **3-6**), while reaction of that with aniline in the presence of pyridine produced 4-aminotetrachloropyridine *via* formation of tetrachloropyridin-4-ylpyridinium chloride **16**, which is cleavage to 4-aminotetrachloropyridine and N-phenylpyridinium chloride **18** by aniline (Scheme **3-7**) [29].

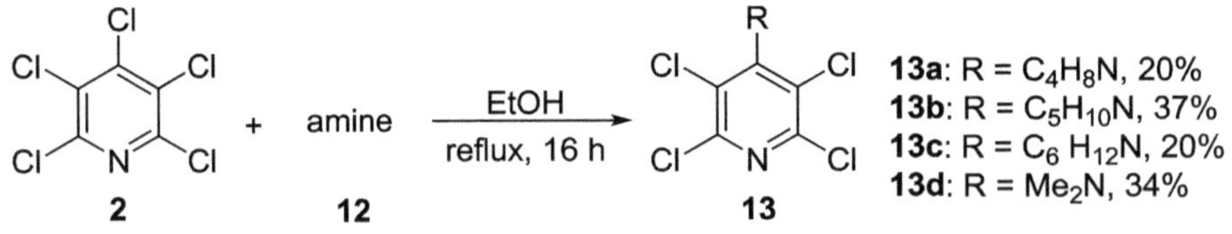

Scheme 3-5. Reaction of pentachloropyridine **2** with aliphatic amines **12**.

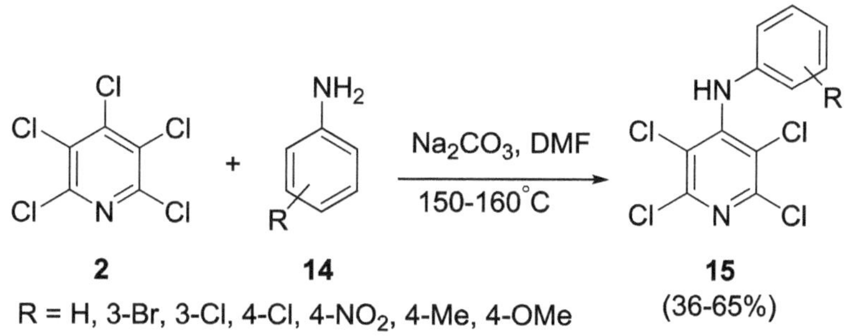

R = H, 3-Br, 3-Cl, 4-Cl, 4-NO$_2$, 4-Me, 4-OMe

Scheme 3-6. Reaction of pentachloropyridine **2** with aromatic amines **14**.

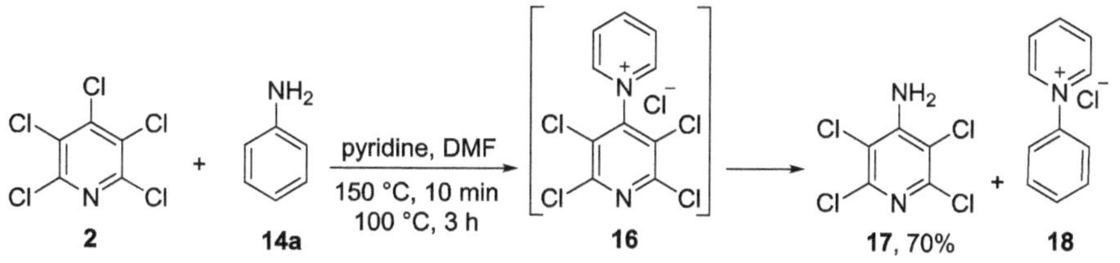

Scheme 3-7. Reaction of aniline **14** with pentachloropyridine **2** in the presence of pyridine.

Heteroarenium molecules are interesting systems from both chemical and biological view [30, 31]. Hearenium substituents able to stabilizing of active anionic species [32 - 34]. Furthermore, polycationic systems can be act as organic oxidants [35]. Mono-, tri-, penta- and decacationic compounds synthesized selectively from polyhalopyridines [36]. Most of replacements have been limited to synthesis of mono- and disubstituted pyridines. Harsh conditions are needed for synthesis of pyridines with more substituents [37]. These salts are useful starting material for site selective synthesis of polysubstituted pyridines [8, 37 - 39].

Heteronium salts **20** and **21**, formed from reaction of pentachloropyridine with 4-(dimethylamino)pyridine (Scheme **3-8**) [40], have been used for multifunctional heterocyclic compounds which inaccessible with other methods [39]. Reaction of salt **20** with n-propyalamine and isopropylamine produced mixture of products (Scheme **3-9**). Reaction of this salt with each of glycine, morpholine and piperidine nucleophiles gave two products (Schemes **3-10** and **3-11**). Reduction of this salt by sodium borohydride at 2-propanol gave 2,3,5,6-tetrachloropyridine in high yield (Scheme **3-12**).

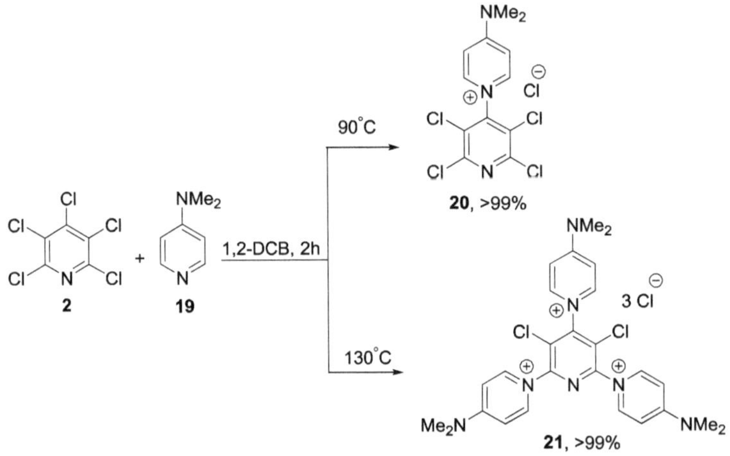

Scheme 3-8. Preparation of heteronium salts **20** and **21** from pentachloropyridine **2**.

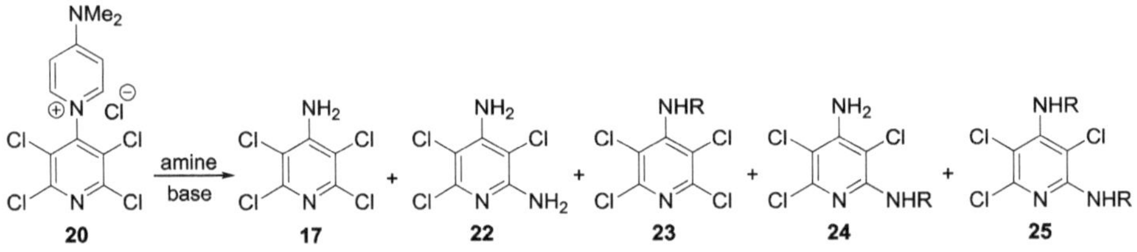

amine / base	**17**	**22**	**23**	**24**	**25**
amine = n-PrNH$_2$ base = NaH, 50°C, 4h				32%	5%
amine = n-PrNH$_2$ base = NaNH$_2$, 50°C, 4h	7%	18%	0	40%	30%
amine = i-PrNH$_2$ base = NaH, 40°C, 4h				37%	5%
amine = i-PrNH$_2$ base = NaNH$_2$, 40°C, 4h	10%	10%	15%	30%	0

Scheme 3-9. Reaction of n-propylamine and isopropylamine with salt **20**.

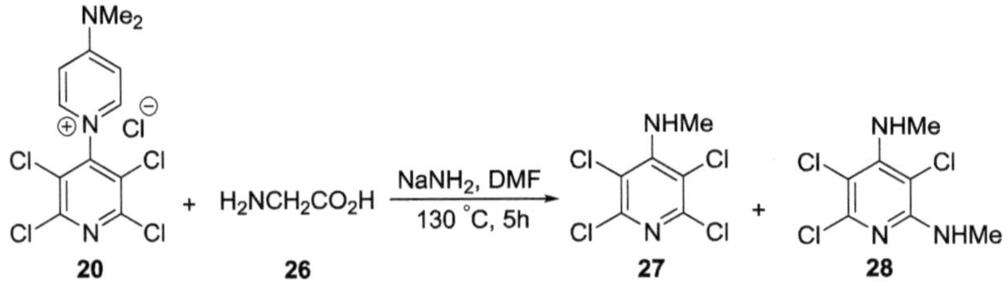

Scheme 3-10. Reaction of glycine with salt **20**.

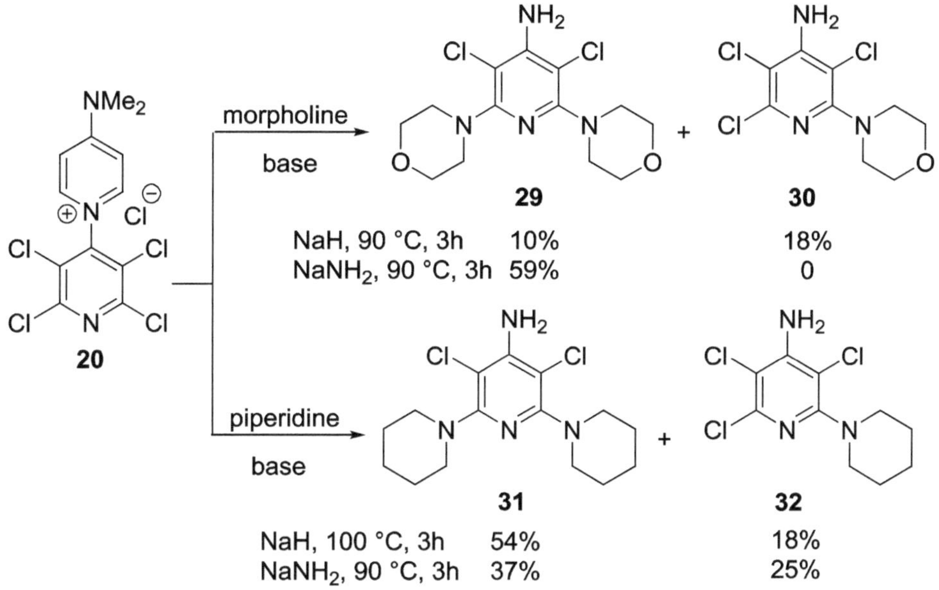

Scheme 3-11. Reaction of morpholine and piperidine with salt **20**.

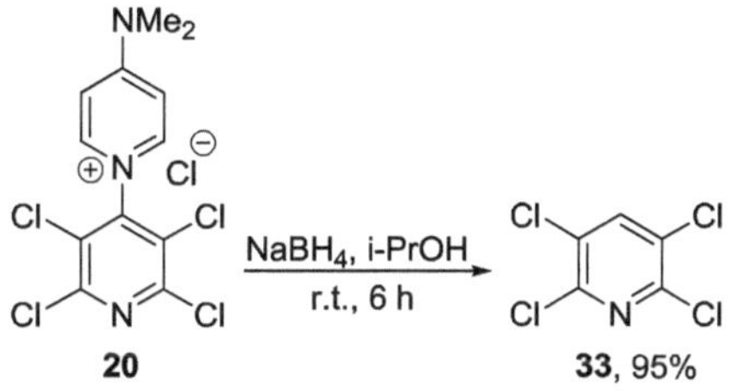

Scheme 3-12. Reduction of salt **20**.

Reaction of heteroarenium salt **20** with *O*-centered nucleophiles such as alkoxides and phenolates depend on reaction conditions leaded to formation of chloropyridines with 4- or 2,4-dialkoxy or phenoxy (Scheme **3-13**) [38]. 2,4,6-trialkoxy or aryloxypyridines produced by reaction of salt **21** with alkoxides and phenolates (Scheme **3-14**). Also, thioethers of chloropyridines obtained by reaction of S nucleophiles with mono- and tricationic pyridinium salts (Schemes **3-15** and **3-16**) [8].

	34	35
MeONa (1eq.) , MeOH, reflux, 6h	51%	
MeONa (5eq.) , MeOH, reflux,3h		55%
EtONa (10 eq.) , EtOH, reflux, 6h		57%
n-PrONa (5 eq.), C$_3$H$_5$OH, r.t., 12 h	28%	
tBuONa (8 eq.), t-BuOH, reflux, 5h	33%	
n-OctONa (1 eq.), DMF, reflux, 18 h	23%	
n-PrONa (15 eq.), n-PrOH, r.t., 12 h	73%	
n-PrONa (10 eq.), n-PrOH, reflux, 24 h		87%
PhOH, NaNH$_2$, DMF, 100°C, 18 h	>99%	
C$_5$H$_4$NOH, NaNH$_2$, DMF, 100°C, 5 h	31%	

Scheme 3-13. Reaction of salt **20** with alkoxides and phenolates.

Scheme 3-14. Reaction of salt **21** with alkoxides and phenolates.

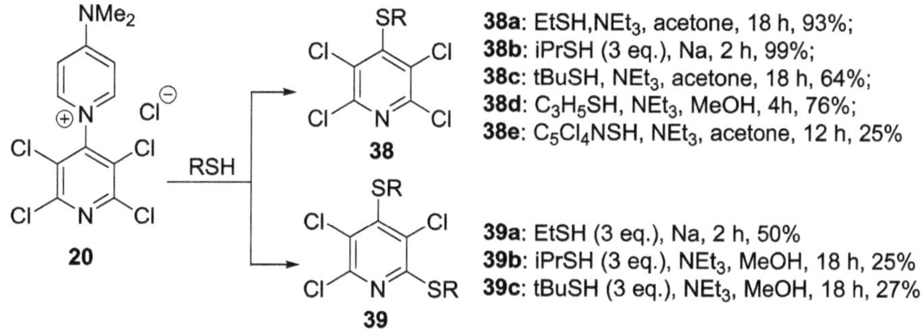

NMe2
Cl
RSH
SR
38
39
20
38a: EtSH,NEt3, acetone, 18 h, 93%;
38b: iPrSH (3 eq.), Na, 2 h, 99%;
38c: tBuSH, NEt3, acetone, 18 h, 64%;
38d: C3H5SH, NEt3, MeOH, 4h, 76%;
38e: C5Cl4NSH, NEt3, acetone, 12 h, 25%
39a: EtSH (3 eq.), Na, 2 h, 50%
39b: iPrSH (3 eq.), NEt3, MeOH, 18 h, 25%
39c: tBuSH (3 eq.), NEt3, MeOH, 18 h, 27%

Scheme 3-15. Reaction of heteronium salt **20** with *S*-centered nucleophiles.

NMe2
3Cl
RSH
Me2N
21
NMe2
SR
RS
40
40a: EtSH (excess.), NEt3, MeOH, 3 h, 80%
40b: iPrSH (excess), MeOH, 3 h, 99%
40c: tBuSH (excess), NEt3, MeOH, 3 h, 70%

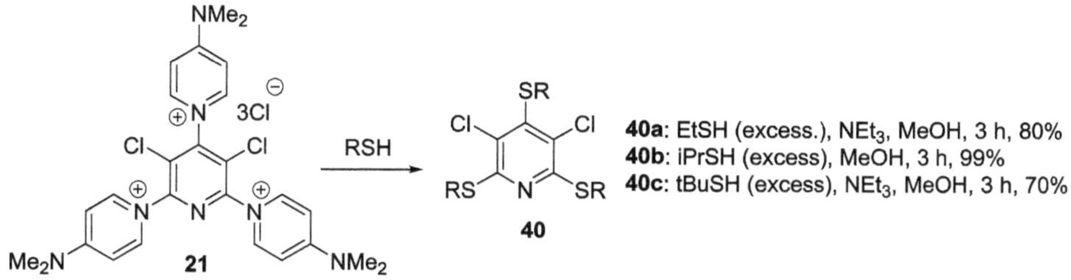

Scheme 3-16. Reaction of heteronium salt **21** with *S*-centered nucleophiles.

Reaction of 2,3,5,6-tetachloropyridine and 4-thioalkyl tetrachloropyridine with heteroaromatic nucleophile such as 4-(dimethylamino)pyridine give bisheteroaromatic salts **41a**-c (Scheme **3-17**) [37]. These salts reacted with *S*-, *N*- and *O*-centered nucleophiles and produced multifunctional puridines (Scheme **3-18**) [37].

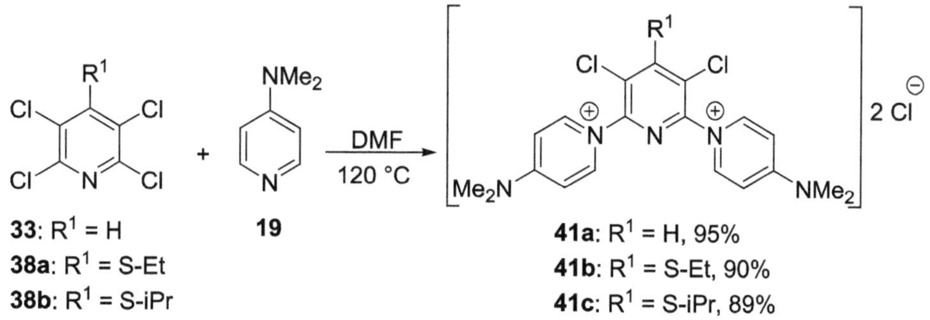

R1
NMe2
DMF
120 °C
2 Cl
Me2N
NMe2
33: R1 = H
38a: R1 = S-Et
38b: R1 = S-iPr
19
41a: R1 = H, 95%
41b: R1 = S-Et, 90%
41c: R1 = S-iPr, 89%

Scheme 3-17. Synthesis of bisheteroaromatic salts **41a-c**.

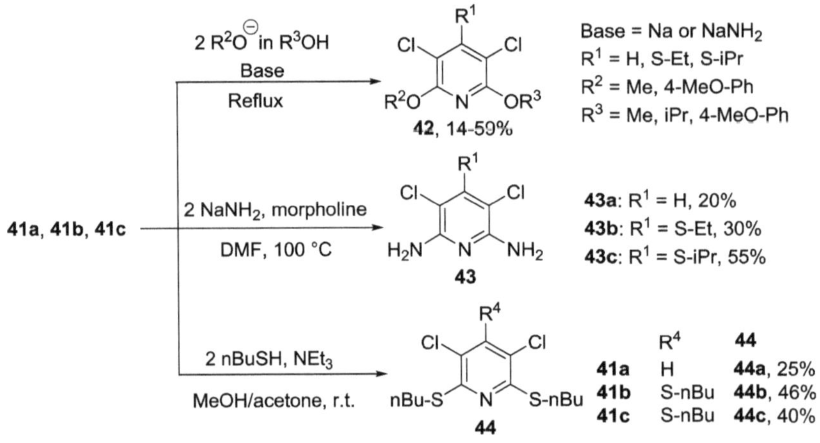

2 R²O⁻ in R³OH
Base
Reflux
Base = Na or NaNH2
R1 = H, S-Et, S-iPr
R2 = Me, 4-MeO-Ph
R3 = Me, iPr, 4-MeO-Ph
42, 14-59%
41a, 41b, 41c
2 NaNH2, morpholine
DMF, 100 °C
43
43a: R1 = H, 20%
43b: R1 = S-Et, 30%
43c: R1 = S-iPr, 55%
2 nBuSH, NEt3
MeOH/acetone, r.t.
44
R4
41a H 44a, 25%
41b S-nBu 44b, 46%
41c S-nBu 44c, 40%

Scheme 3-18. Reaction of various nucleophiles with bisheteroaromatic salts **41a-c**.

Reaction of pentachloropyridine with ammonia in EtOH gives 4-aminotetrachloropyridine as major product and 2-amino derivative (Scheme **3-19**) [14, 15, 20 - 22].

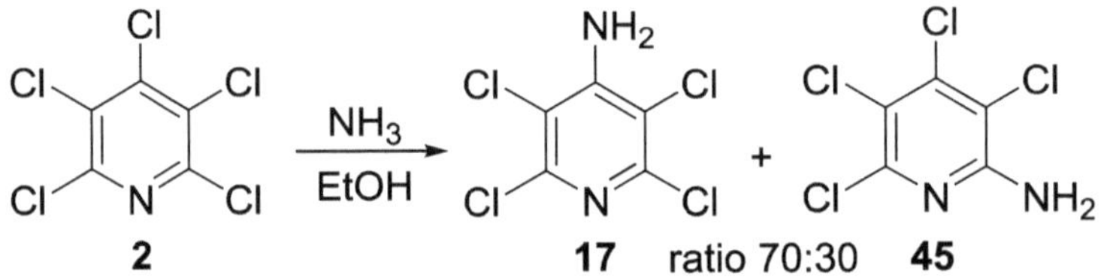

NH3
EtOH
2
17
ratio 70:30
45

Scheme 3-19. Reaction of pentachloropyridine **2** with NH_3.

It is established that the amino group in aminopolyhalopyridines has low nucleophilicity and in most cases is not participated in nucleophilic reactions. 2- and 4-aminotetrachloropyridines have been reacted with sulfur dichloride and produced imino compounds **48** and **51** (Schemes **3-20** and **3-21**), respectively, while sulfur diimides **47** and **50** produced in the presence of dichloroethane at a reagent ratio of 2:1 (Schemes **3-20** and **3-21**). When 2- and 4-aminotetrachloropyridines heated with excess thionyl chloride, tetrachloropyridylthionylimines **46** and **49** obtained in good yield (Schemes **3-20** and **3-21**) [41]. The treatment of phosphorus pentachloride with iminothionyl chlorides **48** and **51,** and thionylimines **46** and **49** has been formed 2- and 4-

trichlorophosphazo-tetrachloropyridines (Schemes **3-22** and **3-23**) [41]. Reaction of either of compounds **46, 47** or **48** with dimethylformamide leaded to formation of formimidamide **54** (Scheme **3-24**). Similarly, formimidamide **55** formed from either of **49, 50** or **51** (Scheme **3-25**). Reaction of **47** and **50** with aromatic aldehyde leaded to formation of benzylidene derivatives **56** and **57**, respectively (Schemes **3-26** and **3-27**) [41].

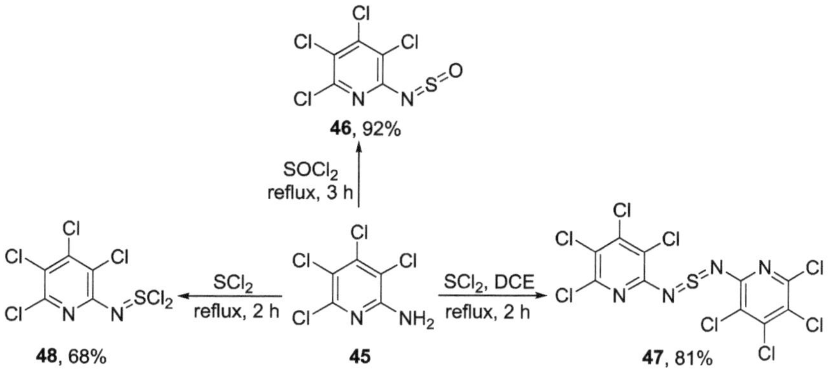

Scheme 3-20. Reaction of 2-aminotetrachloropyridine **45** with SCl_2 and $SOCl_2$.

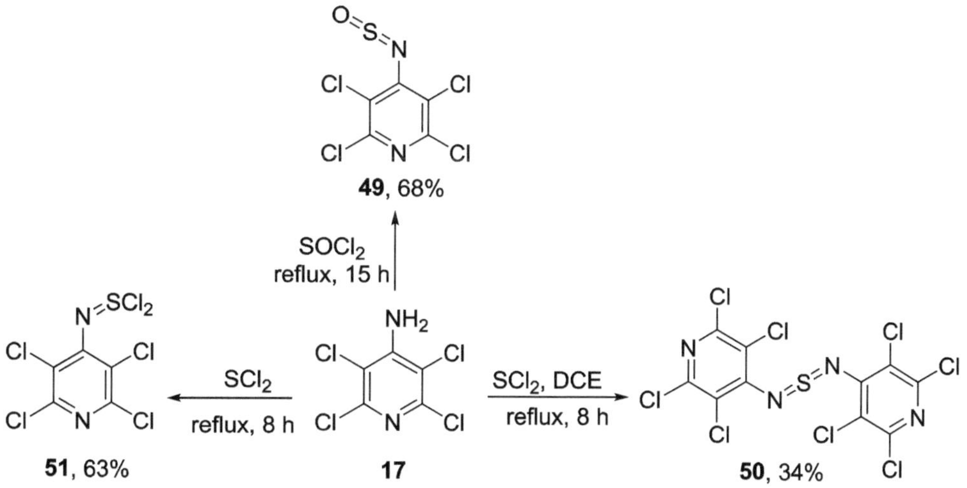

Scheme 3-21. Reaction of 4-aminotetrachloropyridine **17** with SCl_2 and $SOCl_2$.

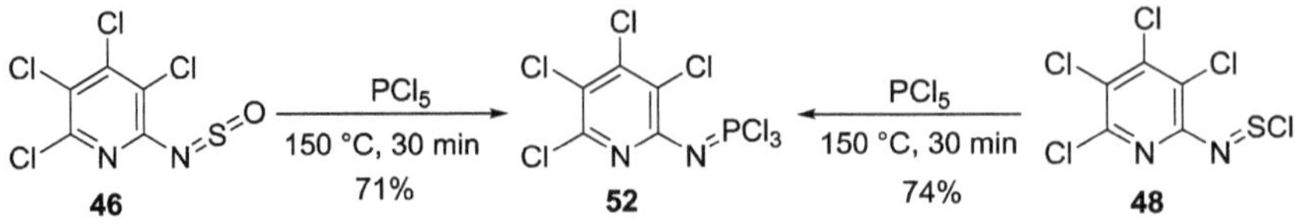

Scheme 3-22. Synthesis of (perchloropyridin-2-yl)phosphorimidoyl trichloride **52**.

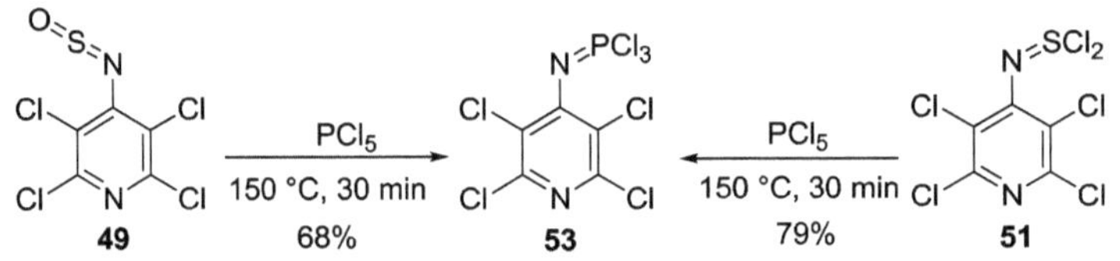

Scheme 3-23. Synthesis of (perchloropyridin-4-yl)phosphorimidoyl trichloride **53**.

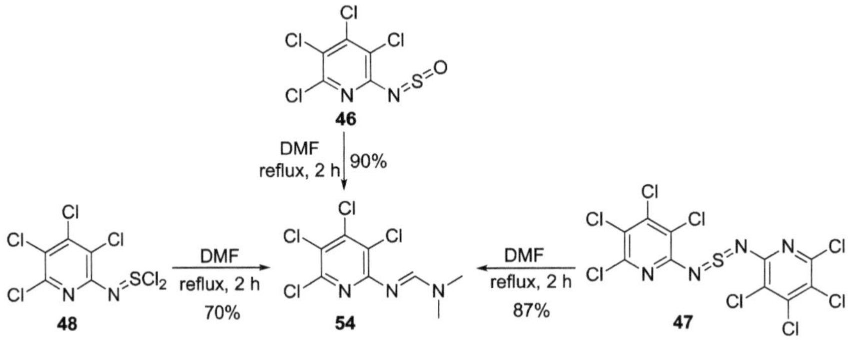

Scheme 3-24. Synthesis of *N,N*-dimethyl-*N'*-(perchloropyridin-2-yl)formimidamide **54**.

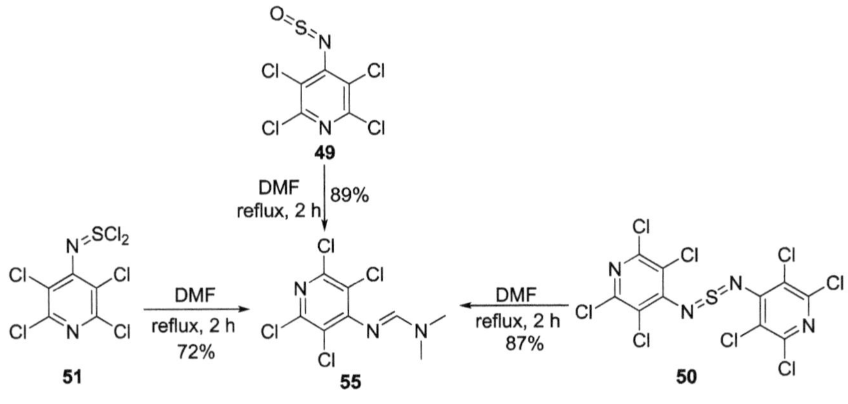

Scheme 3-25. Synthesis of *N,N*-dimethyl-*N'*-(perchloropyridin-4-yl)formimidamide **55**.

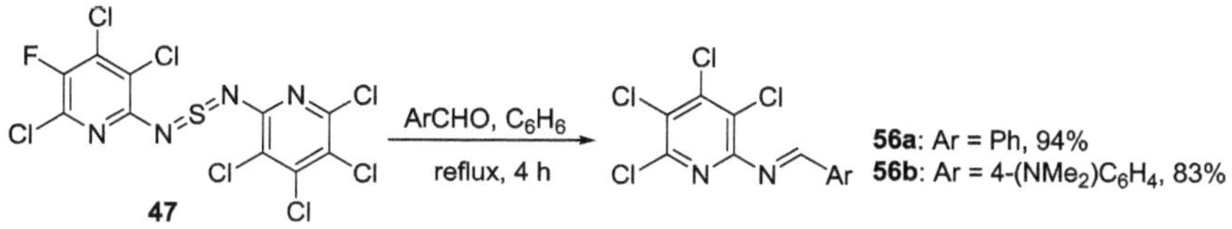

Scheme 3-26. Reaction of sulfur bis(perchloropyridin-2-yl)diimide **47** with benzaldehydes.

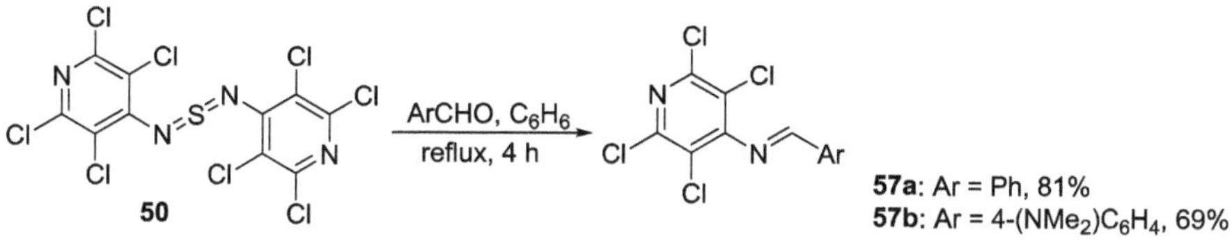

Scheme 3-27. Reaction of sulfur bis(perchloropyridin-4-yl)diimide **50** with benzaldehydes.

The reaction of 4-amino-2,3,5,6-tetrachloropyridine with boiling CCl_4 in the presence of $AlCl_3$ leades to the formation of imidoyldichloride **58** in high yield (Scheme 3-28) [42]. Compound **58** involved readily in nucleophilic reaction (Scheme 3-28) [42]. Its reaction with diethyl amine and piperidine yielded monosubstituted products **59a** and **59b**, while disubstituted product is obtained on reaction with aniline. Two chlorine atoms can be replaced at high temperature and excess amounts of amines. Formamidine **61** has been formed on heating **58** in DMF. Imidoyl **58** is undergoes the Arbuzov reaction on reaction with triethyl phosphite and produced **62**.

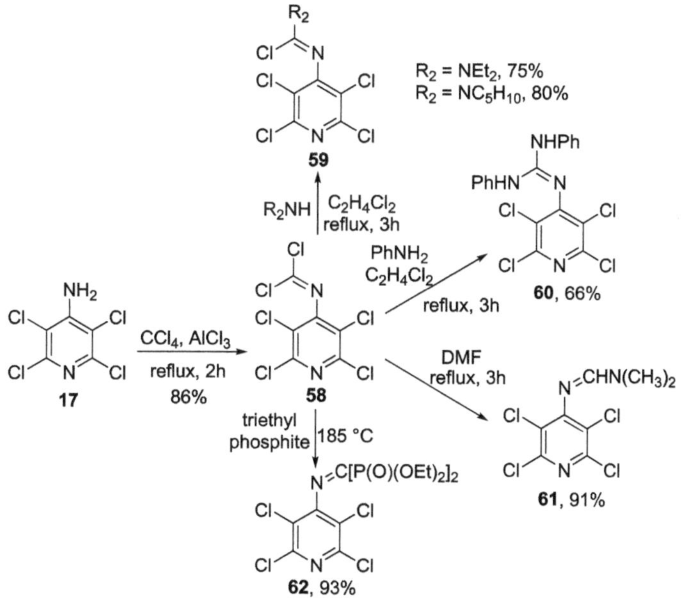

Scheme 3-28. Synthesis and reactions of of imidoyldichloride **58**.

4-nitrotetrachloropyridine prepared by reaction each of 4-(dimethylamino)tetra-chloropyridine, tetrachloro-4-pipyridinopyridine or 4-(methylamino)-tetrachloro-pyridine with TFA and H_2O_2 (30%) at reflux temperature (Scheme **3-29**). Also this compound obtained by oxidation of 4-aminotetrachloropyridine with TFA and H_2O_2 (90%) (Scheme **3-29**) [24]. Nitro group of 2- and 4-nitrotetrachloropyridine replaced easier than chlorine atoms on reaction with nucleophiles. Experimental competition between 4-nitrotetrafluoropyridine and pentachloropyridine showed that 4-nitro compound is more active than pentachloropyridine [24]. Its reaction with *N*- and *O*-centered nucleophiles accompanied with replacing of nitro group (Scheme **3-30**) [24].

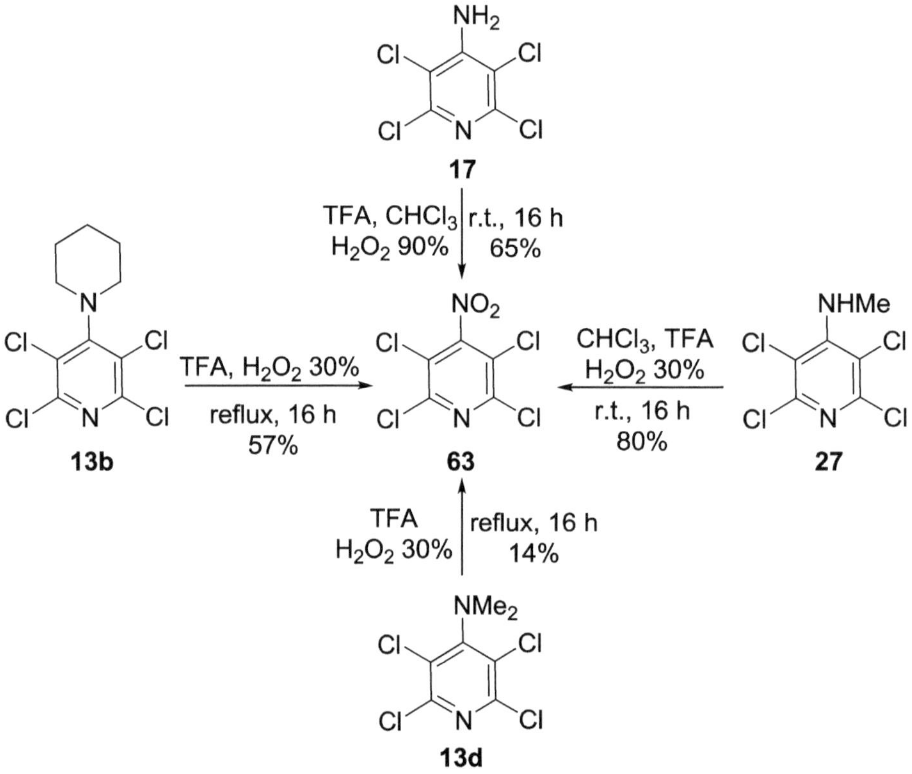

Scheme 3-29. Synthesis of 4-nitrotetrachloropyridine **63**.

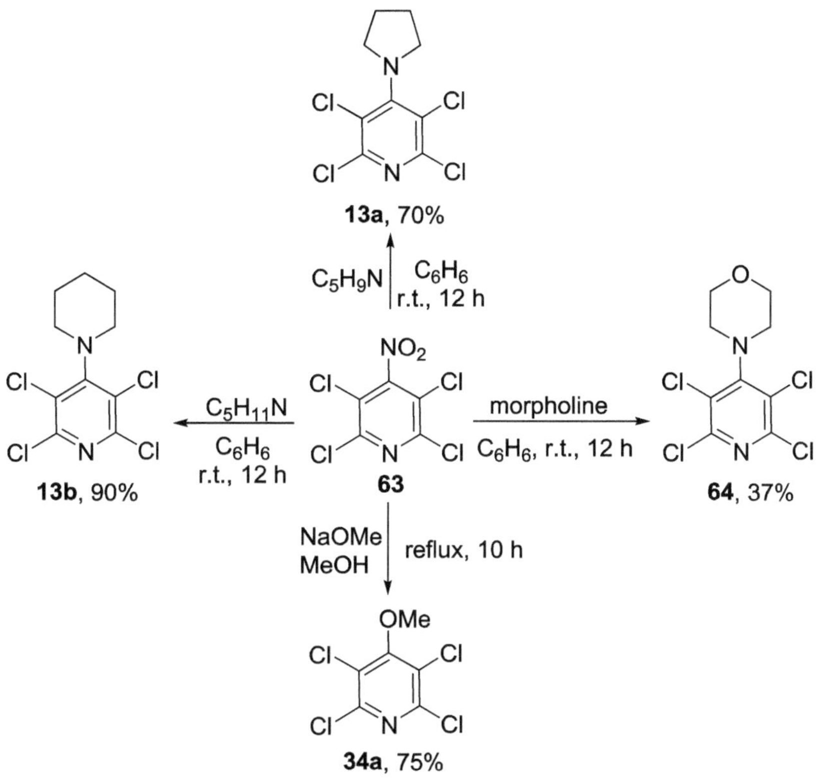

Scheme 3-30. Reaction of 4-nitrotetrachloropyridine **63** with *N*- and *O*-centered nucleophiles.

Reaction of pentachloropyridine with dimethylamine gave majority 2-substituted product at EtOH, while only 2-subtituted product formed in benzene as solvent (Scheme **3-31**) [14, 18, 25]. In comparison with 4-aminotetrachloropyridine, oxidation of tetrachloro-4-dimethylaminopyridine by trifluoroperoxyacetic acid produced 4-amino and 4-nitrosotetrachloropyridine (Scheme **3-32**) [24].

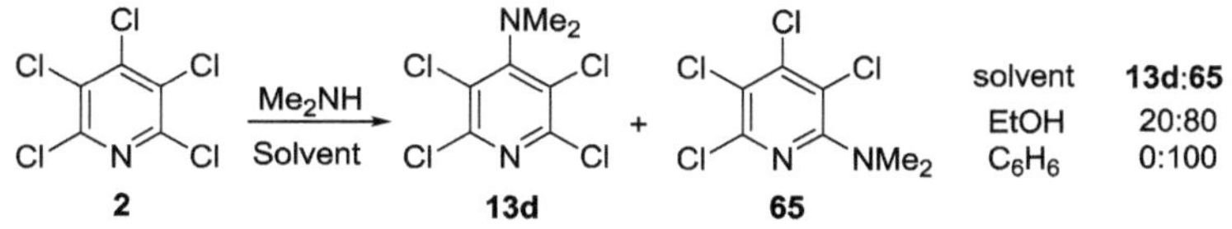

Scheme 3-31. Reaction of pentachloropyridine **2** with dimethylamine.

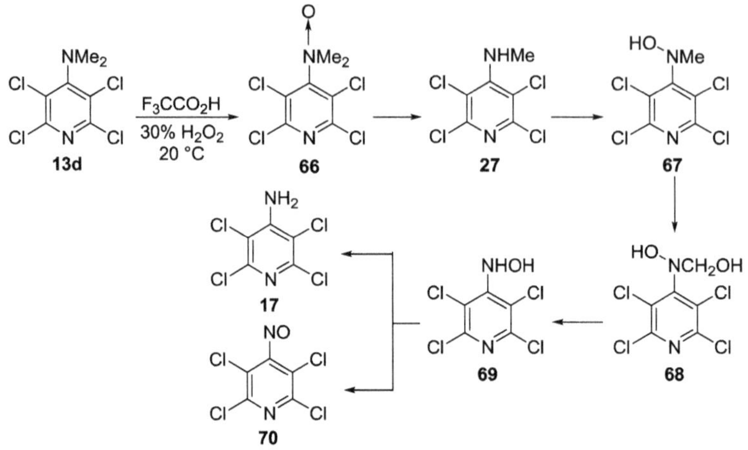

Scheme 3-32. Oxidation of tetrachloro-4-dimethylaminopyridine **13d**.

Reaction of pentachloropyridine with hydrazine produced mainly tetrachloro--hydrazinopyridine (Scheme **3-33**) [15, 23]. This on reaction with copper oxide in hot water converted to 2,3,6-trichlopyridine as major product (Scheme **3-34**). Whereas reaction of tetrachloro-2-hydrazinopyridine with hot solution of copper sulfate produced 2,3,4,5-tetrachloropyridine [23]. Formation of this product explained by hydrogen bonding formed between hydrazine group and ring nitrogen. Its oxidation with H_2O_2 at the presence of TFA gave 2,3,5,6-tetrachloropyridine and 4-hydroxytetrachloropyridine (Scheme **3-35**) [23].

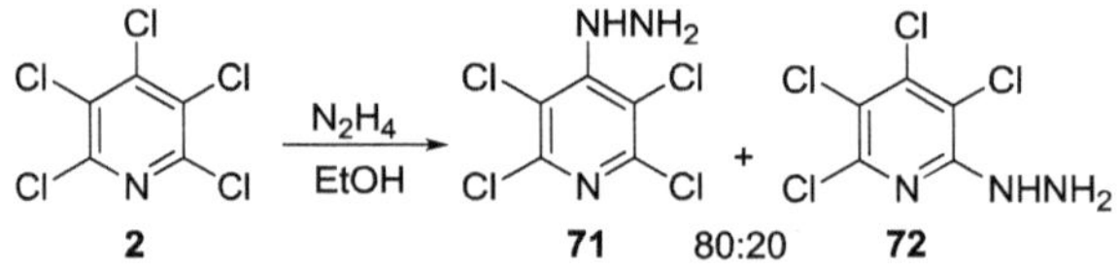

Scheme 3-33. Reaction of pentachloropyridine **2** with hydrazine.

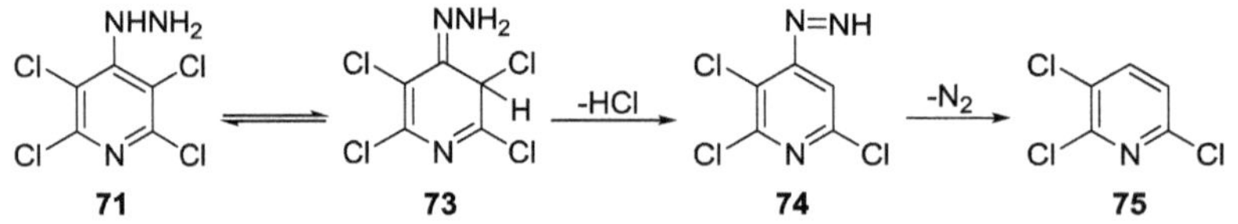

Scheme 3-34. Oxidation of tetrachloro-4-hydrazinopyridine **71**.

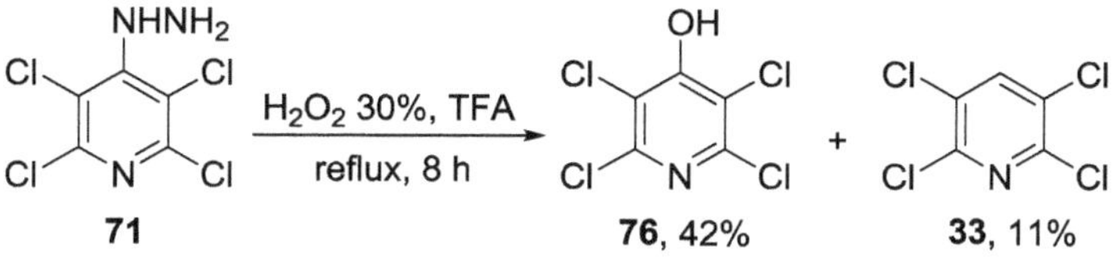

Scheme 3-35. Oxidation of tetrachloro-4-hydrazinopyridine **71** with H_2O_2/TFA.

Tetrachloro-6-hydrazinopyridine in the presence of Ag_2O and MeI produced mixture of products (Scheme **3-36**) [43]. Treatment of tetrachloro-hydrazinopyridine with Br_2 and HBr leads to formation bromotetrachloropyridines **80** and **81** (Schemes **3-37** and **3-38**) [43].

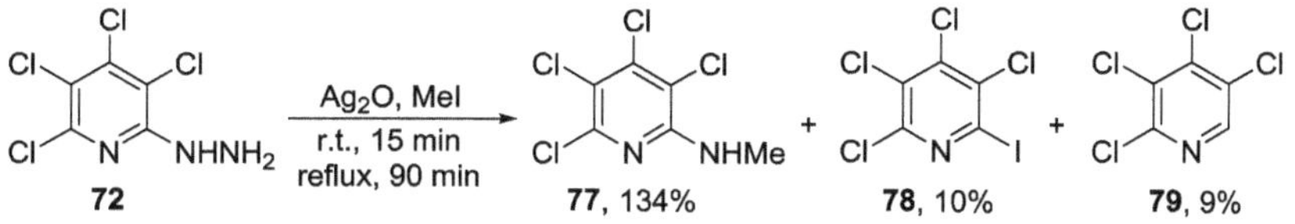

Scheme 3-36. Oxidation of tetrachloro-2-hydrazinopyridine **72** with Ag_2O at the presence of MeI.

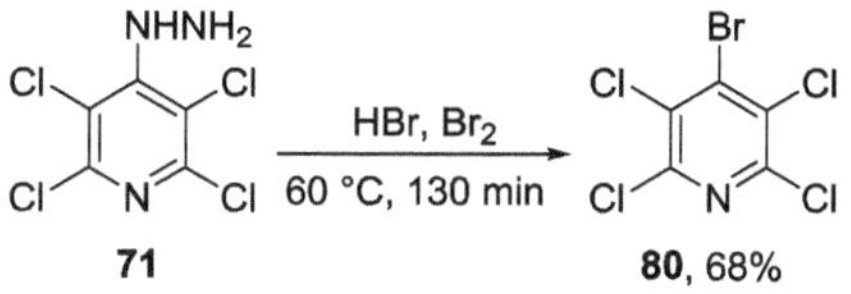

Scheme 3-37. Reaction of tetrachloro-4-hydrazinopyridine **71** with Br_2.

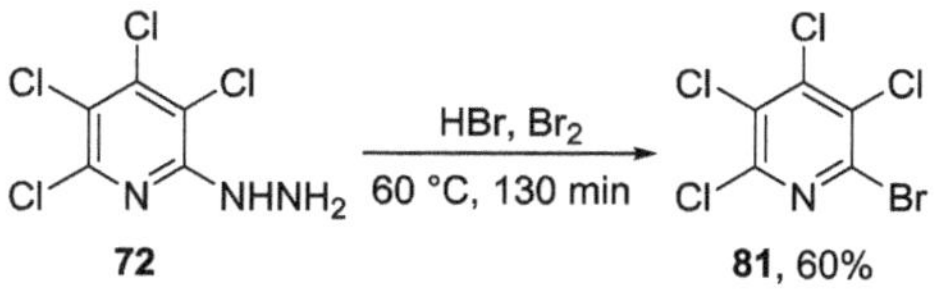

Scheme 3-38. Reaction of tetrachloro-2-hydrazinopyridine **72** with Br_2.

Aromatic azides have interested compounds because of these can be act as 1,3-dipolar systems in cyclization reactions and also can be produce nitrene on pyrolysis or photolysis [44, 45]. Reaction of pentachloropyridine with sodium azide successfully leades to synthesis of 4-azidotetrachloropyridine **82** (Scheme **3-39**) [46]. This compound decomposed in boiling toluene or ortho-xylene. Its reaction with norbornene produced aziridine **85** *via* formation of triazoline **84**, Also, on reactions with triphenylphosphine and aluminum hydride gave iminophosphorane **83** and 4-aminotetrachloropyridine, respectively (Scheme **3-39**) [46].

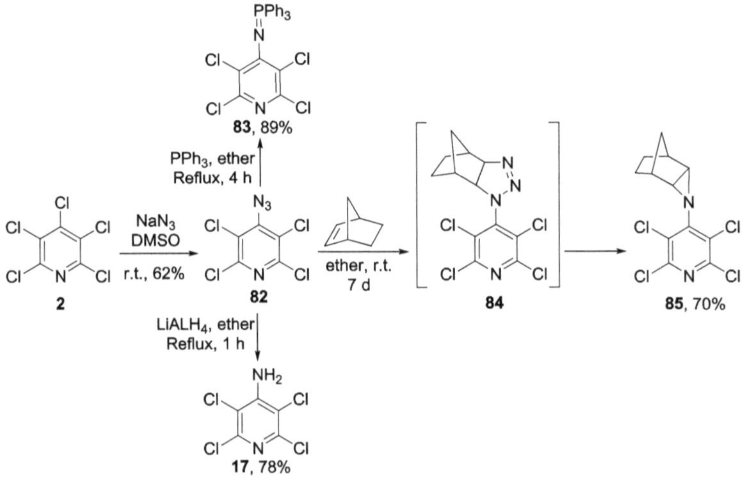

Scheme 3-39. Synthesis and reactions of 4-azidotetrachloropyridine **82**.

Reaction of **2** with four equivalents of sodium azide produced 2,4,6-triazido-3-5-dichloropyridine **86**. This compound reacts selectively with norbornene at 4-azido group, but with dimethyl acetylenedicarboxylate (DMAD) reacts at 2- and 4-azido groups (Scheme **3-40**) [47].

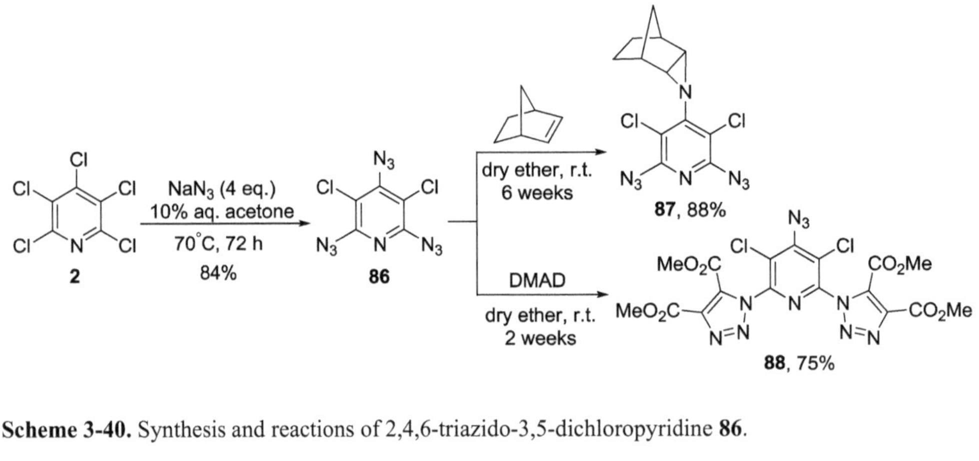

Scheme 3-40. Synthesis and reactions of 2,4,6-triazido-3,5-dichloropyridine **86**.

Pentachloropyridine **2** on reaction with *S,S*-diphenylsulfilimine **89** has been substituted at both 2- and 4-positions, and yielded *N*-perchloropyridyl-*S,S*-diphenylsulfilamines **90** and **91** (Scheme **3-41**) [48].

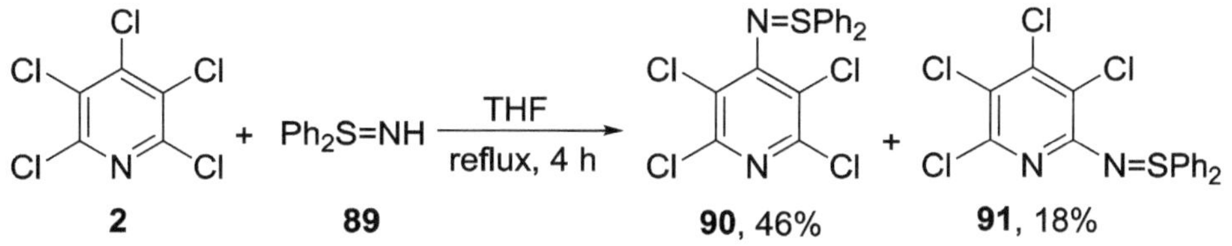

Scheme 3-41. Synthesis of *N*-perchloropyridyl-*S,S*-diphenylsulfilamines **90** and **91**.

Reaction of tetrachloro-4-cyanopyridine **92** with monodentate nitrogen nucleophiles proceeded dominantly at 2-position of pyridine ring (Scheme **3-42**) [49].

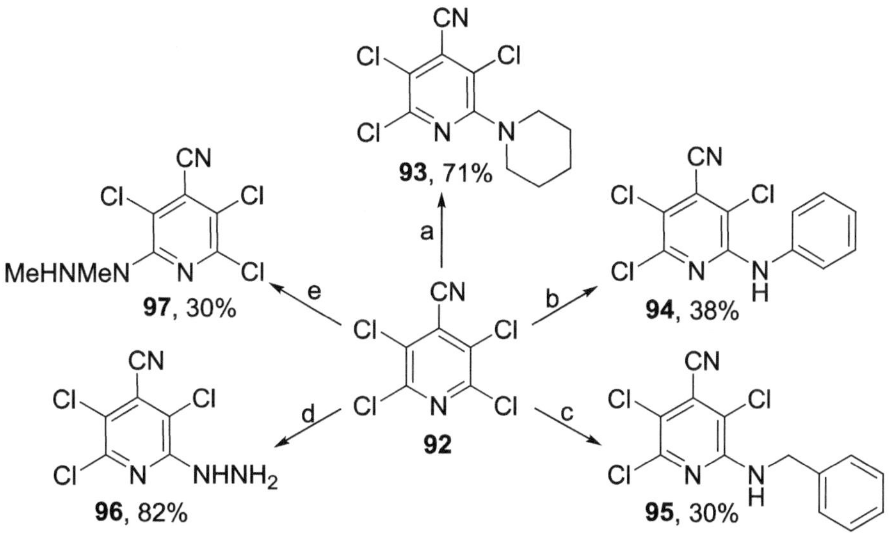

a) toluene, K_2CO_3, reflux, 24 h; b) aniline, ethane-1,2-diol, reflux, 90 min; c) benzylamine, EtOH, reflux, 49 h; d) hydrazine hydrate, r.t., 2 h; e) N,N'-dimethylhydrazine dihydrochloride, $NaHCO_3$ dioxan, reflux, 23 h.

Scheme 3-42. Reaction of tetrachloro-4-cyanopyridine **92** with monodentate nucleophiles.

3.1.2. Reaction of S-centered Nucleophile with Pentachloropyridine

4-mercapto-2,3,5,6-tetrachloropyridine **98** produced from reaction of pentachloropyridine **2** with ethylene glycol in the presence of sodium hydrohide. It converted to 4-methylsulphonyl tetrachloropyridine **100** in two steps (Scheme **3-43**) [28]. This compound reacted at 4-position of ring with less-hindered nucleophiles such as methylamine, sodium cyanide, sodium hydroxide and sodium methoxide, whilst 2-substituted product formed with larger nucleophiles such as dimethylamine, also its reaction with pyrrolidine gave 2- and 4-substituted products (Scheme **3-44**) [50].

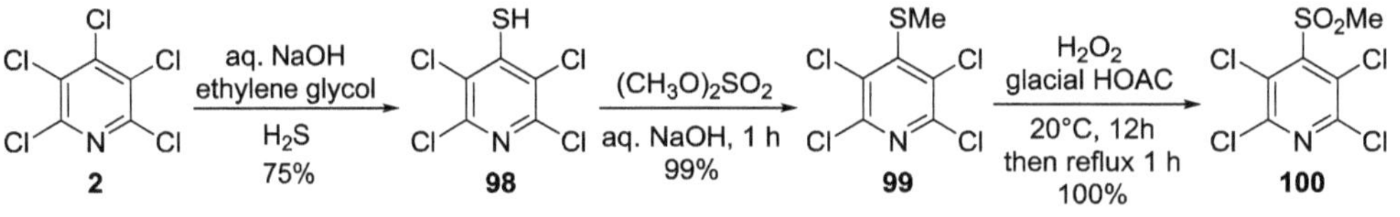
Cl
Cl
Cl
Cl
N
Cl
2
aq. NaOH
ethylene glycol
H2S
75%
SH
98
(CH3O)2SO2
aq. NaOH, 1 h
99%
SMe
99
H2O2
glacial HOAC
20°C, 12h
then reflux 1 h
100%
SO2Me
100

Scheme 3-43. Synthesis of 4-methylsulphonyl tetrachloropyridine **100**.

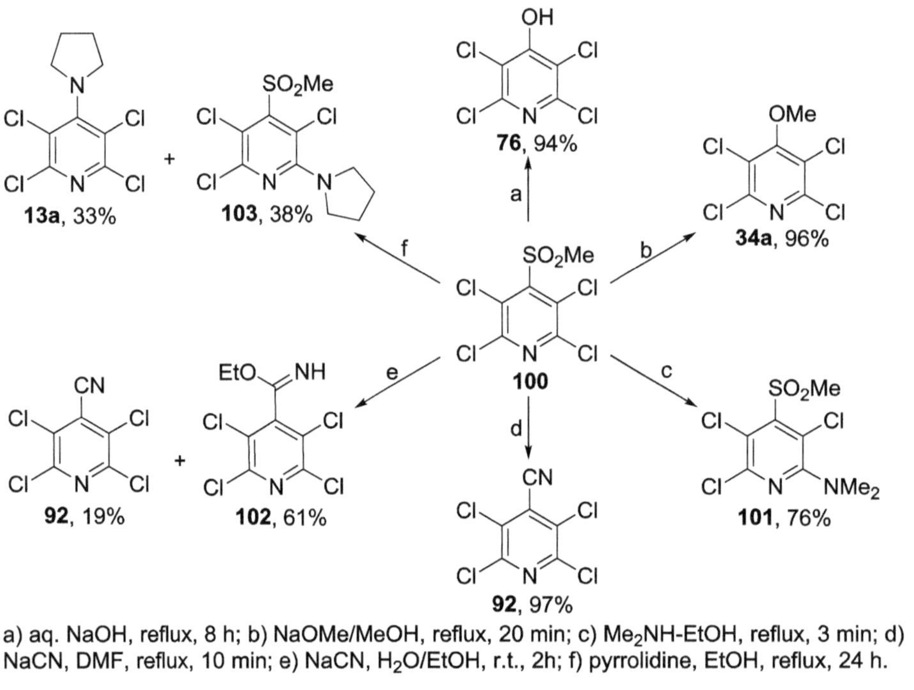
13a, 33%
103, 38%
OH
76, 94%
a
f
SO2Me
b
OMe
34a, 96%
100
c
e
EtO
NH
CN
92, 19%
102, 61%
d
92, 97%
NMe2
101, 76%
a) aq. NaOH, reflux, 8 h; b) NaOMe/MeOH, reflux, 20 min; c) Me2NH-EtOH, reflux, 3 min; d) NaCN, DMF, reflux, 10 min; e) NaCN, H2O/EtOH, r.t., 2h; f) pyrrolidine, EtOH, reflux, 24 h.

Scheme 3-44. Reactions of 4-methylsulphonyl tetrachloropyridine **100**.

Reaction of pentachloropyridine **2** with potassium hydrogensulfide in ethanol produced mainly 4-mercaptotetrachloropyridine **98** and 2,3,5,6-tetrachloro-4-ethoxypyridine **34b** arising attack of ethoxy ion obtained from ethanol to pentachloropyridine (Scheme **3-45**) [51].

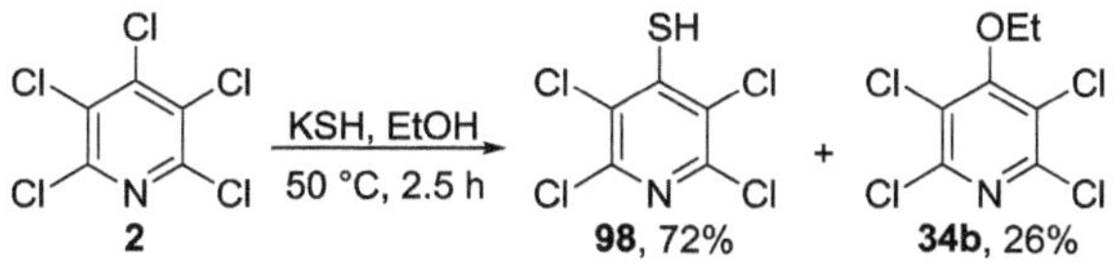

Scheme 3-45. Reaction of pentachloropyridine **2** with KSH in ethanol.

2,3,5,6-tetrachloro-4-pyridyl β-hydroxyethyl sulfone **108** produced from sodium salt of compound **98** during two or three steps (Scheme **3-46**) [51]. Treatment of this sulfone with aqueous sodium bicarbonate solution at room temperature yielded 4-hydroxy-2,3,5,6-tetrachloropyridine **76** (Scheme **3-47**) *via* mechanism showed in Scheme (**3-47**). Reaction of sodium salt **104** with 2-(-nitrophenoxy)ethyl bromide **112** gave sulfide **113**. Oxidation of this sulfide with TFA and 30% H_2O_2 formed sulfone **114**, which converted to vinyl sulfone **115** on heating in DMF (Scheme **3-49**) [51].

Scheme 3-46. Synthesis of 2,3,5,6-tetrachloro-4-pyridyl β-hydroxyethyl sulfone **108**.

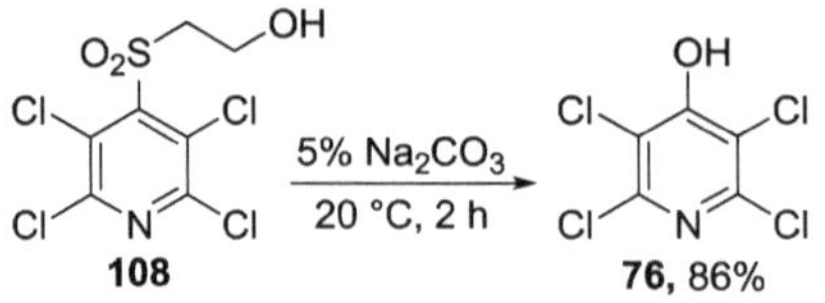

Scheme 3-47. Rearrangement of sulfone **108** to 4-hydroxy-2,3,5,6-tetrachloropyridine **76**.

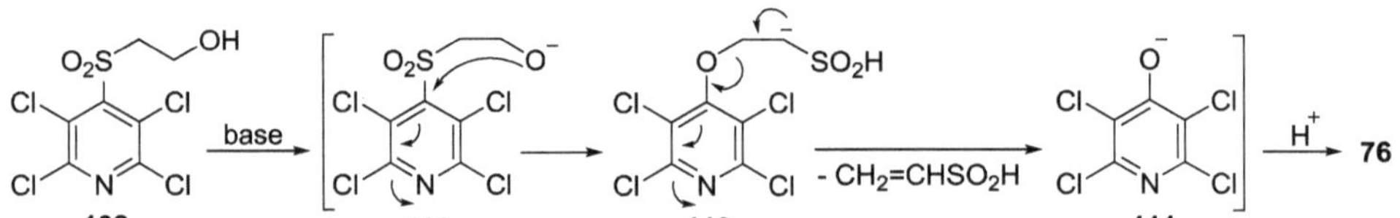

Scheme 3-48. Mechanism formation of 4-hydroxy-2,3,5,6-tetrachloropyridine **76**.

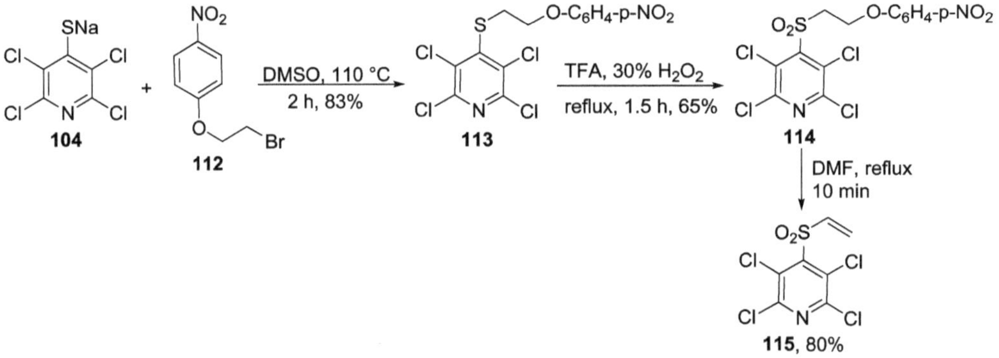

Scheme 3-49. Synthesis of 2,3,5,6-tetrachloro-4-pyridyl vinyl sulfone **115**.

Thiol group of 4-mercaptotetrachloropyridine **98** as nucleophile reacted with methyl iodide, benzyl chlorides and haloacetic acids to produced 4-aryl and 4-alkylthio tetrachloropyrine derivatives (Scheme **3-51**) [52]. Oxidation of these compounds by TFA and H_2O_2 gave corresponding sulphonyl derivatives (Scheme **3-52**) [52]. Compound **116b** on reaction with Cl_2 in carbon tetrachloride converted to tetrachloropyridine-4-sulphenylchloride **120** (Scheme **3-53**) [52].

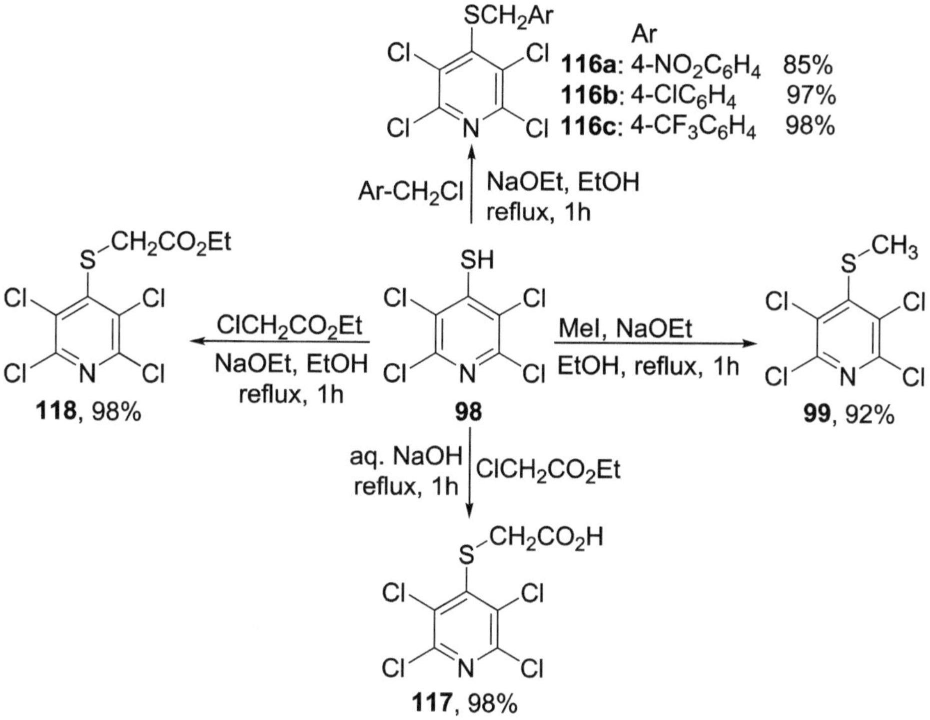

Scheme 3-50. Reactions of 4-mercaptotetrachloropyridine.

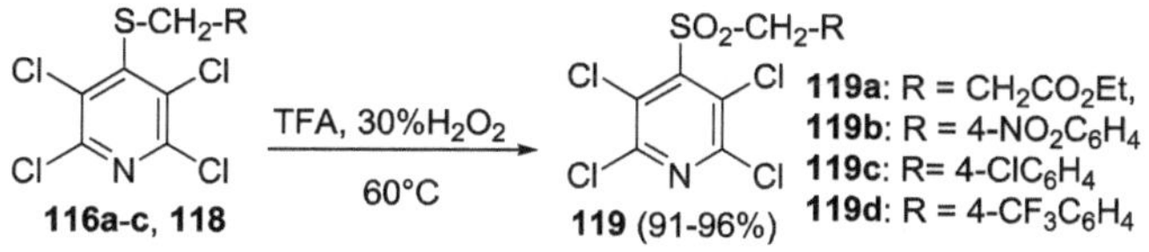

Scheme 3-51. Oxidation of 4-aryl and 4-alkylthio tetrachloropyrine derivatives.

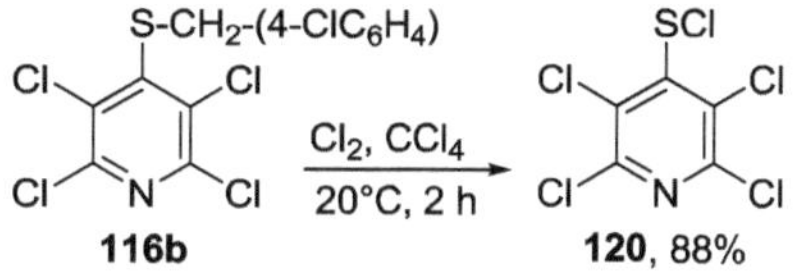

Scheme 3-52. Chlorination of compound **556c**.

Mercapto compounds are interesting molecules for investigation of reaction of thiol group with high active reagents such as xenone difluoride and xenone bisperfluoroalkane carboxylate. Decomposition of xenone bisperfluoroalkane carboxylate **122** leaded to perfluoroalkylation of thiols **98, 121a** and **121b** (Scheme **3-53**) [53].

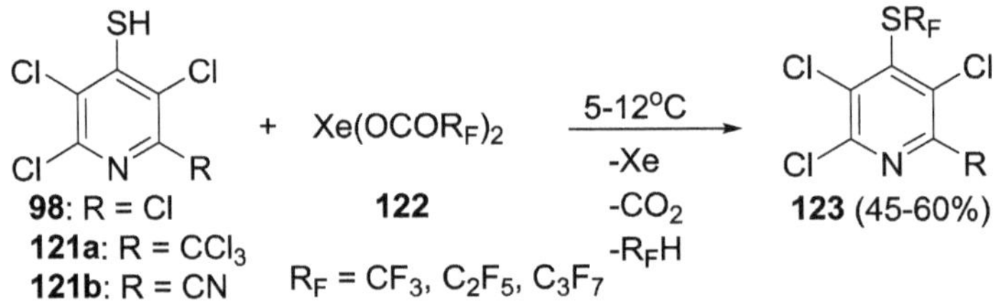

Scheme 3-53. Perfluoroalkylation of perchloropyridine-4-thiols **98** and **121a,b**.

Oxidation of tetrachloropyridine-4-thiol has been carried out by xenone difluoride in aqueous HF and produced 2,3,5,6-tetrachloro-4-fluorosulphonylpyridine and 2,3,5,6-tetrachloro-4-fluorosulphonylpyridine-*N*-oxide **126** (Scheme **3-54**) [53]. Presence of water is necessary for preparation of oxidizing agent.

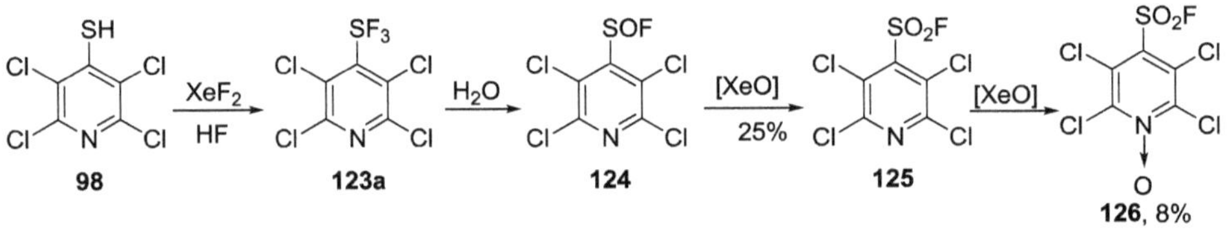

Scheme 3-54. Oxidation of tetrachloropyridine-4-thiol **98**.

Trifluoromethylthio group is replaced easily by *S*-centered nucleophiles such as sodium hydrogensulfide or *N,N*-dimethylthiocarbamate and ethoxy group at solution of EtOH and Et₃N (Scheme **3-54**) [54]. Reaction of compound **123a** with *N*-centered nucleophiles accompanied with competition between chlorine atom and trifluoromethylthio group for replacing (Scheme **3-55**) [54].

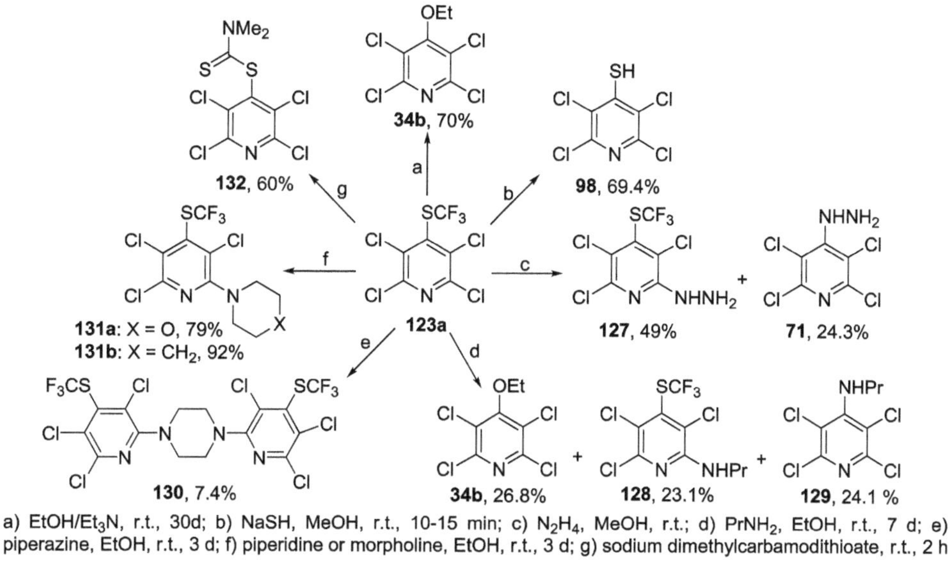

132, 60%   g

34b, 70%   a

98, 69.4%   b

c

131a: X = O, 79%   f
131b: X = CH₂, 92%

123a

127, 49%   **71**, 24.3%

e   d

130, 7.4%

34b, 26.8%   **128**, 23.1%   **129**, 24.1 %

a) EtOH/Et₃N, r.t., 30d; b) NaSH, MeOH, r.t., 10-15 min; c) N₂H₄, MeOH, r.t.; d) PrNH₂, EtOH, r.t., 7 d; e) piperazine, EtOH, r.t., 3 d; f) piperidine or morpholine, EtOH, r.t., 3 d; g) sodium dimethylcarbamodithioate, r.t., 2 h

Scheme 3-55. Reaction of **123a** with *S*-, *O*- and *N*-centered nucleophiles.

p-cresol and *p*-chlorophenol reacted with 2,3,5,6-tetrachloropyridyl-4-sulfenyl chloride **120** from carbon atoms located at the *ortho* position to the hydroxyl group, which could be undergoes various reactions (Scheme **3-56**) [55]. Sulfides **134a** and **134b** upon reaction with *t*-BuOH/K underwent cyclization to ring-fused **135**. Oxidation of **135b** with 30% H₂O₂ in the presence of glacial acetic acid gave sulfone **136** (Scheme **3-57**). In the action of aqueous alkali of the sulfides **134a** and **134b** the spiro Meisenheimer complex **137** formed, which this complex converted to compound **139** on reaction with dimethyl sulfate (Scheme **3-57**). Hydroxy group of **134a** acetylated on treatment acetic anhydride. Compound **140** upon oxidation with 30% H₂O₂ in the presence of acetic acid and in fallowing reaction with 80% H₂SO₄ and HOAc converted to sulfone **141**. This compound transformed into the stable Smiles rearrangement product **142** by the action of sodium hydroxide. Heating of acid **142** to 170 °C leaded to formation of compound **143** (Scheme **3-57**).

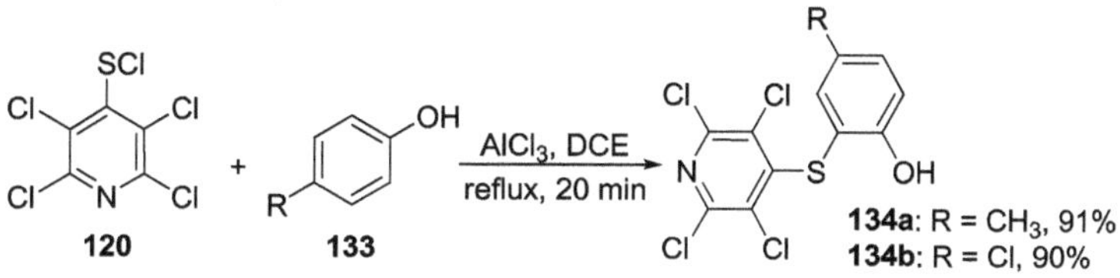

120   +   **133**

AlCl₃, DCE
reflux, 20 min

134a: R = CH₃, 91%
134b: R = Cl, 90%

Scheme 3-56. Reaction of 2,3,5,6-tetrachloropyridyl-4-sulfenyl chloride **120** with phenols **133**.

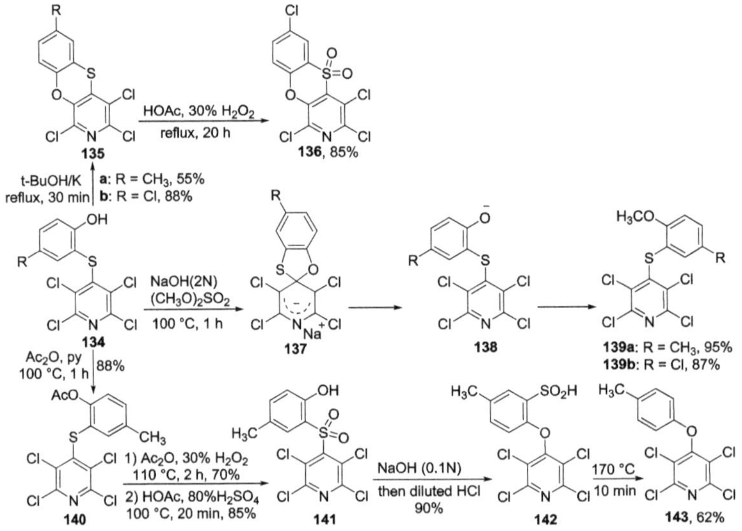

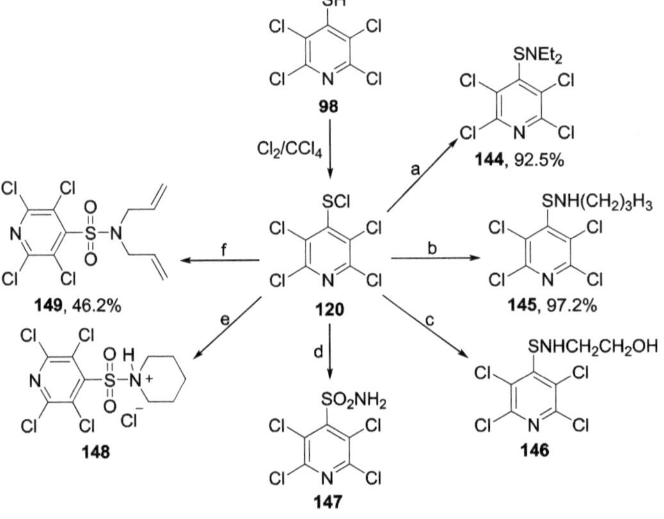

Scheme 3-57. Various reaction of 2-((perchloropyridin-4-yl)thio)phenols **134**.

Tetrachloro-4-pyridinesulfenylchloride **120** is reactive toward *S*-centered nucleophiles and converted to tetracloropyyridine sulfonamides and sulfenamides on treatment with diethyamine, *n*-butylamine, ammonium hydroxide, diallyl amine (Scheme **3-58**) [56]. Also, this compound in reaction with piperidine produced salt **148** (Scheme **3-58**) [56].

a) Et₂NH, r.t., 15 min; b) n-BuNH₂, r.t., c) ethanolamine, C₆H₆, r.t., 2 h;
d) NH₄OH, r.t., 90 min; e) piperidine, r.t., 2.5 h; f) diallyl amine, reflux, 76 °C, 20 min.

Scheme 3-58. Reaction of various *N*-centered nucleophiles with tetrachloro-4-pyridine sulfenyl chloride **120**.

Reaction of tetrachloropyridine-4-sulphenylchloride **120** with alkenes produced 2,3,5,6-tetrachloro-4-((2-chloroalkyl)thio)pyridines, while two products formed at the presence of asymmetric alkenes (Scheme **3-59**) *via* formation of episulfonium ion intermediate **155** (Scheme **3-60**) [57]. Opening approach of this intermediate is dependent on nucleophilicity of sulfur atom.

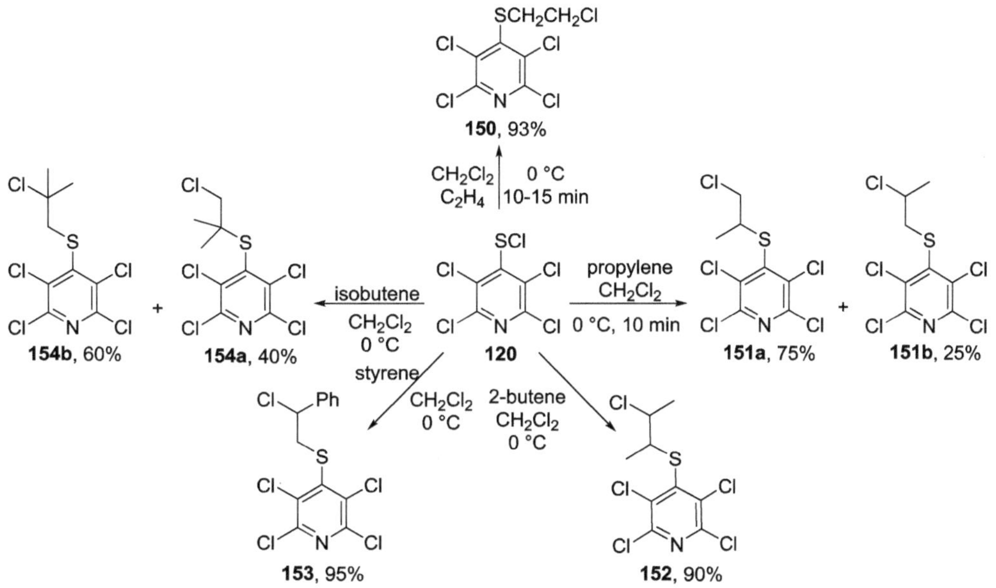

Scheme 3-59. Reaction of tetrachloropyridine-4-sulphenylchloride **120** with alkenes.

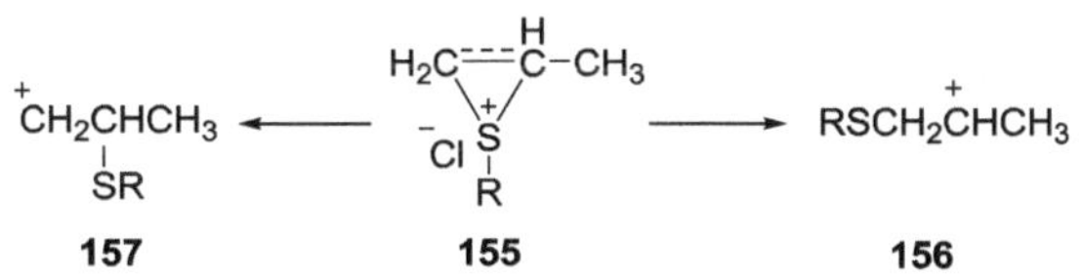

Scheme 3-60. Mechanism of reaction of tetrachloropyridine-4-sulphenylchloride **120** with alkenes.

Nucleophilic reactions of 2,3,5,6-tetrachloro-4-(vinylsulfonyl)pyridine **115** are nucleophile dependent [58]. Primary aliphatic amines and mercaptanes in equimolecular amounts added to double bond, while their excess amounts gave 4-alkylamino- or 4-alkylthiotetrachloropyridine (Scheme **3-61**). Aromatic amines, phenols, thiophenols and alcohols attacked to double bond. Morpholine and piperidine in equimolecular amounts added to double bond and in excess amounts attacked to 2-position of pyridine ring (Scheme **3-61**).

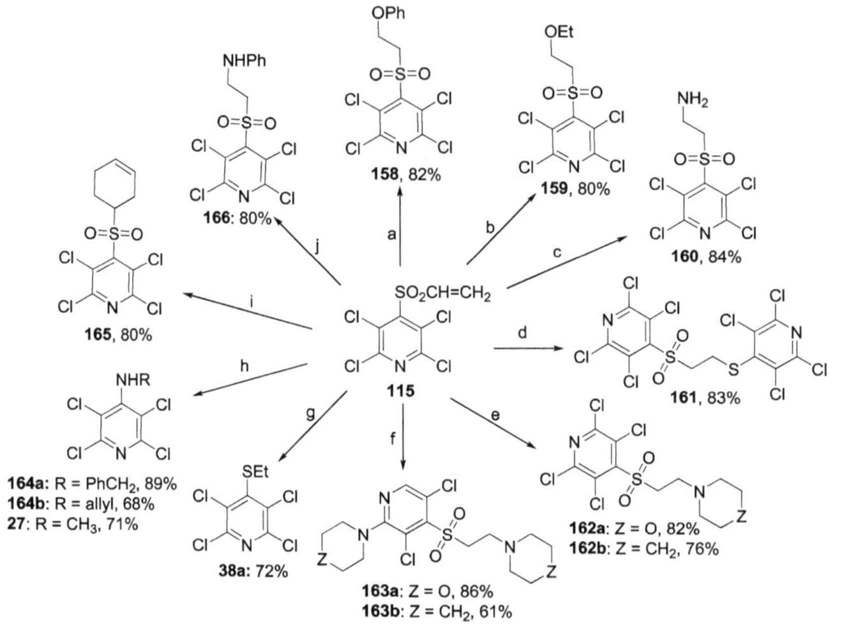
a) PhOH, heptane, 20 °C, 24 h; b) aq. KOH, EtOH, reflux, 5 h; c) ammonia, Et2O; d) 4-mercaptotetrachloropyridine, Et3N, Et2O, 20°C; e) morpholine or piperidine, Et2O, 20 °C, 2 h; f) morpholine or piperidine (3eq.), Et2O, 20 °C, 2h; g) EtSH, Et3N, Et2O, 20 °C, 30 min; h) RNH2, Et2O, 20 °C, 30 min, i) 1,3-butadiene, acetone, 150 °C, 5 h; j) aniline, heptane, reflux, 10 min.

Scheme 3-61. Reaction of various nucleophiles with 2,3,5,6-tetrachloro-4-(vinylsulfonyl)pyridine **115**.

2,3,5,6-tetrachloro-4-(phenylsulfonyl)pyridine **168** have been synthesized by the reaction of sodium phenylsulfnate with pentachloropyridine **2** under optimum reaction condition pentachloropyridine (1 eq.), sodium benzenesulphinate (2 eq.), at room temperature and dimrthylformamide as the solvent (Scheme **3-62**) [59]. Nucleophilic reactions of compound **168** are depended on steric hindrance of nucleophile [59]. Substitution generally is occurred at 4-position of pyridine ring by less steric hindrance nucleophiles (Scheme **3-63**), while mixtures of products (ortho- and para-substituted) are obtained with more steric hindrance cases (Scheme **3-64**).

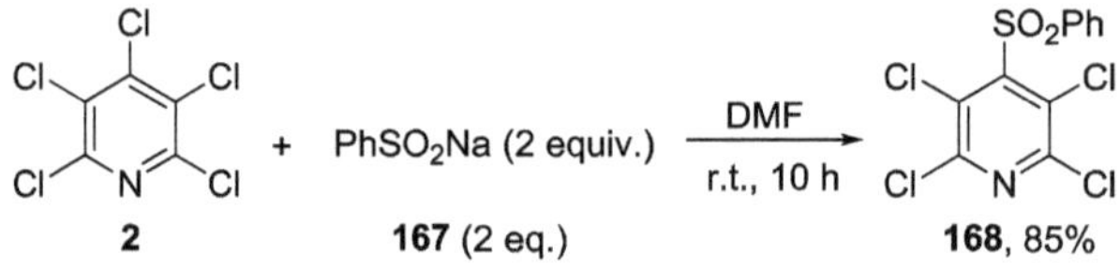
+ PhSO2Na (2 equiv.)
DMF
r.t., 10 h
2
167 (2 eq.)
168, 85%

Scheme 3-62. Synthesis of 2,3,5,6-tetrachloro-4-(phenylsulfonyl)pyridine **168**.

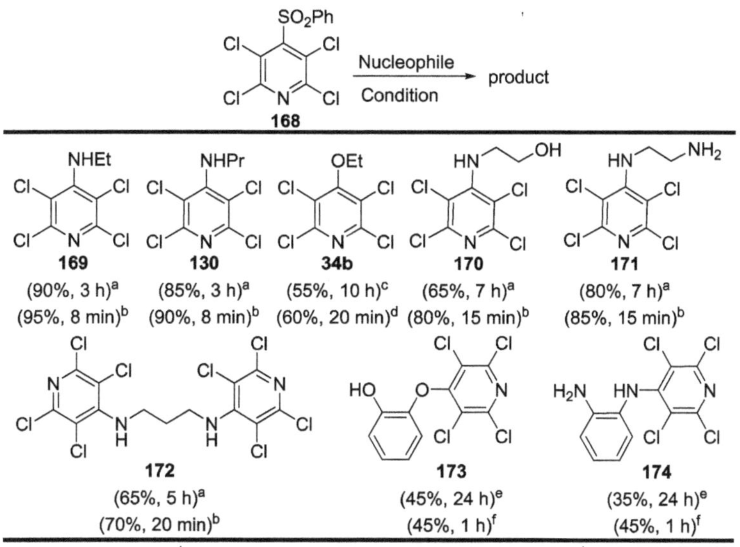

Scheme 3-63. Reaction of 4-phenylsulfonyl-tetrachloropyridine **168** with primary nucleophiles.

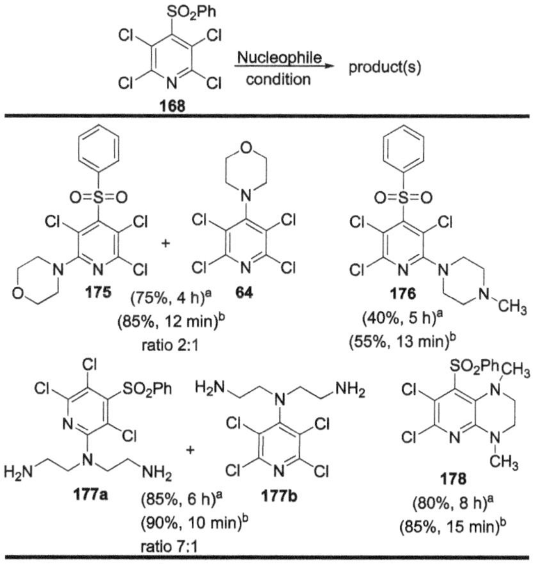

169 (90%, 3 h)[a] (95%, 8 min)[b]

130 (85%, 3 h)[a] (90%, 8 min)[b]

34b (55%, 10 h)[c] (60%, 20 min)[d]

170 (65%, 7 h)[a] (80%, 15 min)[b]

171 (80%, 7 h)[a] (85%, 15 min)[b]

172 (65%, 5 h)[a] (70%, 20 min)[b]

173 (45%, 24 h)[e] (45%, 1 h)[f]

174 (35%, 24 h)[e] (45%, 1 h)[f]

[a] CH$_3$CN, K$_2$CO$_3$, r.t; [b] CH$_3$CN, K$_2$CO$_3$, r.t.))); [c] NaOEt, EtOH, Reflux; [d] NaOEt, EtOH, r.t.,))); [e] CH$_3$CN, K$_2$CO$_3$, reflux; [f] CH$_3$CN, K$_2$CO$_3$, r.t.,))).

Scheme 3-64. Reaction of **168** with secondary amines.

175 (75%, 4 h)[a] (85%, 12 min)[b] ratio 2:1 **64**

176 (40%, 5 h)[a] (55%, 13 min)[b]

177a (85%, 6 h)[a] (90%, 10 min)[b] ratio 7:1 **177b**

178 (80%, 8 h)[a] (85%, 15 min)[b]

[a] CH$_3$CN, K$_2$CO$_3$, r.t; [b] CH$_3$CN, K$_2$CO$_3$, r.t.)))

Reaction of pentachloropyridine **2** with potassium ethylxanthate **179** is solvent dependent [60, 61]. Compound **180** has been formed in ethanol, while compound **38a** has been produced in acetone (Scheme **3-65**).

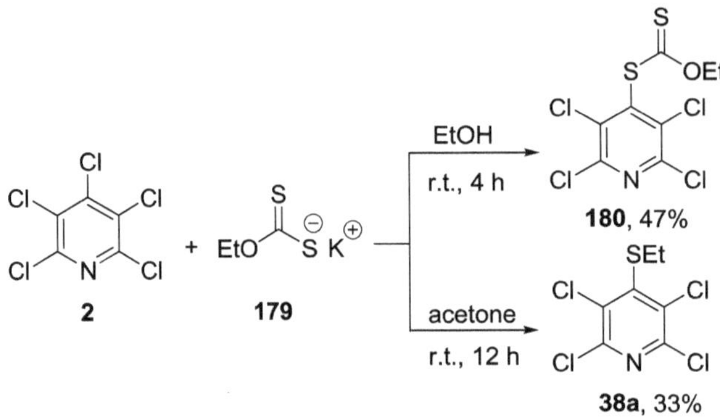

Scheme 3-65. Reaction of pentachloropyridine **2** with potassium ethylxanthate **179**.

Reaction of tetrachloro-4-cyanopyridine **92** with potassium ethylxanthate yielded 2,5-dichloro-3,5-bis(ethylthio)-4-cyanopyridine with losing of COS [60, 61]. Tetrachloro-2 and 3-cyanopyridines on reaction with **179** produced mixture of products resulting of substitution at *meta* and *para* positions of ring nitrogen (Scheme **3-66**) [60, 61].

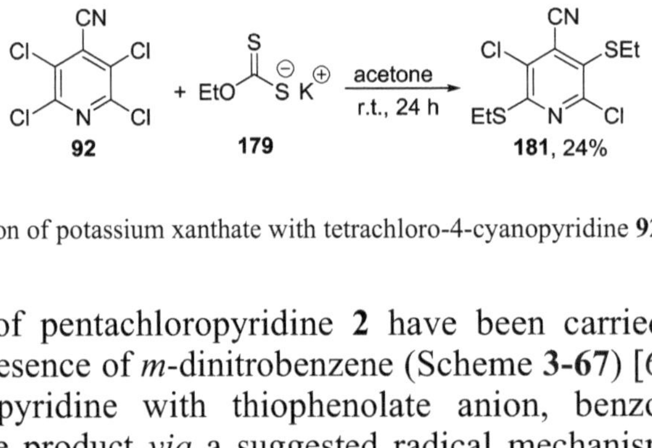

Scheme 3-66. Reaction of potassium xanthate with tetrachloro-4-cyanopyridine **92**.

Persulfuration of pentachloropyridine **2** have been carried out using thiolate anions in the presence of *m*-dinitrobenzene (Scheme **3-67**) [62]. In persulfuration of pentachloropyridine with thiophenolate anion, benzothienopyridine **184** obtained as side product *via* a suggested radical mechanism (Scheme **3-68**).

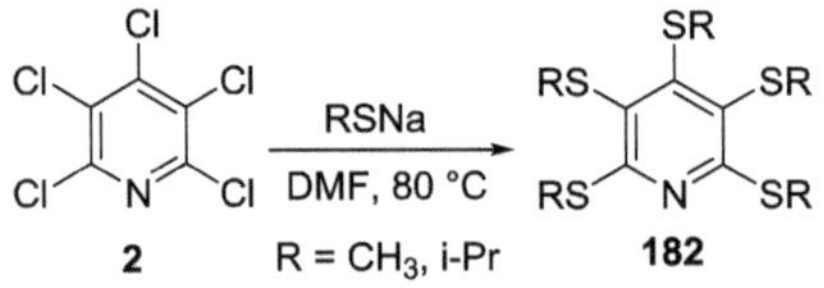

Scheme 3-67. Persulfuration of pentachloropyridine **2** using alkylthiolate anions.

Cl
Cl
Cl
Cl
N
Cl
2
PhSH
DMI, NaH, 20 °C
SPh
PhS
SPh
PhS
N
SPh
183
+
S
PhS
PhS
N
SPh
184

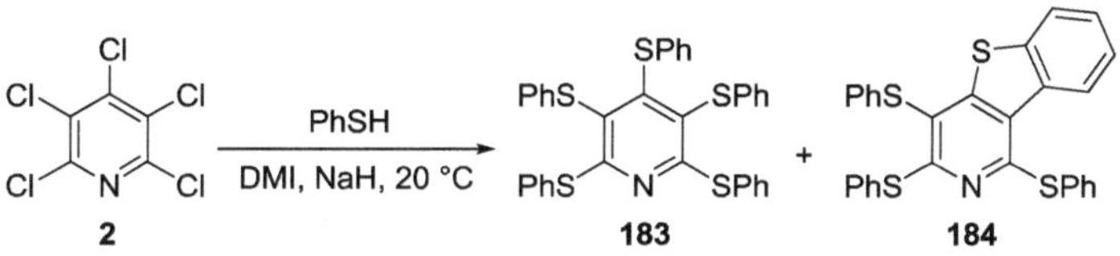

Scheme 3-68. Reaction of thiophenol with pentachloropyridine **2**.

4-amino-3,6-dichloropicolinic acid (aminopyralid) and 4-amino-3,5,6-trichloropicolinic acid (picloram) are plant growth regulator herbicides [17]. One type of internal standard for registration studies is an analog of the test material including at least one or more stable isotopes. These compounds have been synthesized from pentachloropyridine in several steps (Scheme **3-69**) [17]. Picloram-1-^{15}N-2,6-$^{13}C_2$**188** produced in several steps in high yield from pentachloropyridine-1-^{15}N-2,6-$^{13}C_2$. Electrochemical reduction picloram-1-^{15}*N*-2,6-$^{13}C_2$ in an aqueous solution containing sodium hydroxide yielded aminopyralid-1-^{15}*N*-2,6-$^{13}C_2$**190** (Scheme **3-70**).

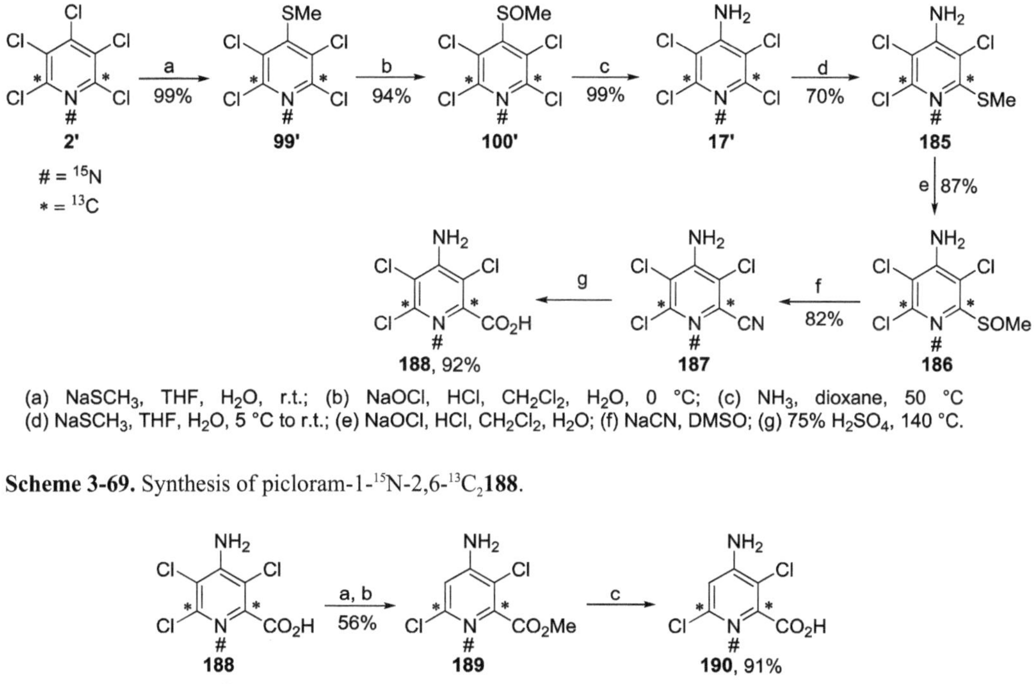

2'
= 15N
* = 13C
a
99%
SMe
99'
b
94%
SOMe
100'
c
99%
NH2
17'
d
70%
SMe
185
e 87%
SOMe
186
f
82%
CN
187
g
CO2H
188, 92%
(a) NaSCH3, THF, H2O, r.t.; (b) NaOCl, HCl, CH2Cl2, H2O, 0 °C; (c) NH3, dioxane, 50 °C
(d) NaSCH3, THF, H2O, 5 °C to r.t.; (e) NaOCl, HCl, CH2Cl2, H2O; (f) NaCN, DMSO; (g) 75% H2SO4, 140 °C.

Scheme 3-69. Synthesis of picloram-1-^{15}N-2,6-$^{13}C_2$**188**.

NH2
CO2H
188
a, b
56%
CO2Me
189
c
CO2H
190, 91%
= 15N
* = 13C
(a) e-, -13 V, NaOH, NaCl, H2O; (b) CH3OH, H2SO4 cat.;
(c) LiOH, THF, H2O, r.t., 2 h.

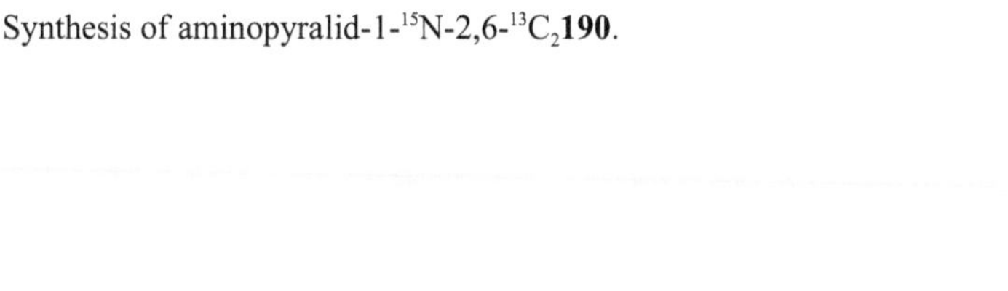

Scheme 3-70. Synthesis of aminopyralid-1-^{15}N-2,6-$^{13}C_2$**190**.

Reaction of 2,3,5,6-tetrachloro-4-(pyridylthio)thiocyanate **191**, which that formed from tetrachloro-4-pyridylsulfenylchloride with an alkali metal thiocyanate, with NaCN results in the formation of 2,3,5,6-tetrachloro-4-(thiocyanato) pyridine **192** (Scheme **3-71**) [63].

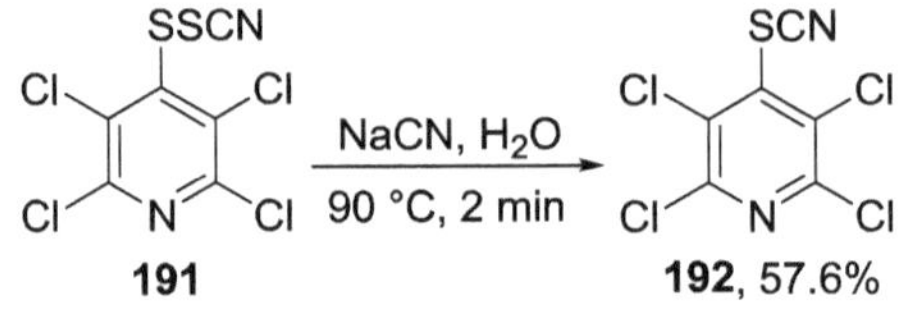

Scheme 3-71. Synthesis of 2,3,5,6-tetrachloro-4-(thiocyanato) pyridine **192**.

3.1.3. Reaction of C-centered Nucleophile with Perchloropyridines

2-cyanotetrachloropyridine **194** has been obtained from heating mixture of pentachloropyridine **2** and KF in 18-crown-6-ether and sulfolane and subsequent reaction with NaCN in DMSO (Scheme **3-72**) [64].

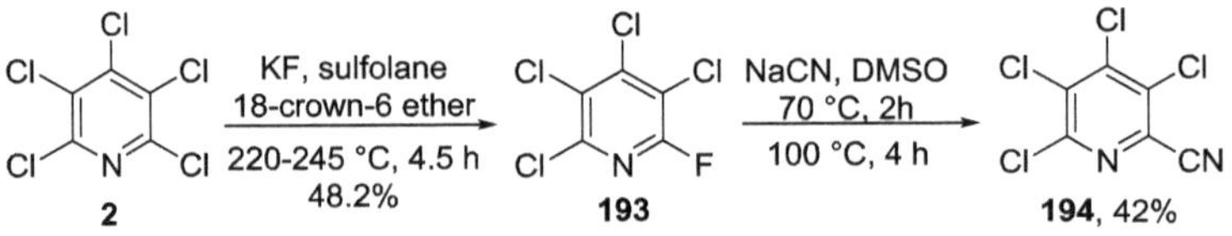

Scheme 3-72. Synthesis of 2-cyanotetrachloropyridine **194**.

Organomagnesium compounds replaced at 4-position of pyridine ring in reaction with pentachloropyridine **2** and produced 4-alkyltetrachloropyridines **195** (Scheme **3-73**) [65].

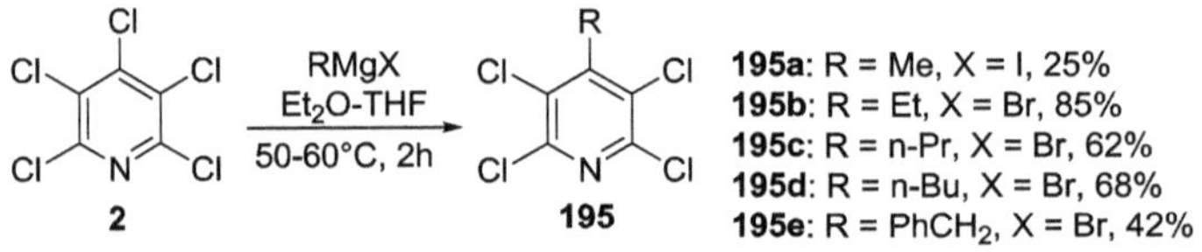

Scheme 3-73. Reaction of pentachloropyridine **2** with organomagnesium compounds.

3.2. Reaction of Perchloropyridines with Bidentate Nucleophiles

Products of pentachloropyridine reaction with bifunctional nucleophiles are interest due to their possible biological activity and because of these products can undergo intramolecular nucleophilic substitution and produce novel heterocyclic compounds [6]. Reaction of pentachloropyridine **2** with ethane-1,2-diamine and dodecane-1,12-diamine give products resulting replacement at 4-position of pyridine ring (Scheme **3-74**) [66].

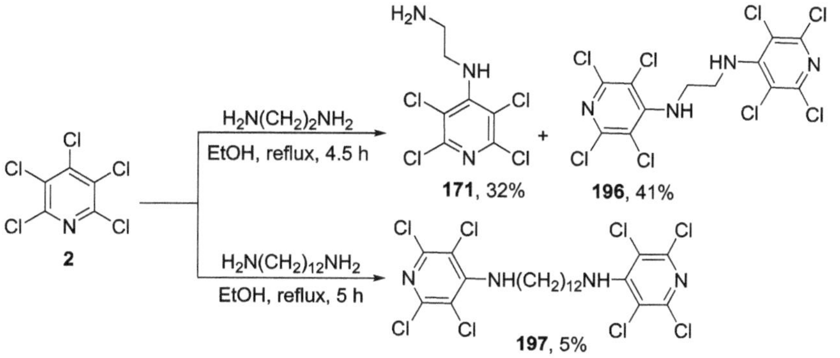

Scheme 3-74. Reaction of pentachloropyridine with aliphatic diamines.

It is established that reaction of *N*-aryl formamides **198** with pentachloropyridine **2** depend on the nature of the aromatic ring substituent (Scheme **3-75**) [67]. When substituent on benzene ring is an electron releasing group, nucleophilic attack is accomplished by oxygen atom and when it is an electron-withdrawing group, attack to pentafluoropyridine occurred by nitrogen site. Proposed mechanism for formation of product **15** is shown in Scheme (**3-76**). The first step in these reactions is the expected nucleophilic attack by the nitrogen of formamide, to give the first formed intermediate **201**, which under reaction conditions converted rapidly to the main product **15** and formyl chloride. Formyl chloride cannot be isolated, because it decomposes to carbon monoxide (CO) and hydrogen chloride (HCl).

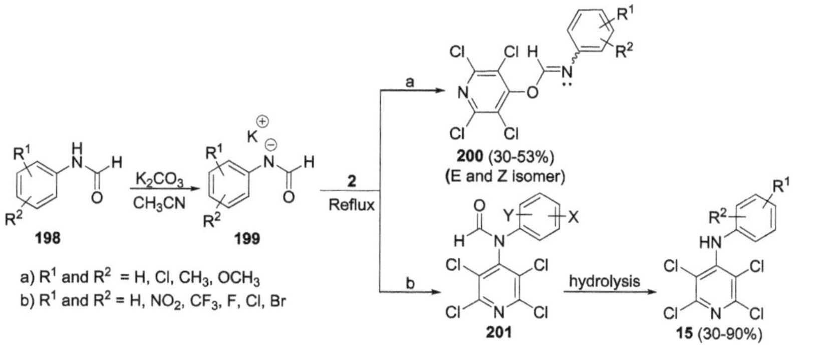

Scheme 3-75. Reaction of formamides **198** with pentachloropyridine **2**.

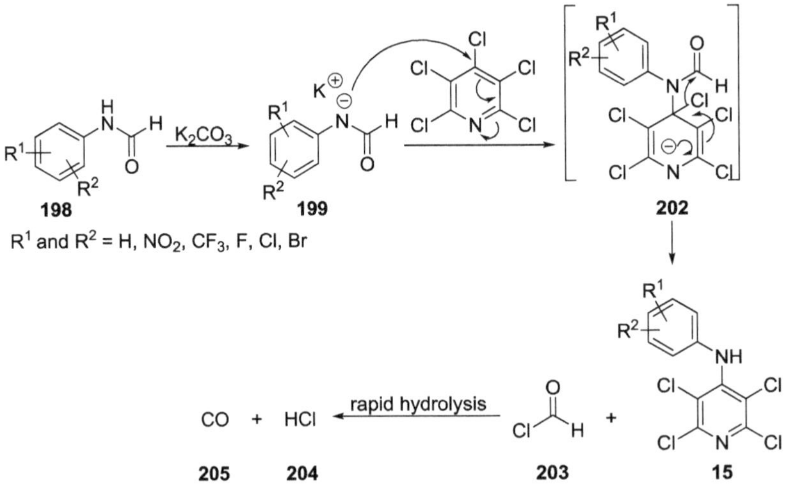

R^1 and R^2 = H, NO_2, CF_3, F, Cl, Br

Scheme 3-76. Proposed explanation for formation **15**.

Pyrimidine-2(5H)-thione and quinazoline-2(1H)-thione derivatives **206** are efficient binucleophiles for synthesis heterocyclic compounds. Cyclocondensation of these compounds with pentachloropyridine **2** leads to formation of fused trichloro-thiazolo[3,2-*a*]pyrimidine and thiazolo[2,3-*b*] quinazoline systems **207** (Scheme **3-77**) *via* nucleophilic attack at 4-position of pyridine ring by S atom followed by an intermolecular cyclization at 3-position of pyridine ring by the nucleophilic attack of nitrogen atom [68].

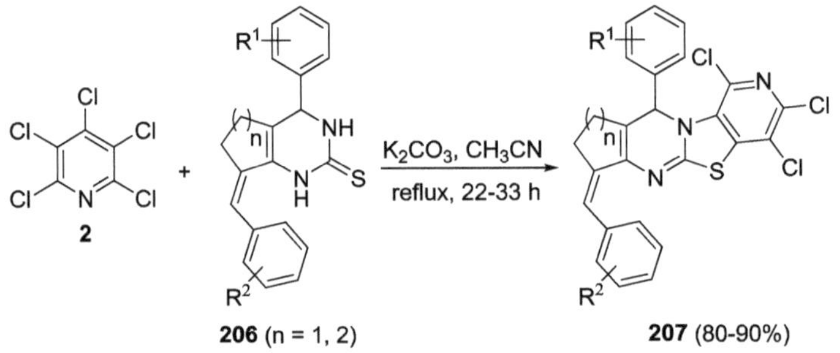

Scheme 3-77. Synthesis of trichloro thiazolo[3,2-*a*]pyrimidine and thiazolo[2,3-*b*]quinazoline derivatives **207**.

Similar to pentafluoropyridine, pyridine-2-ol **208c** reacted with pentachloro-pyridine **2** from both N and O sites, while pyridine-4-ol and pyridine-3-ol reacted essentially from *N* and *O* sites with pentachloropyridine, respectively (Scheme **3-78**) [69].

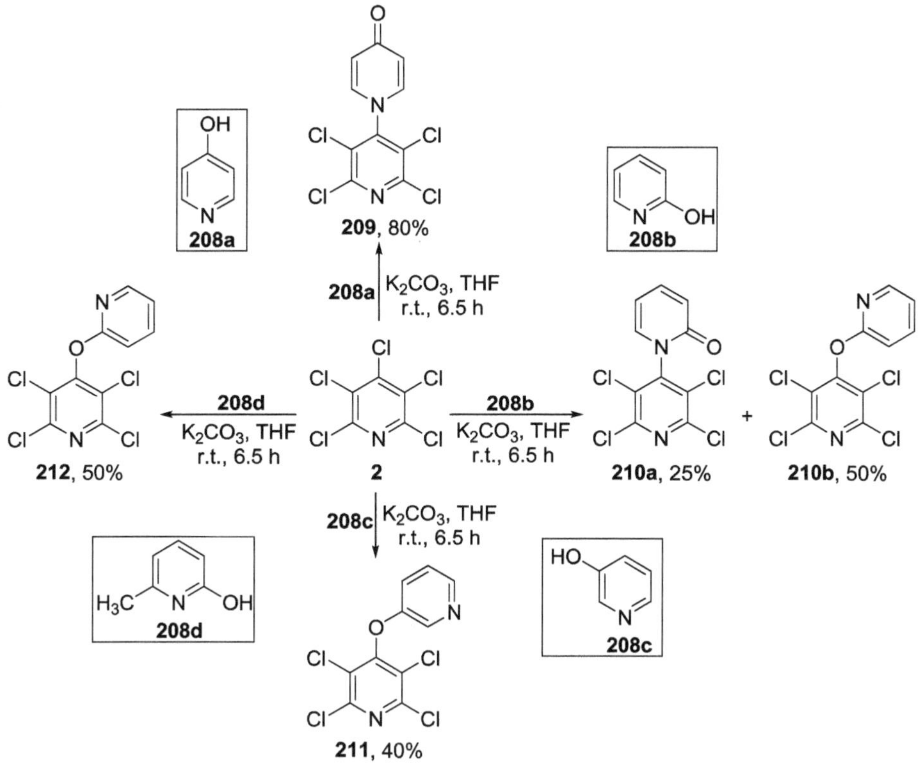

Scheme 3-78. Reactions of pyridinols **208** with pentachloropyridine **2**.

Pentachloropyridine **2** has been substituted selectively at 4-position by *S* atom of 4,6-diaminopyrimidine-2(1H)-thione **213** to gave 2-[(2,3,5,6-Tetrachloropyrid-n-4-yl)sulfanyl]pyrimidine-4,6-diamine **214** (Scheme **3-79**) [70].

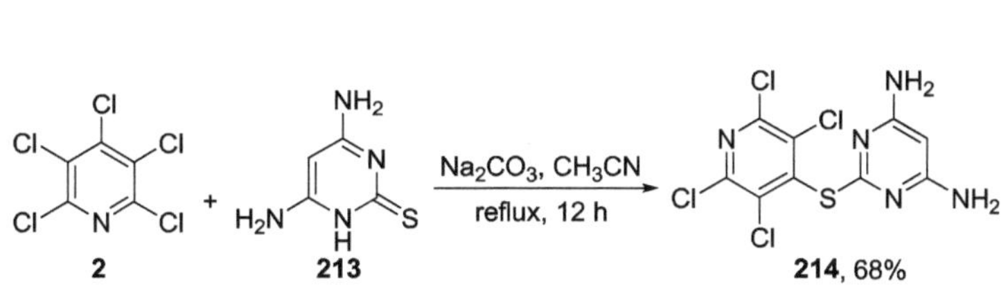

Scheme 3-79. Reaction of 4,6-diaminopyrimidine-2(1H)-thione **213** with pentachloropyridine **2**.

Reaction of 2,3,5,6-tetrachloro-4-(phenylsulfonyl)pyridine **168** with 4,6-diaminopyrimidine-2(1H)-thione **213** has been yielded 2-[(2,3,5,-tetrachloropyridin-4-yl)sulfanyl]pyrimidine-4,6-diamine **214** from nucleophilic attack of *S* atom at the 4-position of pyridine ring and egression of SO_2Ph group (Scheme **3-80**) [70].

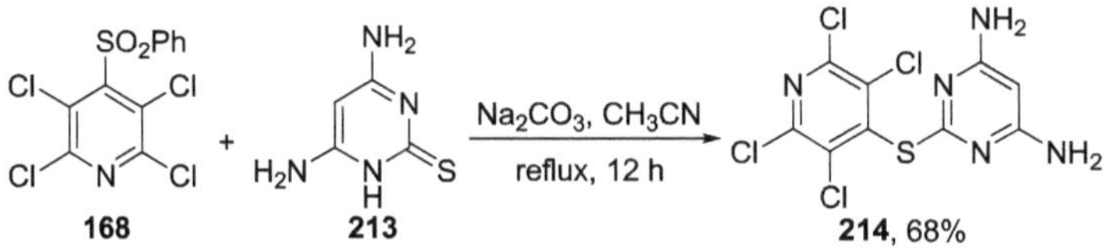

Scheme 3-80. Reaction of 4,6-diaminopyrimidine-2(1H)-thione with 2,3,5,6-tetrachloro-4-(phenylsulfon-l)-pyridine.

Diethyl malonate as ambident nucleophile reacted with pentachloropyridine **2** from *C* site and gave tetrachloropyridine-4-yl malonate **215** (Scheme **3-81**) [71]. This on acid hydrolysis and then heating produced 4-methyltetrachloropyridine **195a**, which on oxidation by potassium permanganate yielded 2,3,5,6-tetrachloroisonicotinic acid **219** (Scheme **3-81**) [71]. Also, its treatment with sodium hydroxide and then heating produced 3,5,6-trichloro-4-methylpyridin-2-ol **217** (Scheme **3-81**).

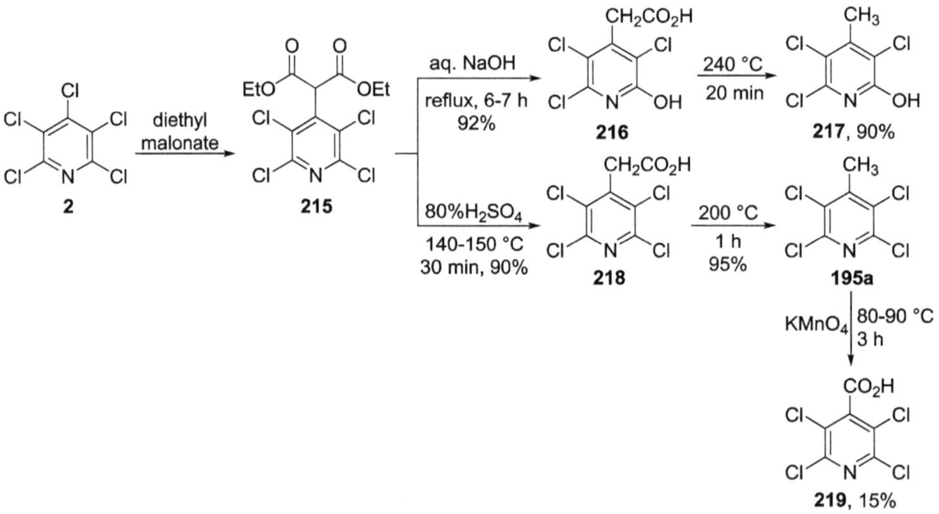

Scheme 3-81. Hydrolysis of tetrachloropyridine-4-yl malonate **215**.

Reaction of pentachloropyridine **2** with sodioacetoacetic ester in ethanol occurred at 4-position of pyridine ring *via* nucleophic attack of *C* atom and produced ethyl 2,3,5,6-tetrachloro-4-pyridylacetoacetate **221** as major product, while in dioxane occurred at 2-position of pyridine ring and gave ethyl 3,4,5,6-tetrachloro-2-pyridylacetoacetate **222** as major product (Scheme **3-82**) [72].

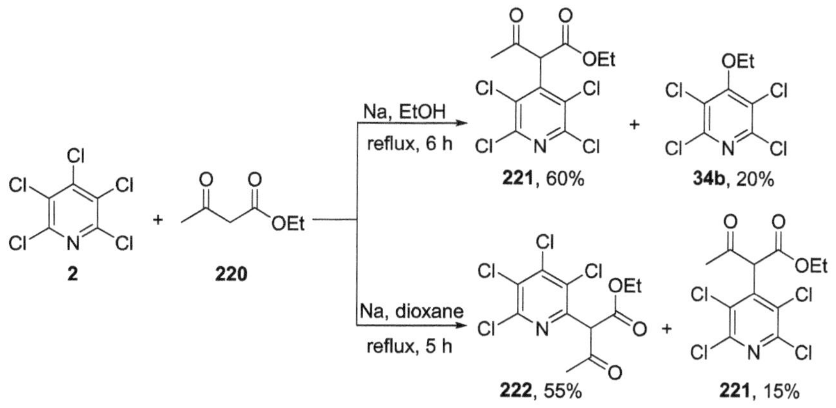

Scheme 3-82. Reaction of pentachloropyridine **2** with sodioacetoacetic ester.

Ester **221** on treatment with 80% sulfuric acid has been converted to 4-acetony--2,3,5,6-tetrachloropyridine **223**. This oxidized to 2,3,5,6-tetrachloroisonicotinic acid **219** by reaction with potassium permanganate at the presence of HOAc and 25% H_2SO_4 while has been converted to 2-ethoxy-4-methyl-3-5,6-trichloropyridine **224** by reaction with Na/EtOH (Scheme **3-83**) [72].

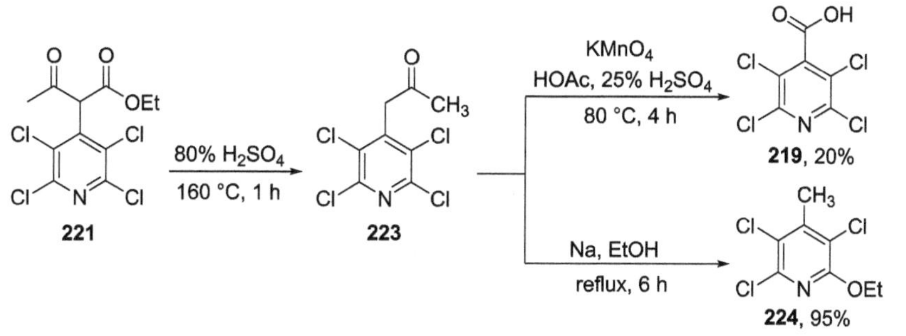

Scheme 3-83. Synthesis of 2,3,5,6-tetrachloroisonicotinic acid **219** and 2-ethoxy-4-methyl-3-5,6-trichloropyridine **224**.

Action of 25% KOH with **221** gave 2-hydroxy-3,5,6-trichloropyridi-e-4-pyridylacetic acid, which converted to 2-hydroxy-4-methyl-3-5,6-trichloropyridine **217** on heating (Scheme **3-84**) [72].

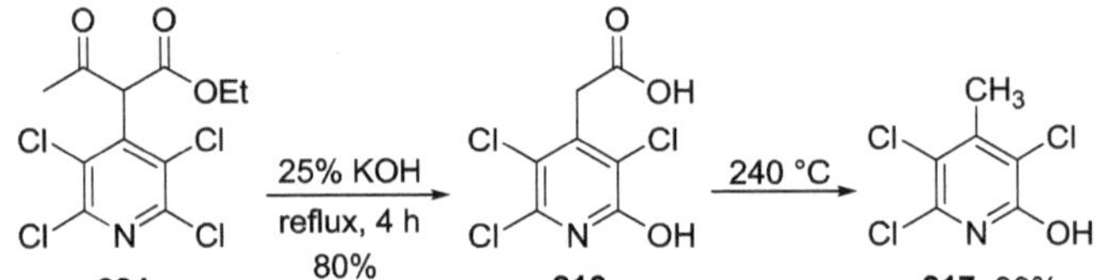

Scheme 3-84. Synthesis of 2-hydroxy-4-methyl-3,5,6-trichloropyridine **217**.

Heating of ester **222** with 80% H_2SO_4 has been gave 3,4,5,6-tetrachloro-2-pyridylacetic acid **225**, while yielded ethyl 3,4,5,6-tetrachloro-2-pyridylacetate **227** on action with 80% H_2SO_4 at 20 °C (Scheme **3-85**) [72]. Proposed mechanism for formation of **218** has been shown in Scheme (**3-86**). Compound **218** on heating has been converted to compound **225**, followed by heating and gave compound **226**.

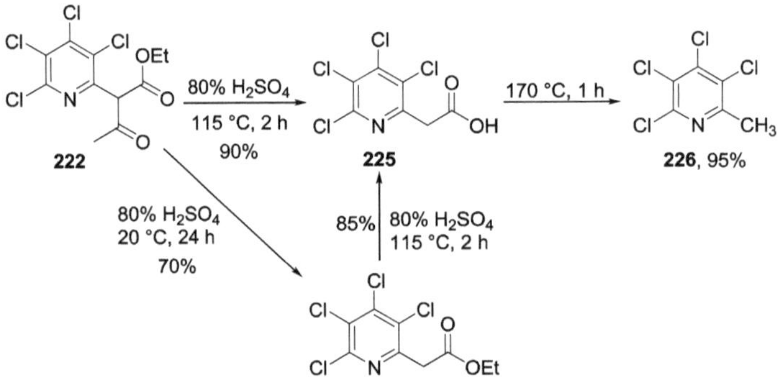

Scheme 3-85. Synthesis of 2-methyl-3,4,5,6-tetrachloropyridine **226**.

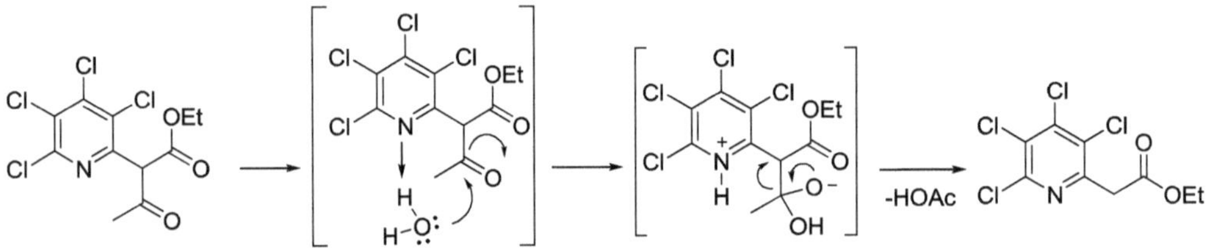

Scheme 3-86. Proposed amidation mechanism for formation compound **218**.

Both 2- and 3-positions of tetrachloro-4-cyanopyridine **92** are active toward nucleophilic attack. Its reaction with bidentate nucleophiles leaded to formation of ring-fused heterocyclic systems (Scheme **3-87**) [49].

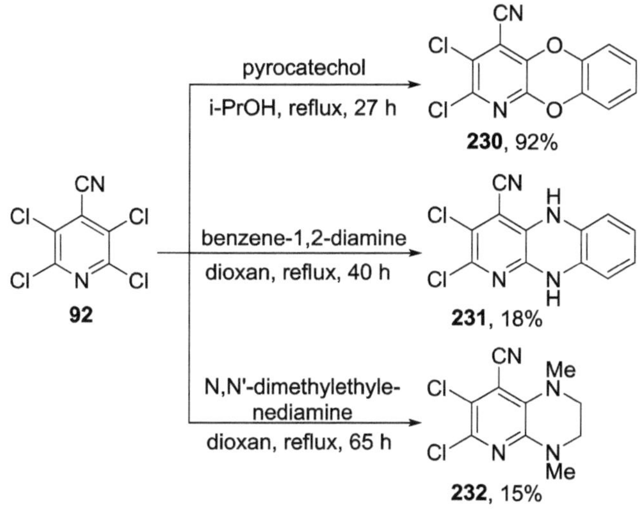

Scheme 3-87. Reaction of tetrachloro-4-cyanopyridine **92** with bidentate nucleophiles.

Reaction of tetrachloro-4-cyanopyridine **92** with 1-(diethylamino)cyclohexene compounds **233a-d** produced tetrahydro-5H-pyrido[3,2-*b*]indoles **234** and tetrahydro-9H-pyridi[2,3-*b*]indoles **235** as major products arising attack both *C* and *N* atoms of enamine (Scheme **3-88**) [73].

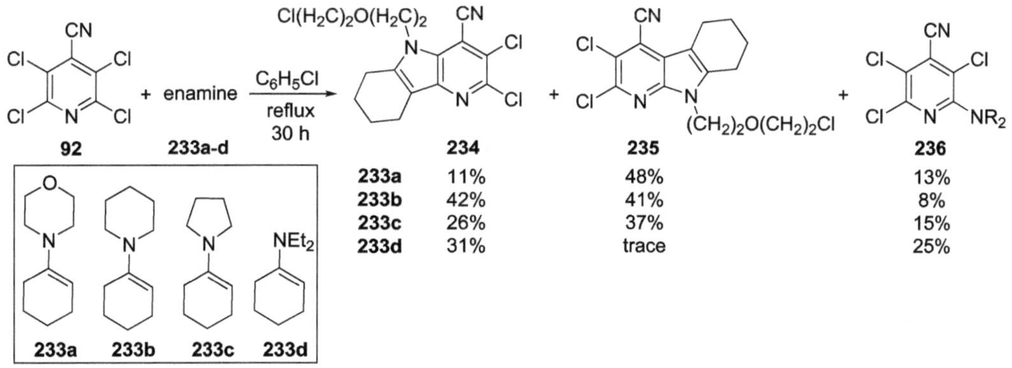

	234	**235**	**236**
233a	11%	48%	13%
233b	42%	41%	8%
233c	26%	37%	15%
233d	31%	trace	25%

Scheme 3-88. Reaction of enamines **233a-d** with tetrachloro-4-cyanopyridine **92**.

4. CROSS-COUPLING REACTIONS OF PERCHLOROPYRIDINES

Synthesis of polyfunctional pyridines has attracted considerable interest and efficient methods that have been developed for synthesis of these compounds. Cross-coupling reactions make possible inserting the desired substituent on pyridine. In last years, site selective cross-coupling reactions of perhaloheterocycles have been considered [74 - 78]. Reaction of pentachloropyridine **2** with arylboronic acids **237** produced pentaarylpyridines **238** *via* Suzuki–Miyaura cross-coupling (Scheme **3-89**) [79]. In addition, pyridines with different substituents synthesized selectively from this process (Schemes **3-90** and **3-91**).

Ar = Ph, 4-MeC$_6$H$_4$, 4-EtC$_6$H$_4$, 4-t-BuC$_6$H$_4$, 4-(MeO)C$_6$H$_4$, 4-PhC$_6$H$_4$, 4(vinyl)C$_6$H$_4$, 4-FC$_6$H$_4$, 4-(CF$_3$)C$_6$H$_4$, 4-(CF$_3$O)C$_6$H$_4$, 3-(MeO)C$_6$H$_4$, 3-(NO$_2$)C$_6$H$_4$, 2-thienyl,

Scheme 3-89. One step synthesis of pentaarylpyridines **238**.

Ar^1 = Ph, 4-MeC$_6$H$_4$, 4-EtC$_6$H$_4$, 4-t-BuC$_6$H$_4$, 4-(MeO)C$_6$H$_4$, 3-(MeO)C$_6$H$_4$, 3-MeC$_6$H$_4$, 2-(MeO)C$_6$H$_4$
Ar^2 = Ph, 4-EtC$_6$H$_4$, 4-(MeO)C$_6$H$_4$, 3-(MeO)C$_6$H$_4$, 4-(CF$_3$)C$_6$H$_4$

Scheme 3-90. Site selective synthesis of pentaarylpyridines **240**.

Scheme 3-91. Site selective arylation of 4-aryltetrachloropyridines **241a,b**.

Sonogashira cross-coupling of pentachloropyridine **2** with acetylene derivatives **247** produced pentaalkynylpyridine compounds **248** (Scheme **3-92**) [80].

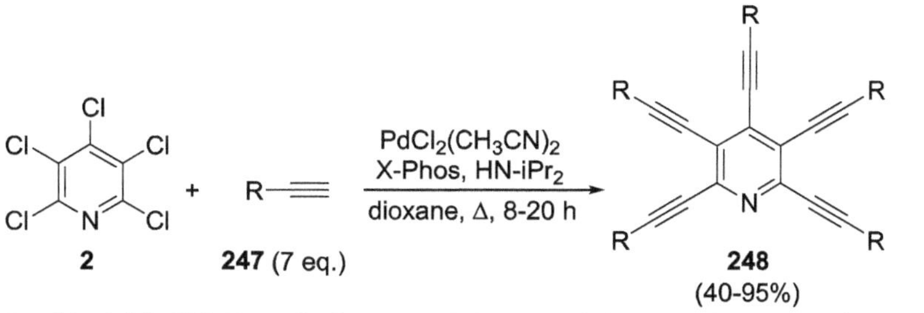

R = Ph, 4-(MeO)C_6H_4, 4-tBuC_6H_4, 4-FC_6H_4, 2-MeC_6H_4, 3-MeC_6H_4, 4-MeC_6H_4, 4-(C_9H_{11}O)C_6H_4, 3-thienyl, C_4H_9

Scheme 3-92. One-step synthesis of pentaalkynylpyridines **248**.

2,3,5,6-tetrachloropyridine **33** has been utilized as good precursor for synthesis of various tetraalkynyl and tetraalkenylpyridine compounds in excellent yields by palladium-catalyzed cross-coupling reactions in one-pot procedures (Schemes **3-93** and **3-94**) [78].

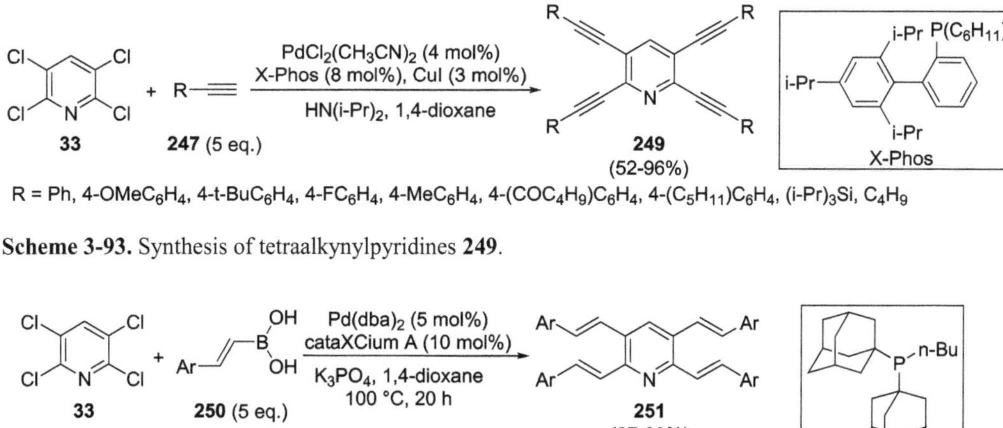

R = Ph, 4-OMeC_6H_4, 4-t-BuC_6H_4, 4-FC_6H_4, 4-MeC_6H_4, 4-(COC_4H_9)C_6H_4, 4-(C_5H_{11})C_6H_4, (i-Pr)$_3$Si, C_4H_9

Scheme 3-93. Synthesis of tetraalkynylpyridines **249**.

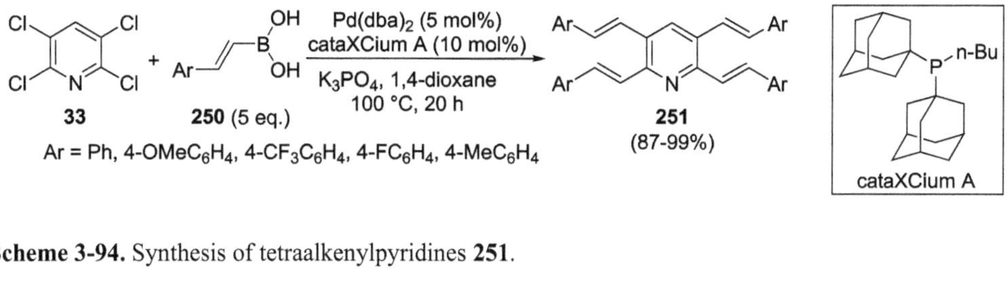

Ar = Ph, 4-OMeC_6H_4, 4-CF$_3$$C_6H_4$, 4-F$C_6H_4$, 4-Me$C_6H_4$

Scheme 3-94. Synthesis of tetraalkenylpyridines **251**.

The reaction of 2,3,5,6-tetrachloropyridines **33** with alkynes proceeded with very good site selectivity in favour of 2- and 6-positions of pyridine ring *via* Sonogashira cross-coupling and produced 2,6-dialkynyl derivatives **253-255** (Schemes **3-95** to **3-97**) [81]. The selectivity explained by the fact that 2- and 6-

positions are less electron rich than 3- and 5-positions, and the fact that the oxidative addition of Pd(0) catalysed cross-coupling reactions of polyhalogenated substrates proceeds by predominant attack at the more electron poor position [81]. Furthermore, tetraalkynylated pyridines provided in good to excellent yields from tetrachloropyridines and 3,5-dichloro-2,6-dialkynylpyridines *via* this method (Schemes **3-98** and **3-99**.

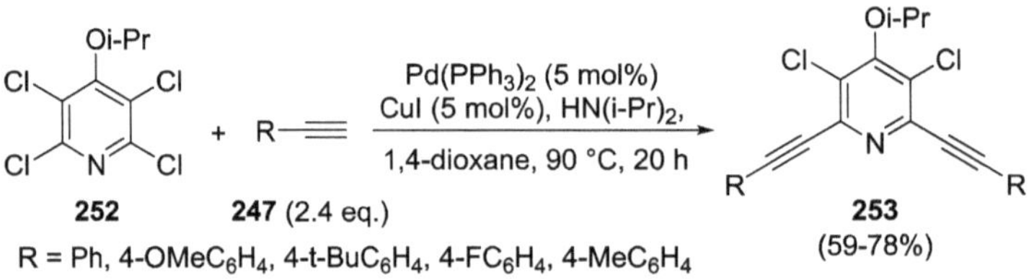

Scheme 3-95. Synthesis of 3,5-dichloro-4-isopropoxy-2,6-bis(arylethynyl)-pyridines **253**.

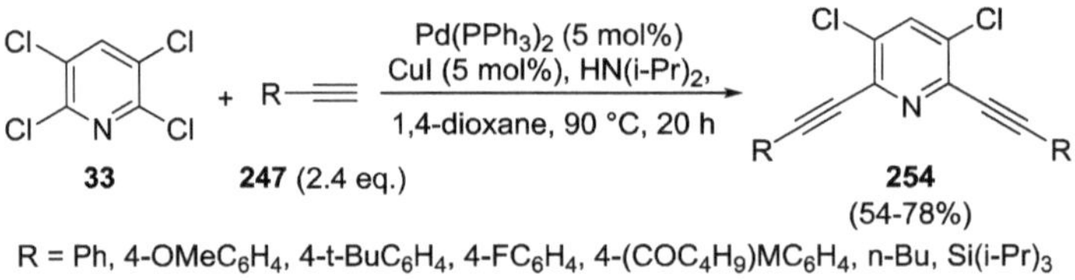

Scheme 3-96. Synthesis of 3,5-dichloro-2,6-dialkynylpyridines **254**.

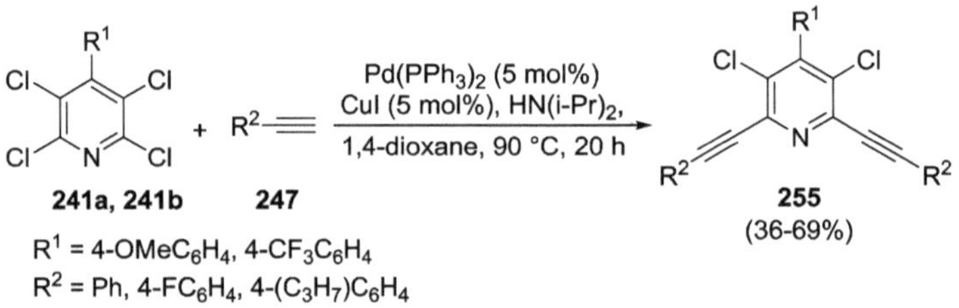

Scheme 3-97. Synthesis of 3,5-dichloro-4-aryl-2,6-bis(arylethynyl)-pyridines **255**.

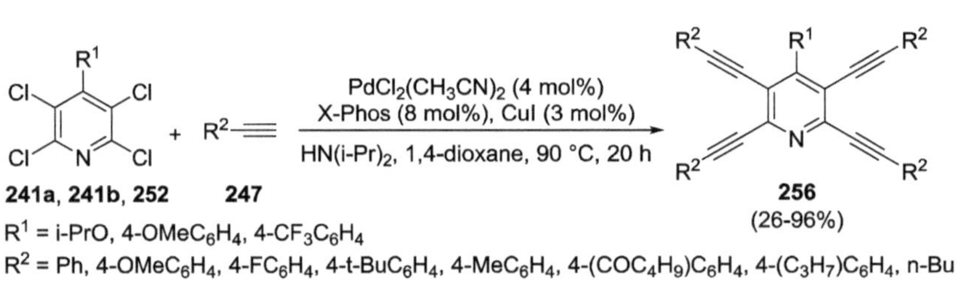

Scheme 3-98. Synthesis of 2,3,5,6-tetraalkynylpyridines from tetrachloropyridines **256**.

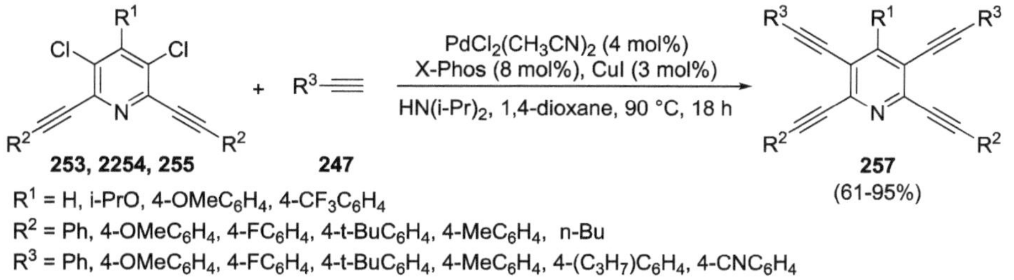

PdCl2(CH3CN)2 (4 mol%)
X-Phos (8 mol%), CuI (3 mol%)
HN(i-Pr)2, 1,4-dioxane, 90 °C, 18 h
253, 2254, 255
247
257
(61-95%)
R1 = H, i-PrO, 4-OMeC6H4, 4-CF3C6H4
R2 = Ph, 4-OMeC6H4, 4-FC6H4, 4-t-BuC6H4, 4-MeC6H4, n-Bu
R3 = Ph, 4-OMeC6H4, 4-FC6H4, 4-t-BuC6H4, 4-MeC6H4, 4-(C3H7)C6H4, 4-CNC6H4

Scheme 3-99. Synthesis of 2,3,5,6-tetraalkynylpyridines from 3,5-dichloro-2,6-dialkynylpyridines **257**.

5. BROMINATION OF PENTACHLOROPYRIDINE

Pentachloropyridine **2** on treatment with sodium bromide in DMF as solvent gave 4-bromotetrachloropyridine **80** in 31% yield (Scheme **3-100**). Also, it produced from pentachloropyridine in two steps in 68% yield (Scheme **3-100**) [43].

NaBr, DMF
31%
1) N2H4.H2O, EtOH
Na2CO3, reflux, 5 h
2) HBr, Br2, 60 °C, 30 min
68%
2
80
2

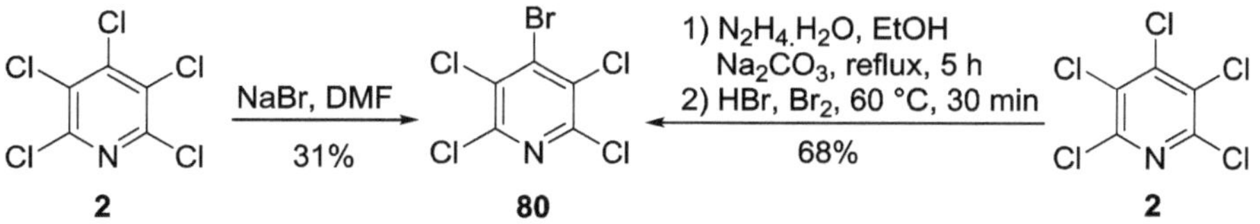

Scheme 3-100. Synthesis of 4-bromotetrachloropyridine **80**.

Nucleophilic substitutions of 4-bromotetrachloropyridine **80** have carried out exclusively by replacement of bromine atom with nucleophiles [29, 82]. Thilos in the reaction with 4-bromotetrachloropyridine **80** have been replaced bromine and produced 4-arylthiotetrachloropyridine derivatives **259** (Scheme **3-101**) [82]. In a similar manner, it substituted at 4-position on reaction with aromatic amines [29].

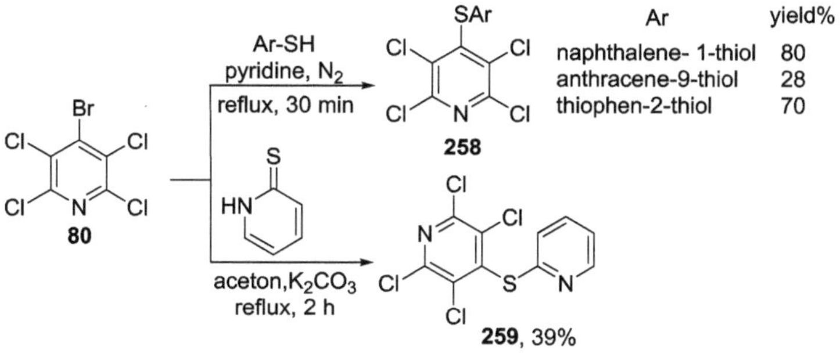

Ar-SH
pyridine, N2
reflux, 30 min
Ar yield%
naphthalene- 1-thiol 80
anthracene-9-thiol 28
thiophen-2-thiol 70
80
258
aceton,K2CO3
reflux, 2 h
259, 39%

Scheme 3-101. Reactions of 4-Bromotetrachloropyridine **80** with thaiols.

Reaction of 4-bromotetrachloropyridine **80** with piperidine gave mixture of 2- and 4-substituted products, while with n-BuLi yielded 2,3,5,6-tetrachloropyrdine **33** (Scheme **3-102**) [23].

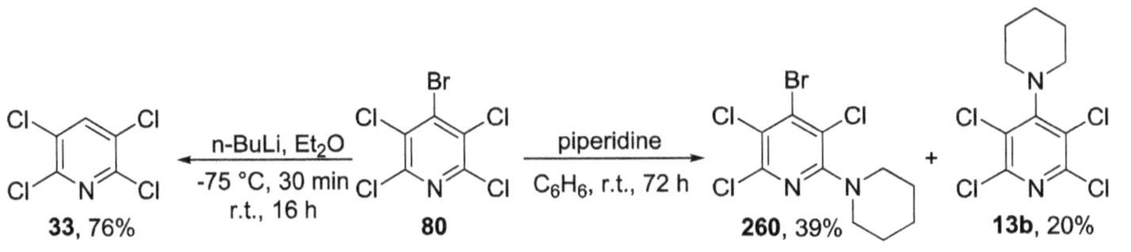

Scheme 3-102. Reaction of 4-bromotetrachloropyridine **80** with piperidine and n-BuLi.

4-bromotetrachloropyridine **80** converted to tetrachloro-4-iodopyridine **261** on treatment with n-BuLi and iodine, respectively (Scheme **3-103**) [43]. 4-iodotetrachloropyrdine reacted with piperidine at both 2- and 4-positions of pyridine ring (Scheme **3-104**) [23]. It converted to ctachloro-4,4'-bipyridyl **263** at the presence of copper (Scheme **3-104**) [23].

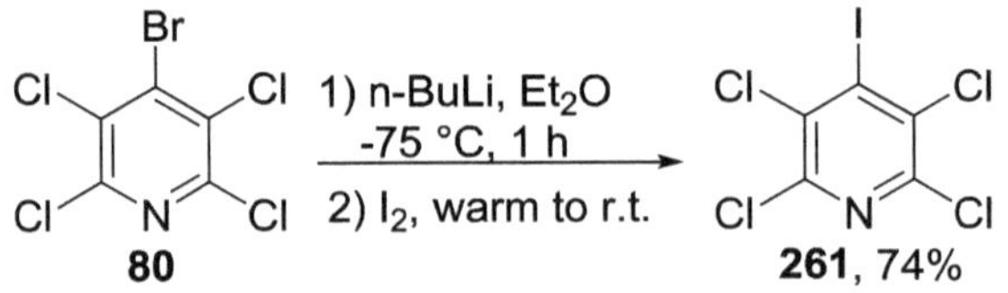

Scheme 3-103. Synthesis of tetrachloro-4-iodopyridine **261**.

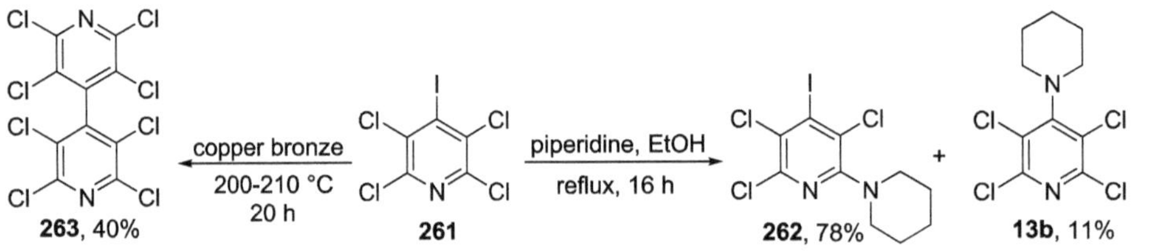

Scheme 3-104. Some reactions of 4-iodotetrachloropyridine **261**.

6. OXIDATION OF POLYCHLOROPYRIDINES

Oxidation of pentachloropyridine **2** by hot trifluoroperoxyacetic acid [25], by mixture of 87% hydrogen peroxide, sulfuric acid and trifluoroacetic acid [5] or by mixture of concentrated sulphuric acid, acetic acid and 90% hydrogen peroxide [83] produced pentachloropyridine-*N*-oxide **264** in 20%, 72% and 85% yields, respectively (Scheme **3-105**).

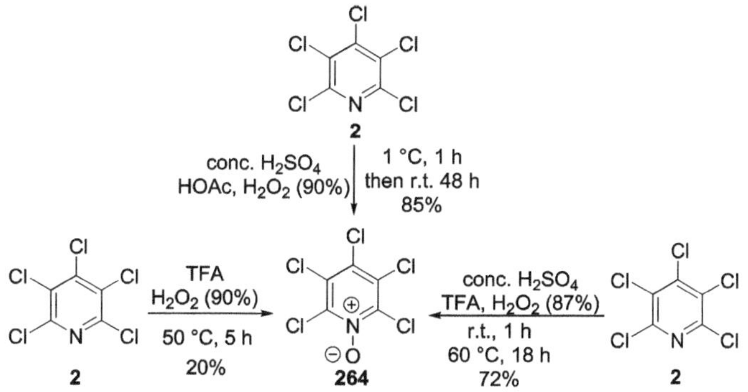

Scheme 3-105. Synthesis of pentachloropyridine-N-oxide **264**.

Pentachloropyridine-*N*-oxide **264** reacted with ammonia, methylamine, sodium acetate, sodium hydroxide and potassium hydrogensulfide at 2-position and produced corresponding 2-substituted tetrachloropyridine-*N*-oxide derivatives (Scheme **3-106**) [24, 84]. Whereas its reaction with hydrazine hydrate and phosphorus trichloride gave 2-substituted tetrachloropyridines (Scheme **3-106**) [23, 84]. Reaction of **264** with phosphorus pentasulfide and thiourea produced tetrachloropyridine-4-thiol **98** and bis(tetrachloro-2-pyridyl)disulfide **268**, respectively (Scheme **3-106**) [84].

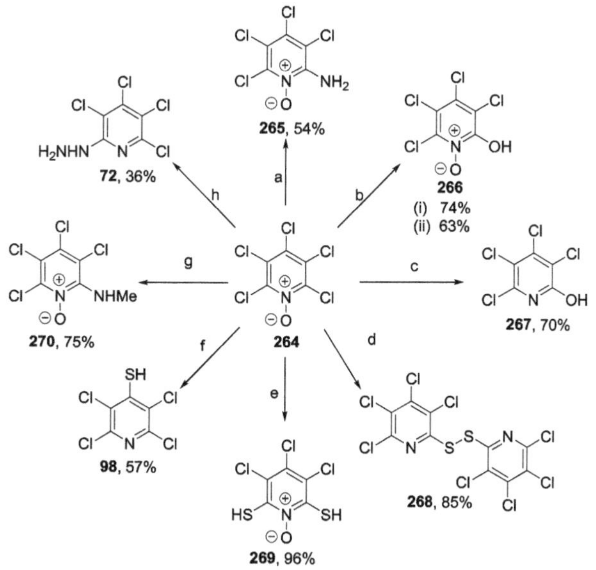

a) aq. NH$_3$, DMF, r.t., 2 h; b) (i) NaOAc, Ac$_2$O, reflux, 24 h or (ii) NaOH, EtOH, r.t., 48 h; c) PCl$_3$, CHCl$_3$, reflux, 30 min; d) thiourea, EtOH, reflux, 2 h; e) KSH, ethylene glycol, r.t., overnight; f) P$_2$S$_5$, 60°C, 10 min; g) MeNH$_2$, dioxane, r.t., 16 h; h) hydrazine hydrate, EtOH, reflux, 2 h.

Scheme 3-106. Reactions of pentachloropyridine-*N*-oxide **264**.

Enamines not reacted with pentachlopyridine in benzene or toluene, but reacted with pentachloropyridine-*N*-oxide **264** because of this compound is more active than pentachloropyridine (Scheme **3-107**) [85].

enamine	solvent	product (yield/%) 271 + 272	273 + 274	275 or 276
233a	toluene	-	-	39
233d	benzene	50	0	9
	toluene	17	6	46
233e	toluene	-	-	11
233f	toluene	7	0	0

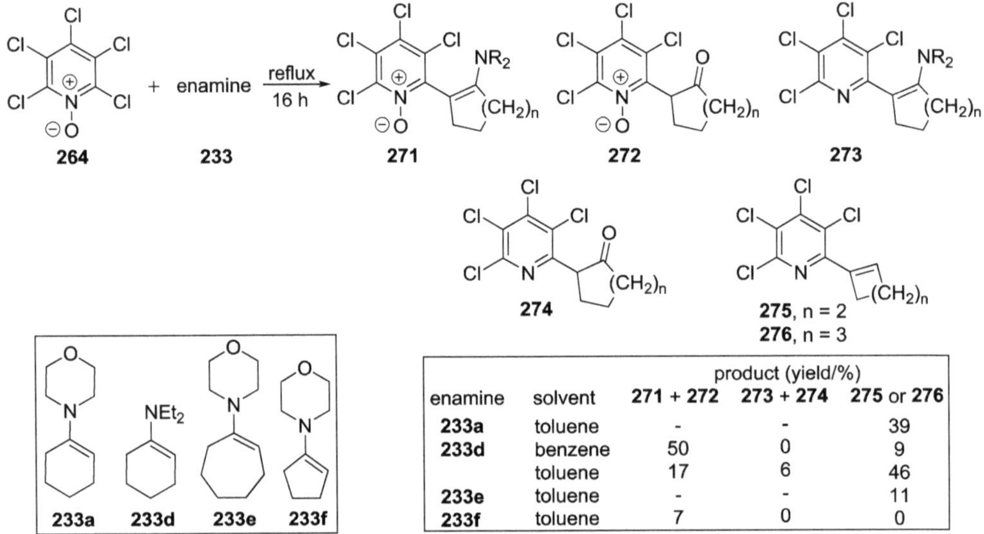

Scheme 3-107. Reactions of enamines **233** with pentachloropyridine-N-oxide **264**.

Oxidation of tetrachloro-4-methoxypyridine **34a** by mixture of hydrogen peroxide, concentrated sulfuric acid and acetic acid, and by produced tetrachloro-4-hydroxypyridine-*N*-oxide **277** in 50% yield, while with polyphosphoric acid at the presence of hydrogen peroxide gave tetrachloro-4-methoxypyridine-*N*-oxide **278** in 80% yield (Scheme **3-108**) [5].

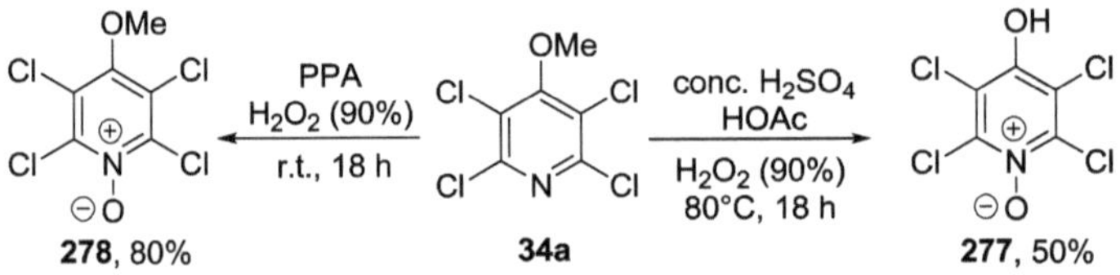

Scheme 3-108. Oxidation of tetrachloro-4-methoxypyririne **j**.

Nucleophilic substitution of sodium dimethyldithiocarbamate on pentachloropyridine-*N*-oxide **264** occurred at 2-position of pyridine ring and formed intermediate **280**, which undergoes a 5-exo trig rearrangement to the thermodynamically more stable derivative **281** (Scheme **3-109**) [86]. Compound

281 on heating decomposed to the radicals **282** and **283** (Scheme **3-109**).

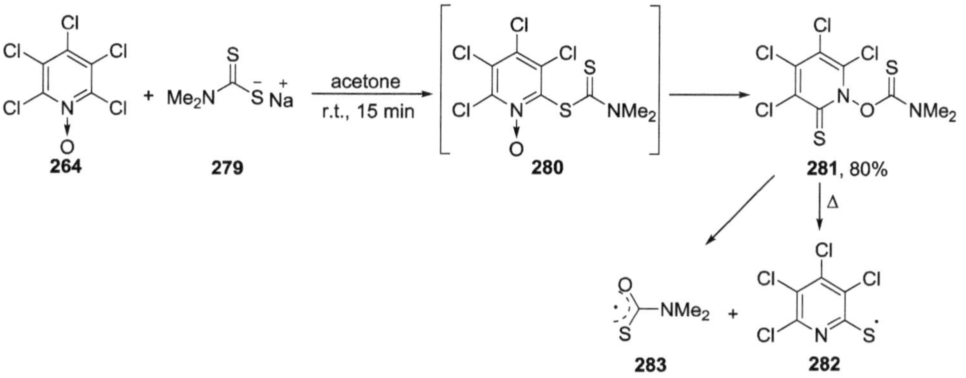

Scheme 3-109. Reaction of pentachloropyridine N-oxide **264** with sodium dimethyldithiocarbamate **279**.

Compound **281** is unstable on heating and produced various products depending on solvent [86]. In chloroform, the recombination of the radicals **282** and **283** have been occurred and gave compound **284** (Scheme **3-110**). In ethyl acetate, disulfide **268** have been formed *via* recombination of two mole of radical **282** (Scheme **3-110**). In acetone, radical $CH_3CH_2{}^{\cdot}$, formed from the reaction of radical **283** with acetone, with radical **282** combined and produced *S*-acetonyl derivative **285** (Scheme **3-110**).

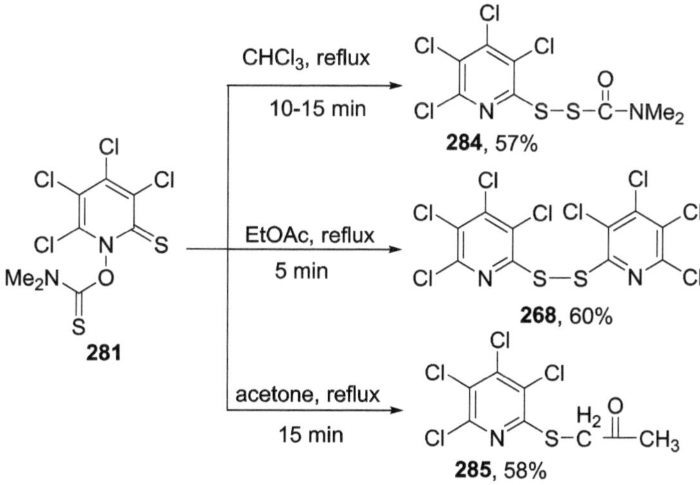

Scheme 3-110. Refluxing compound **281** in various solvents.

Pentachloropyridine-N-oxide **264** on reaction with methyl fluorosulphonate produced salt **287** at high yield. This salt in the presence of water and aq. sodium azide converted to 2-pyridone **288** and triazide **86** (Scheme **3-111**) [4].

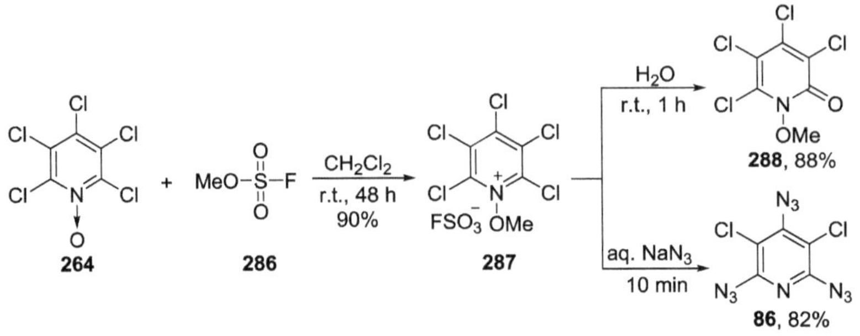

Scheme 3-111. Synthesis and reactions of salt **287**.

Heating of pentachloropyridine-N-oxide **264** in dimethyl sulphate yielded N-methoxytetrachloro-2-pyridone **288** (Scheme **3-112**) [4].

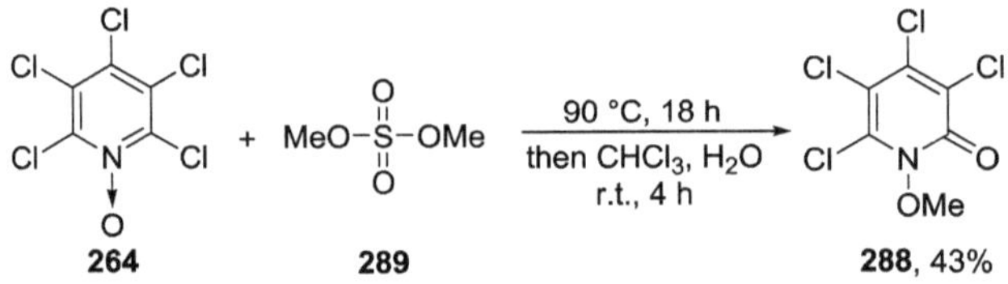

Scheme 3-112. Reaction of pentachloropyridine-N-oxide **264** with dimethyl sulphate.

7. REDUCTION OF POLYCHLOROPYRIDINES

Chloropyridines used as a chemical basis for synthesis of several pesticides and many efforts have been carried out for resolve of their preparation problem in large scale. 2,3,5,6-tetrachloropyridine **33** obtained from reduction of pentachloropyridine **2** with zinc powder at the presence of ammonium chloride in 97.6% yield and at the presence of ammonium methylphosphonic acid methyl ester **290** in 80.4% yield (Scheme **3-113**) [87].

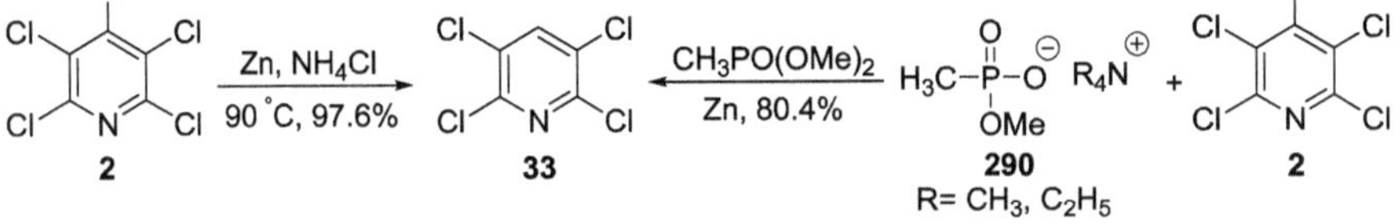

Scheme 3-113. Synthesis of 2,3,5,6-tetrachloropyridine **33**.

Electrolytical reduction of pentachloropyridine carried out at 4-position of pyridine ring. Reaction of pentachloropyridine **2** with excess of lithium aluminum hydride at 60°C produced 2,3,5,6-tetrachloropyridine **33** as major product, whereas 2,3,6-trichloropyridine **296** obtained as major product at room temperature (Scheme **3-114**) [88]. Lithium borohydride and lithium aluminum hydride reduced pentachloropyridine **2** to 2,3,5,6-tetrachloropyridine **33** *via* 1,4- and 3,4-additions, respectively (Scheme **3-115**) [88].

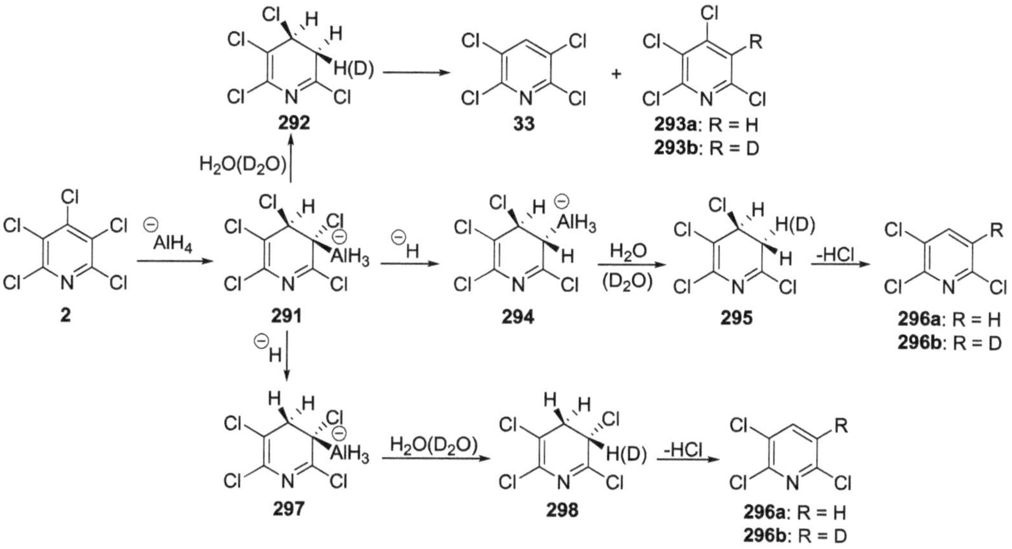

Scheme 3-114. Reduction of pentachloropyridine by lithium aluminum hydride.

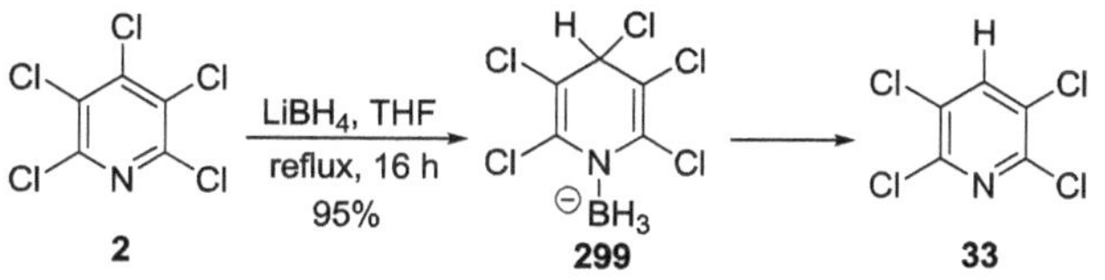

Scheme 3-115. Reduction of pentachloropyridine by lithium borohydride.

8. ALKYLATION OF POLYCHLOROPYRIDINES

Polychloropyridines have considerable low basicity because of the strong inductive effect of the chlorine atoms and usually are resistance toward *N*-alkylation. However, methyl fluorosulphonate has been successfully reacted with pentachloropyridine **2**, tetrachloro-2-fluoropyridine **193** in the absence of a solvent and gave corresponding *N*-methylated pyridinium fluorosulphonates **300** in good yields (Scheme **3-116**) [4]. The strong inductive effect of the positively charged nitrogen atom activated the 2(6)-positions of ring toward nucleophilic substitution (Scheme **3-117**) [4].

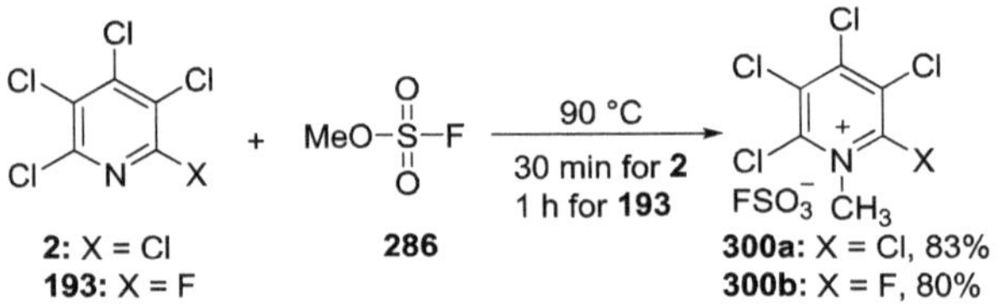

Scheme 3-116. *N*-methylation of perchloropyridines **2** and **193**.

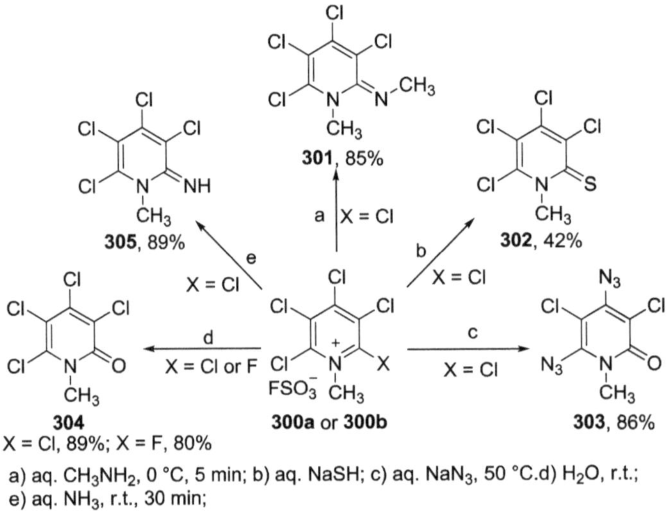

a) aq. CH_3NH_2, 0 °C, 5 min; b) aq. NaSH; c) aq. NaN_3, 50 °C.d) H_2O, r.t.; e) aq. NH_3, r.t., 30 min;

Scheme 3-117. Reactions of salts **300a** and **300b** with nucleophiles.

N-ethylpentachloropyridinium fluoroborate **306** has been formed by reaction of pentachloropyridine with triethyloxonium fluoroborate, followed by treatment with water and produced 2-pyridone **307** (Scheme **3-118**) [4].

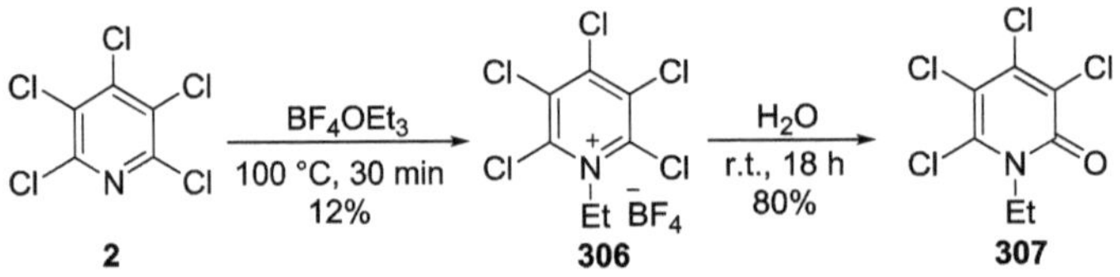

Scheme 3-118. Synthesis of *N*-ethyltetrachloro-2-pyridone **307**.

9. PHOTOCHEMICAL REACTIONS OF POLYCHLOROPYRIDINES

Irradiation of pentachloropyridine **2** in diethyl ether have been leaded to replacement of β-halogen with hydrogen atom (Scheme **3-119**) [82]. Photolysis of 4-bromotetrachloropyridine **80** and tetrachloro-4-iodopyridine **261** in diethyl ether have been accompanied with elimination of bromine and iodine atoms, respectively (Scheme **3-120**) [82].

2 **293**, 40%

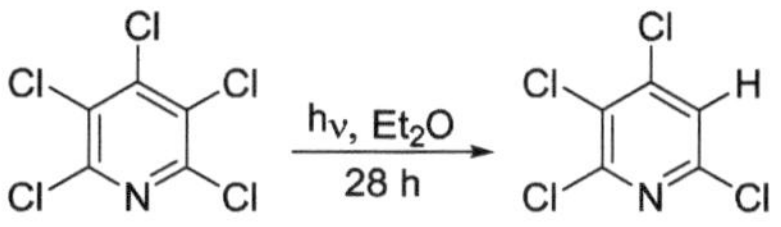

Scheme 3-119. Photolysis of pentachloropyridine **2** in ether.

80: X = Br
261: X = I

X	time/h	**33**	**308**
Br	71	17%	6%
I	19	87%	-

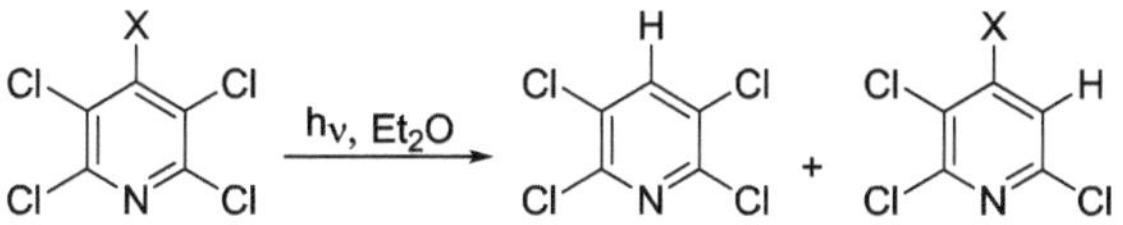

Scheme 3-120. Photolysis of tachloropyridines **80** and **261** in ether.

Photolysis of **261**, **78** and **310** in benzene have been leaded to replacement of iodine with phenyl group (Schemes **3-121** to **3-123**) [82].

261 **241c**, 74%

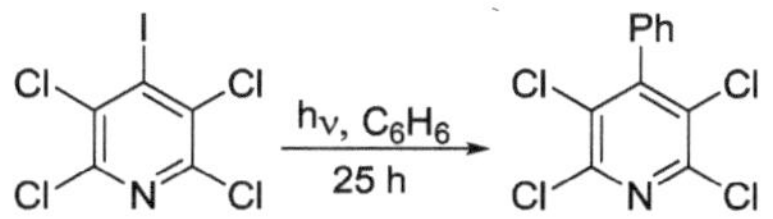

Scheme 3-121. Photolysis of tetrachloro-4-iodopyridine **261** in benzene.

78 **309**, 40%

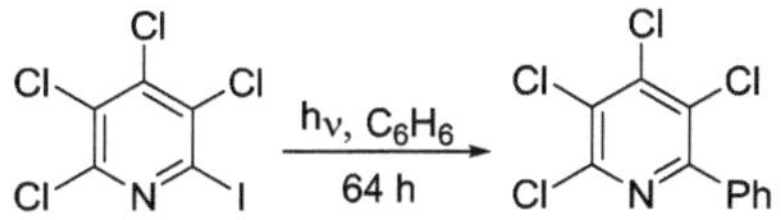

Scheme 3-122. Photolysis of tetrachloro-2-iodopyridine **78** in benzene.

Scheme 3-123. Photolysis of tetrachloro-3-iodopyridine **310** in benzene.

Photolysis of 4-aryl and heteroarylthiotetrachloropyridines **38e** and **312** have been leaded to cyclization at 3-position of pyridine ring and formation corresponding ring-fused systems **313-317** (Scheme **3-124**). Also photolysis of 4-aryloxy and 4-arylaminotetrachloropyridines, and 2-aryloxy and 2-arylaminotetrachloropyridines have been gave corresponding ring-fused products (Schemes **3-125** and **3-126**) [82].

Scheme 3-124. Photolysis of 4-aryl and heteroarylthiotetrachloropyridines **38e** and **312**.

Scheme 3-125. Photolysis of 4-aryloxy and arylaminotetrachloropyridines **15a** and **34g**.

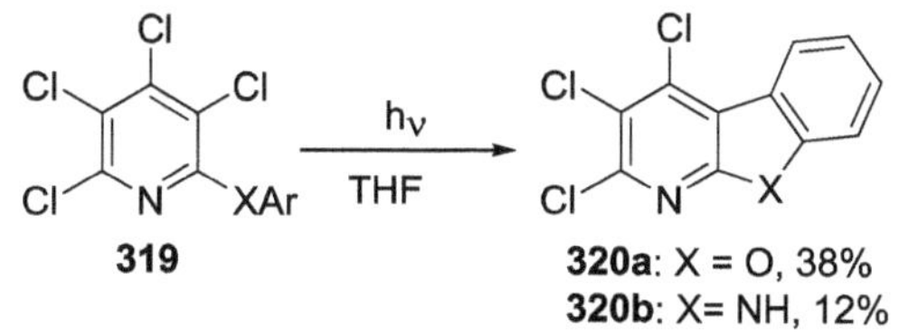

Scheme 3-126. Photolysis of 2-aryloxy and arylaminotetrachloropyridines **319**.

10. ORGANOMETALLIC REAGENTS OF PERCHLOROPYRIDINE

Pentachloropyridine reacted with magnesium in THF at -10°C and produced tetrachloro-4-pyridylmagnesium chloride **321**. The reaction of pentachloropyridine with magnesium is more selective than its reactions with organolithium reagents and therefore Grignard reagent derived from pentachloropyridine is probably the preferred organometallic reagent for the synthesis of 4-substituted tetrachloropyridine derivatives (Table **3-3**) [6].

Table 3-3. Products obtained from tetrachloro-4-pyridylmagnesium chloride 321.

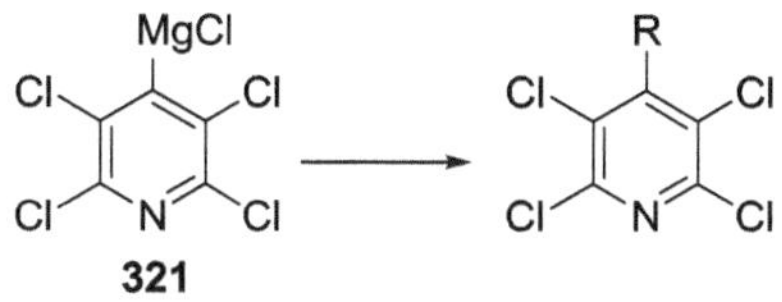

Code	R	Reagent	Yield (%)	Ref.
33	H	Acid	46.5, 88	[6, 89]
219	CO_2H	CO_2	14, 35-40	[6, 89]
322	CHMeOH	MeCHO	30	[6]
323	CPh_2OH	Ph_2CO	42	[90]
195b	Et	EtI	54	[91]
263	C_5Cl_4N	C_5Cl_5N	32	[91]
324	$SiMe_3$	$ClSiMe_3$	80	[90, 92, 93]
325	$SiPh_3$	$ClSiPh_3$	50	[91, 93]
326	$SiMePh_2$	$ClSiMePh_2$	52	[93]
327	$SiMe_2Ph$	$ClSiM_2Ph$	65	[92, 93]
328	$SiPh_2(CH=CH_2)$	$ClSiPh_2(CH=CH_2)$	35	[93]
329	$SiMe_2H$	$ClSiMe_2H$	75	[92, 93]
330	SiMePhH	ClSiMePhH	55	[93]

(Table 3-3) cont.....

Code	R	Reagent	Yield (%)	Ref.
331	$SiPh_2H$	$ClSiPh_2H$	61	[93]
332	$Si(C_5Cl_4N)R_2{}^a$	Cl_2SiR_2	40	[93]
333	$Si(C_5Cl_4N)_2R^a$	Cl_3SiR	40-50	[93]

[a] R = tetrachloro-4-pyridyl

Pentachloropyridine has been underwent metal-halogen exchange reaction on reaction with methyl- [6, 91] *n*-butyl- [89, 91, 92, 94, 95] and phenyllithium [6, 91]. Reaction of pentachloropyridine with *n*-butyllithium is solvent dependent. Tetrachloro-2-pyridyl lithium obtained as major product in hydrocarbon solvents such as benzene or methylcyclohexane and tetrachloro-4-pyridyl lithium produced at ether in 78% yield. Mixture of products have been obtained from reaction of tetrachloro-4-pyridyl lithium **334** with benzonitrile (Scheme **3-127**) [96, 97]. Some reactions of tetrachloro-4-pyridyl-lithium **334** are summarized in Table **3-4**.

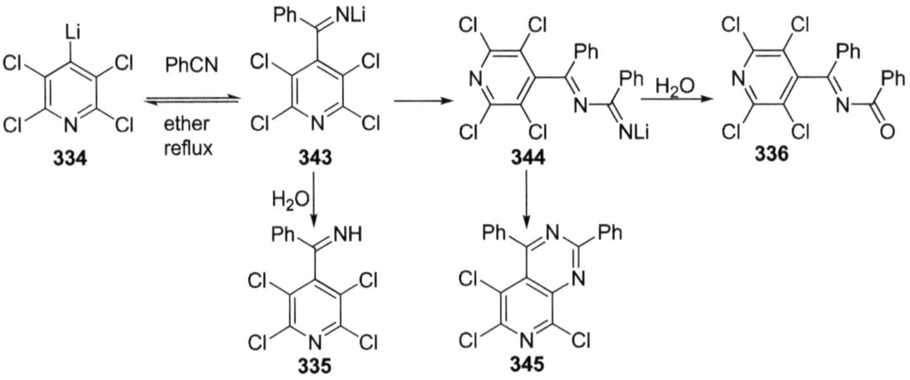

Scheme 3-127. Reaction of tetrachloro-4-pyridyl lithium **334** with benzonitrile.

Table 3-4. Products obtained from tetrachloro-4-pyridyllithium 334.

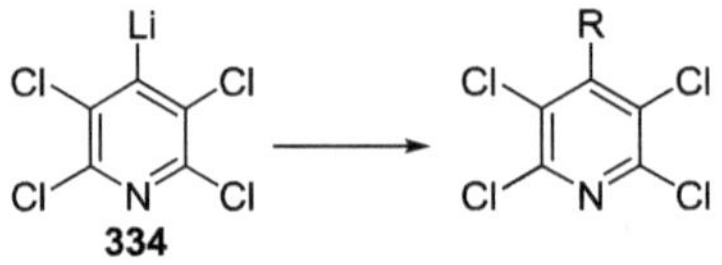

Code	R	Reagent	Yield (%)	Ref.
33	H	Acid	-	[89]
195a	Me	Me_2SO_4	64	[98]
219	CO_2H	CO2	69[a], 86	[99, 100]
323	CPh_2OH	Ph_2CO	65	[90]

(Table 3-4) cont.....

Code	R	Reagent	Yield (%)	Ref.
335	CPh=NH	PhCN	-	[96, 97]
336	CPh=NCOPh	PhCN	-	[96, 97]
324	$SiMe_3$	$ClSiMe_3$	-	[90 - 92]
329	SiMe2H	$ClSiMe_2H$	-	[92]
327	SiMe2Ph	$ClSiMe_2Ph$	-	[92]
263	C5Cl4N	$TiCl_4$	-	[101]
337	HgC5Cl4N	$HgCl_2$	12	[89]
338	HgCl	$HgCl_2$	-	[89]
339	PPh_2	$ClPPh_2$	57	[102]
340	$PPh(C_5Cl_4N)$	Cl_2PPh	52	[102]
341	$P(C_5Cl_4N)_2$	PCl_3	40	[102]
342	Cu	Cu_2I_2 or MeCu	-	[94, 103]

[a] A mixture of tetrachloro-4-carboxypyridine (85-90%), ahd tetrachloro-2-carboxypyridine (10-15%).

Tetrachloro-4-pyridyl copper **342** can be prepared by reaction of both tetrachloro-4-pyridyl lithium and the corresponding Gringard reagent with CuCl or CuI [94, 103 - 105], by reaction of lithium compound with MeCu [94], or by reaction of 2,3,5,6-tetrachloropyridine [94, 105] or tetrachloro-4-iodopyridine [94] with Me_2CuLi. Its reactions with electrophilic compounds produced 4-substituted tetrachloropyridines **195b** [103], **346** [103, 104], **347** [105], **33** and **241c** [103], **348** [106], **349** [94] and **350** [94, 104] (Scheme **3-128**).

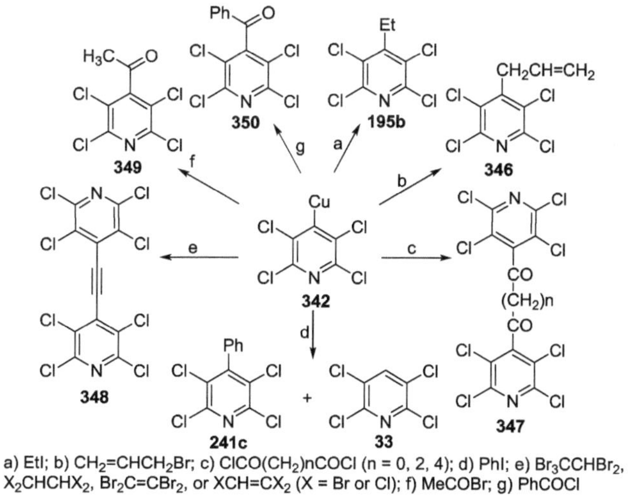

349
350
195b
346
342
348
241c
33
347
a) EtI; b) CH2=CHCH2Br; c) ClCO(CH2)nCOCl (n = 0, 2, 4); d) PhI; e) Br3CCHBr2, X2CHCHX2, Br2C=CBr2, or XCH=CX2 (X = Br or Cl); f) MeCOBr; g) PhCOCl

Scheme 3-128. Reactions of tetrachloro-4-pyridyl copper **342**.

Efforting for direct preparation of tetrachloro-4-pyridyl copper from pentachloropyridine at the presence copper leads to formation of mixture of products including 2,3,4,5-tetrachloropyridine, 2,3,4,6-tetrachloropyridine, 2,3,5,6-tetrachloropyridine, and tetrachloro-4-dimethylaminopyridine (Scheme 3-129) [107].

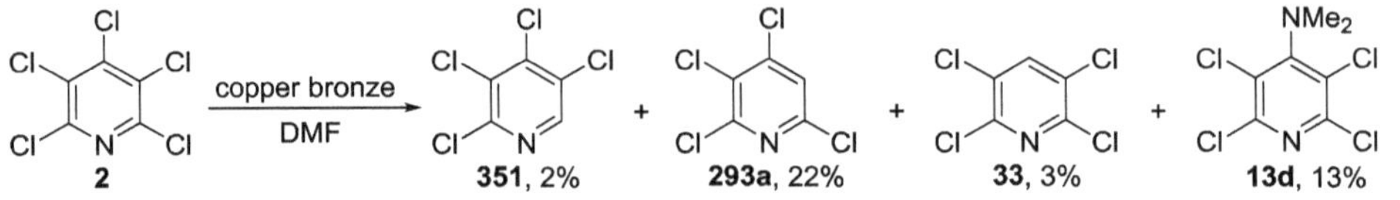

Scheme 3-129. Reaction of pentacloropyridine **2** with copper bronze.

Tetrachloropyridines obtained from above reaction are susceptible nucleophilic substitution reactions, so that reactions of 2,3,5,6-tetrachloropyridine **33** [108, 109], 2,3,4,5-tetrachloropyridine **330** [6, 109 - 115], and 2,3,4,6-tetrachloropyridine **293a** [116] carried out at α-position (Scheme **3-130**), both α- and γ-positions (Scheme **3-131**) and α- and γ-positions (Scheme **3-132**) than ring nitrogen, respectively. 2,3,5,6-tetrachloropyridine can be used as a precursor for preparation of pentachloropyridine at the presence of polyhalomethanes as a halogenation sources (Scheme **3-133**) [117].

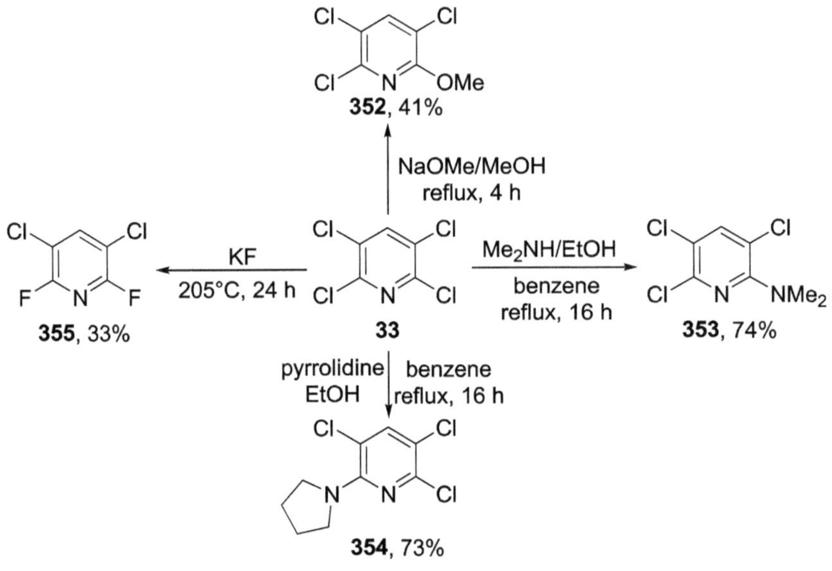

Scheme 3-130. Nucleophilic substitution reactions of 2,3,5,6-tetrachloropyridine **33**.

a) NaOMe, MeOH, 70-80°C; b) NaOEt, EtOH, reflux; c) NaSMe, monoglyme, reflux; d) KSMe, EtOH, reflux; e) NaSH, EtOH, 65°C; f) aq. NH$_3$ under pressure, 180°C or NH$_3$, DMSO; g) NaCH(CO$_2$Et)$_2$, EtOH, reflux; h) NaOMe, MeOH, under pressure, 200-250°C; i) aq. NaOH, reflux

Scheme 3-131. Nucleophilic reaction of 2,3,4,5-tetrachloropyridine **330**.

Scheme 3-132. Nucleophilic reaction of 2,3,4,6-tetrachloropyridine **293a**.

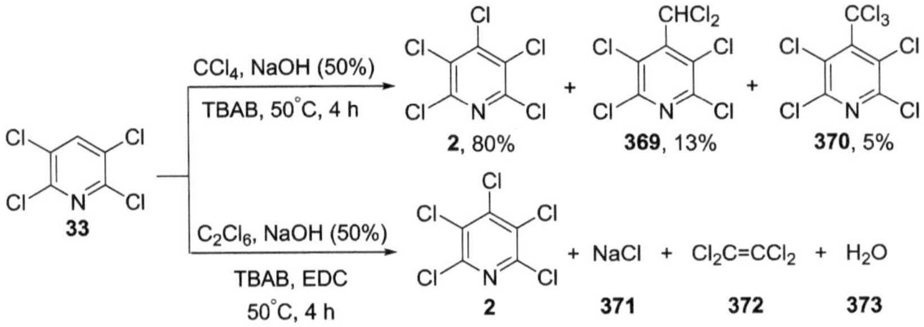

Scheme 3-133. Chlorination of 2,3,5,6-tetrachloropyridine **33**.

REFERENCES

[1] Sell, W.J.; Dootson, F.W. XCVIII.—Studies on citrazinic acid. Part V. *J. Chem. Soc. Trans.*, **1897**, *71*, 1068-1084.
[http://dx.doi.org/10.1039/CT8977101068]

[2] Sell, W.J.; Dootson, F.W. XLV.—The chlorine derivatives of pyridine. Part I. *J. Chem. Soc. Trans.*, **1898**, *73*, 432-441.
[http://dx.doi.org/10.1039/CT8987300432]

[3] Ager, E.; Suschitzky, H. Reactions of polyhalogenopyridines with methyl fluorosulphonate. *J. Fluor. Chem.*, **1973**, *3*(2), 230-232.
[http://dx.doi.org/10.1016/S0022-1139(00)84167-6]

[4] Ager, E.; Suschitzky, H. Polyhalogeno-aromatic compounds. Part XXV. Quaternisation of polyhalogenopyridines and reactions of the pyridinium salts. *J. Chem. Soc., Perkin Trans. 1*, **1973**, 2839-2841.
[http://dx.doi.org/10.1039/p19730002839]

[5] Chivers, G.; Suschitzky, H. Polyhalogeno-aromatic compounds. Part XXI. A novel reagent system for the N-oxidation of weakly basic N-heteroaromatic compounds. *J. Chem. Soc. C: Organ.*, **1971**, 2867-2871.

[6] Suschitzky, H., Ed. *Polychloroaromatic compounds*; Plenum Press: London, New York, **1974**.

[7] Kyriacou, D. *Method for the preparation of tetra-halo-4-(alkylsulfonyl) pyridines*; Google Patents, **1974**.

[8] Schmidt, A.; Mordhorst, T. Synthesis of pyridine-thioethers *via* mono-and tricationic pyridinium salts. *Z. Naturforsch. B,* **2005**, *60*(6), 683-687.
[http://dx.doi.org/10.1515/znb-2005-0613]

[9] Matolcsy, G.; Nádasy, M.; Andriska, V. *Pesticide chemistry*; Elsevier, **1988**, Vol. 32, .

[10] Ranjbar-Karimi, R.; Davoodian, T.; Mehrabi, H. Utility of pentachloropyridine in organic synthesis. *Journal of the Iranian Chemical Society,* **2020**.

[11] Chambers, R. D.; Hutchinson, J.; Musgrave, W. K. R. 691. Polyfluoro-heterocyclic compounds. Part I. The preparation of fluoro-, chlorofluoro-, and chlorofluorohydro-pyridines. *J. Chem. Soc. (Resumed),* **1964**, (0), 3573-3576.

[12] den Hertog, H., Jr; Wibaut, J. On the bromination of pyridine in the gaseous phase at elevated temperatures. A new method for the preparation of 2-bromopyridine and 2, 6-dibromopyridine. *Recl. Trav. Chim. Pays Bas,* **1932**, *51*(4), 381-388.
[http://dx.doi.org/10.1002/recl.19320510412]

[13]   Banks, R. E.; Haszeldine, R. N.; Latham, J. V.; Young, I. M. 95. Heterocyclic polyfluoro-compounds. Part VI. Preparation of pentafluoropyridine and chlorofluoropyridines from pentachloropyridine. *J. Chem. Soc. (Resumed)*, **1965**, *0*, 594-597.

[14]   Flowers, W.T.; Haszeldine, R.N.; Majid, S.A. Synthesis and reactions of pentachloropyridine. *Tetrahedron Lett.*, **1967**, *8*(26), 2503-2505.
[http://dx.doi.org/10.1016/S0040-4039(00)90842-6]

[15]   Roedig, A.; Grohe, K. Eine neue Synthese des Perchlorpyridins. *Chem. Ber.*, **1965**, *98*(3), 923-927.
[http://dx.doi.org/10.1002/cber.19650980334]

[16]   Roedig, A.; Märkl, G. Zur Konstitution der verschiedenen Verbindungen $C_5C_{14}O_2$. Über die Perchlorderivate von Cyclopenten-(1)-dion-(3.5), Pyron-(2) und Protoanemonin. *Justus Liebigs Ann. Chem.*, **1960**, *636*(1), 1-18.
[http://dx.doi.org/10.1002/jlac.19606360102]

[17]   Johnson, P.L.; Pearson, N.R.; Schuster, B.; Cobb, J. Synthesis of stable isotopes of auxinic herbicides 4-amino-3,5,6-trichloropicolinic acid and 4-amino-3,6-dichloropicolinic acid. *J. Labelled Comp. Radiopharm.*, **2009**, *52*(9), 382-386.
[http://dx.doi.org/10.1002/jlcr.1613]

[18]   Roberts, S.; Suschitzky, H. Nucleophilic reactions of pentachloropyridine 1-oxide and pentachloropyrine. *Chem. Commun. (Camb.)*, **1967**, (17), 893-894.

[19]   Roberts, S. M.; Suschitzky, H. Polychloroaromatic compounds. Part I. Oxidation of pentachloropyridine and its NN-disubstituted amino-derivatives with peroxyacids. *J. Chem. Soc. C: Organ.*, **1968**, (0), 1537-1541.

[20]   Sell, W.; Dootson, F. LXVI.—Chlorine derivatives of pyridine. Part VI. Orientation of some chloraminopyridines. *J. Chem. Soc. Trans.*, **1900**, *77*, 771-774.
[http://dx.doi.org/10.1039/CT9007700771]

[21]   Den Hertog, H.; Maas, J.; Kolder, C.; Combe, W. The action of acid chlorides on 4-chloro-and 4-hydroxypyridine-n-oxide and some of their derivatives. *Recl. Trav. Chim. Pays Bas*, **1955**, *74*(1), 59-68.
[http://dx.doi.org/10.1002/recl.19550740108]

[22]   Sell, W.; Dootson, F. LXXXII.—Chlorine derivatives of pyridine. Part II. Interaction of ammonia and pentachloropyridine. Constitution of glutazine. *J. Chem. Soc. Trans.*, **1898**, *73*, 777-783.
[http://dx.doi.org/10.1039/CT8987300777]

[23]   Collins, I.; Roberts, S.; Suschitzky, H. Polyhalogeno-aromatic compounds. Part XVI. The preparation and reactions of polyhalogenophenyl-and polyhalogenopyridyl-hydrazines. *J. Chem. Soc. C: Organ.*, **1971**, 167-174.

[24]   Roberts, S.; Suschitzky, H. Polychloroaromatic compounds. Part IV. Oxidation of 2-and 4-N-alkylaminotetrachloropyridines and nucleophilic substitution of tetrachloronitropyridines. *J. Chem. Soc. C: Organ.*, **1968**, 2844-2848.

[25]   Roberts, S.; Suschitzky, H. Polychloroaromatic compounds. Part I. Oxidation of pentachloropyridine and its NN-disubstituted amino-derivatives with peroxyacids. *J. Chem. Soc. C: Organ.*, **1968**, 1537-1541.

[26]   Roedig, A.; Grohe, K.; Klatt, D. Synthese von Pyridinderivaten aus Perchlorpentadiensäurenitril und Alkoholaten. *Chem. Ber.*, **1966**, *99*(9), 2818-2821.
[http://dx.doi.org/10.1002/cber.19660990914]

[27]   Ager, E.; Iddon, B.; Suschitzky, H. Reactions of n-butyl-lithium with 2, 3, 5, 6-tetrachloro-4-mercapto-and 2, 3, 5, 6-tetrachloro-4-methylmercapto-pyridine. *Tetrahedron Lett.*, **1969**, *10*(19), 1507-1510.
[http://dx.doi.org/10.1016/S0040-4039(01)87926-0]

[28]   Ager, E.; Iddon, B.; Suschitzky, H. Polyhalogenoaromatic compounds. Part XI. Some reactions of 2, 3, 5, 6-tetrachloro-4-mercapto-and 2, 3, 5, 6-tetrachloro-4-methylthiopyridine. *J. Chem. Soc. C: Organ.,* **1970**, (1), 193-197.

[29]   Ivashchenko, Y.N.; Moshchitskii, S.; Sologub, L.; Zalesskii, G. The reaction of pentachloropyridine with aromatic amines. *Chem. Heterocycl. Compd.,* **1970**, *6*(7), 895-897.
[http://dx.doi.org/10.1007/BF00471684]

[30]   Spitzner, D. *Methoden der Organischen Chemie*; Thieme: Stuttgart, Germany, **1994**, E7b, .

[31]   Weissberger, A. *E. C. T., The Chemistry of Heterocyclic Compounds, Pyridine and Its Derivatives: Supplement*; Wiley-Interscience: New York, **1974**, Vol. 14, .

[32]   Waterman, K.C.; Streitwieser, A., Jr Pyridinium-1-yl carbons: 1, 2, 3, 3-tetrakis [4-(dimethylamino) pyridinium-1-yl] cyclopropene tetrachloride and 1, 1, 2, 3, 3-pentakis [4-(dimethylamino) pyridinium-1-yl] allylide tetrachloride. *JACS,* **1984**, *106*(13), 3874-3875.
[http://dx.doi.org/10.1021/ja00325a035]

[33]   Schmidt, A.; Kindermann, M.K.; Vainiotalo, P.; Nieger, M. Charge-Separated Modified Nucleobases. On π-Interactions and Hydrogen Bonding of Self-Complementary Cationic and Betainic Uracils. *J. Org. Chem.,* **1999**, *64*(26), 9499-9506.
[http://dx.doi.org/10.1021/jo991125t]

[34]   Schmidt, A. Synthesis and characterization of stable betainic pyrimidinaminides. *J. Heterocycl. Chem.,* **2002**, *39*(5), 949-956.
[http://dx.doi.org/10.1002/jhet.5570390515]

[35]   Weiß, R.; May, R.; Pomrehn, B. Ladung und Potential: Arene als Oxidantien. *Angew. Chem.,* **1996**, *108*(11), 1319-1321.
[http://dx.doi.org/10.1002/ange.19961081118]

[36]   Schmidt, A.; Mordhorst, T. Syntheses and properties of di-and tricationic hetarenium-substituted pyrimidines. *Z. Naturforsch. B,* **2006**, *61*(4), 396-405.
[http://dx.doi.org/10.1515/znb-2006-0405]

[37]   Schmidt, A.; Mordhorst, T.; Nieger, M. Heteroarenium salts in synthesis. Highly functionalized tetra- and pentasubstituted pyridines. *Tetrahedron,* **2006**, *62*(8), 1667-1674.
[http://dx.doi.org/10.1016/j.tet.2005.11.065]

[38]   Schmidt, A.; Mordhorst, T. Synthesis of alkoxy-substituted pyridines from mono- and tricationic pyridinium salts. *Synthesis,* **2005**, *2005*(05), 781-786.
[http://dx.doi.org/10.1055/s-2005-861827]

[39]   Schmidt, A.; Namyslo, J.C.; Mordhorst, T. Reactions of 4-(dimethylamino) pyridinium activated pentachloropyridine with nitrogen nucleophiles and hydride. *Tetrahedron,* **2006**, *62*(29), 6893-6898.
[http://dx.doi.org/10.1016/j.tet.2006.04.091]

[40]   Schmidt, A.; Mordhorst, T.; Habeck, T. Synthesis of new pyridines with oligocations and oxygen nucleophiles. *Org. Lett.,* **2002**, *4*(8), 1375-1377.
[http://dx.doi.org/10.1021/ol0256926] [PMID: 11950366]

[41]   Kukhar', V.P.; Matsnev, V.V.; Pavlenko, N.G.; Pavlenko, A.F. Reaction of aminotetrachloropyridines with sulfur chlorides. *Chem. Heterocycl. Compd.,* **1978**, *14*(10), 1104-1106.
[http://dx.doi.org/10.1007/BF00469950]

[42]   Sologub, L.; Kisilenko, A.; Vdovenko, S. Synthesis and intramolecular electron interactions in tetrachloro-4-pyridylcarbonimidoyl dichloride and its derivatives. *Chem. Heterocycl. Compd.,* **1983**, *19*(6), 641-643.
[http://dx.doi.org/10.1007/BF00523077]

[43]   Mack, A.G.; Suschitzky, H.; Wakefield, B.J. Polyhalogenoaromatic compounds. Part 39. Synthesis of the bromoand lodo-tetrachloropyridines. *J. Chem. Soc., Perkin Trans. 1,* **1979**, 1472-1474.

[http://dx.doi.org/10.1039/p19790001472]

[44] Patai, S. *The chemistry of alkenes*; Interscience: London, **1963**.

[45] Patai, S. *The chemistry of the azido group*; Interscience: London, **1971**.

[46] Bernard, I.; Chivers, G.; Cremlyn, R.; Mootoosamy, K. The synthesis and reactions of some polychloroaromatic azides, sulphonyl azides and sulphonohydrazides. *Aust. J. Chem.*, **1974**, *27*(1), 171-178.
[http://dx.doi.org/10.1071/CH9740171]

[47] Chapyshev, S.V. Regioselective cycloaddition of the dimethyl ester of acetylenedicarboxylic acid to 2,4,6-triazidopyridines. *Chem. Heterocycl. Compd.*, **2001**, *37*(7), 861-866.
[http://dx.doi.org/10.1023/A:1012451508449]

[48] Claridge, P. R.; W. Millar, R.; P. B. Sandall, J.; Thompson, C., Preparation of a series of N-aryl-S-S-diphenylsulfilimines by nucleophilic attack of S,S-diphenyl-sulfilimine on activated halogenoaromatic compounds. *J. Chem. Res. Synop.*, **1999**, (8), 520-520.
[http://dx.doi.org/10.1039/a901862j]

[49] Dainter, R.S.; Julia, L.; Suschitzky, H.; Wakefield, B.J. Polyhalogenoaromatic compounds. Part 48. Reactions of tetrachioro-4-cyanopyridine with mono-and di-functional nucleophiles. *J. Chem. Soc., Perkin Trans. 1,* **1982**, 2897-2900.
[http://dx.doi.org/10.1039/p19820002897]

[50] Ager, E.; Iddon, B.; Suschitzky, H. Polyhalogeno-aromatic compounds. Part XXII. Some reactions of tetrachloro-4-methylsulphonylpyridine and related compounds. *J. Chem. Soc., Perkin Trans. 1,* **1972**, 133-138.
[http://dx.doi.org/10.1039/p19720000133]

[51] Moshchitskii, S.; Sologub, L.; Kovalevskaya, T.; Kisilenko, A. Rearrangement of 2, 3, 5, 6-tetrachloro-4-pyridyl β-hydroxyethyl sulfone. *Chem. Heterocycl. Compd.*, **1978**, *14*(12), 1334-1337.
[http://dx.doi.org/10.1007/BF00487401]

[52] Moshchitskii, S.; Zalesskii, G.; Ivashchenko, Y.N.; Yagupol'skii, L. Chlorination and oxidation of some sulfurcontaining tetrachloropyridine derivatives. *Chem. Heterocycl. Compd.*, **1972**, *8*(8), 988-992.
[http://dx.doi.org/10.1007/BF00476330]

[53] Sipyagin, A.; Pomytkin, I.; Pal'tsun, S.; Aleinikov, N. Reaction of polyhalopyridines 4. Reaction of mercaptopolychloropyridines with fluorine-containing xenon compounds. *Chem. Heterocycl. Compd.*, **1994**, *30*(1), 52-55.
[http://dx.doi.org/10.1007/BF01164732]

[54] Sipyagin, A.; Pal'tsun, S.; Pomytkin, I.; Aleinikov, N. Reactions of polyhalopyridines 5. Reaction of 2, 3, 5, 6-tetrachloro-4-trifluoromethylthiopyridine with nucleophilic reagents. *Chem. Heterocycl. Compd.*, **1994**, *30*(1), 56-59.
[http://dx.doi.org/10.1007/BF01164733]

[55] Moshchitskii, S.; Kovalevskaya, T.; Sologub, L.; Pavlenko, A.; Kukhar, V. Smiles rearrangement of tetrachloropyridyl methyl-hydroxyphenyl sulfone. *Chem. Heterocycl. Compd.*, **1979**, *15*(10), 1085-1088.
[http://dx.doi.org/10.1007/BF00471904]

[56] Domenico, P. *Polyhalo-4-pyridine sulfen and sulfonamides*; Google Patents, **1974**.

[57] Sologub, L.; Moshchitskii, S.; Ivashchenko, Y.N.; Levchuk, Y.N. Reaction of 2, 3, 5, 6-tetrachloropyridine-4-sulfenyl chloride with olefins. *Chem. Heterocycl. Compd.*, **1972**, *8*(4), 468-472.
[http://dx.doi.org/10.1007/BF00477425]

[58] Moshchitskii, S.; Sologub, L.; Ivashchenko, Y.N.; Yagupol'skii, L. Reaction of 2, 3, 5, 6-tetrachlor--4-pyridyl vinyl sulfone with nucleophilic agents. *Chem. Heterocycl. Compd.*, **1972**, *8*(12), 1482-1485.
[http://dx.doi.org/10.1007/BF00471835]

[59] Ranjbar-Karimi, R.; Poorfreidoni, A. 4-Phenylsulfonyl-2,3,5,6-tetrachloropyridine: synthesis and synthetic utility. *J. Iran. Chem. Soc.,* **2017**, *14*(4), 933-941.
[http://dx.doi.org/10.1007/s13738-016-1043-3]

[60] Sipyagin, A.; Kolchanov, V.; Lebedev, A.; Karakhanova, N. Reactions of polyhalogenopyridines. 14. Reaction of isomeric dichlorocyanopyridines and pentachloropyridine with potassium ethylxanthate. *Chem. Heterocycl. Compd.,* **1997**, *33*(11), 1306-1314.
[http://dx.doi.org/10.1007/BF02320333]

[61] Sipyagin, A.; Kolchanov, V.; Aliev, Z.; Karakhanova, N.; Lebedev, A. Reactions of polyhalogenopyridines. 15. Reaction of isomeric tetrachlorocyanopyridines and pentachloropyridine with potassium isopropyltrithiocarbonate. *Chem. Heterocycl. Compd.,* **1998**, *34*(3), 297-307.
[http://dx.doi.org/10.1007/BF02290720]

[62] Testaferri, L.; Tiecco, M.; Tingoli, M.; Bartoli, D.; Massoli, A. The reactions of some halogenated pyridines with methoxide and methanethiolate ions in dimethylformamide. *Tetrahedron,* **1985**, *41*(7), 1373-1384.
[http://dx.doi.org/10.1016/S0040-4020(01)96539-1]

[63] Domenico, P. *Halopyridyl thiocyanates*; Google Patents, **1974**.

[64] Orvik, J.A.; Fung, A.P.; Love, J.; Dietsche, T.J. *Preparation of 2-cyano-6-chloropyridine compounds*; Google Patents, **1988**.

[65] Ivashchenko, Y.N.; Moshchitskii, S.; Eliseeva, A. Reactions of pentachloropyridine with organomagnesium compounds. *Chem. Heterocycl. Compd.,* **1970**, *6*(1), 54-56.
[http://dx.doi.org/10.1007/BF00475424]

[66] Moran, D.; Patel, M.N.; Tahir, N.A.; Wakefield, B.J. Polyhalogenoaromatic compounds. Part XXXIV. Reactions of pentachloropyridine and 3, 5-dichlorotrifluoropyridine with aliphatic diamines. *J. Chem. Soc., Perkin Trans. 1,* **1974**, 2310-2313.
[http://dx.doi.org/10.1039/p19740002310]

[67] Poorfreidoni, A.; Ranjbar-Karimi, R.; Kia, R. Regiochemistry of nucleophilic substitution of pentachloropyridine with N and O bidentate nucleophiles. *New J. Chem.,* **2015**, *39*(6), 4398-4406.
[http://dx.doi.org/10.1039/C5NJ00418G]

[68] Darehkordi, A.; Fazli-Zafarani, S.M.; Kamali, M. Direct Synthesis of Trichloro-thiazolo [3, 2-a] pyrimidine and Thiazolo [2, 3-b] quinazoline Derivatives. *J. Heterocycl. Chem.,* **2017**, *54*(4), 2287-2296.
[http://dx.doi.org/10.1002/jhet.2816]

[69] Ranjbar-Karimi, R.; Davodian, T.; Mehrabi, H. Reactions of pyridin-2-ol, pyridin-3-ol, and pyridin--ol with pentafluoro-and pentachloropyridine. *Chem. Heterocycl. Compd.,* **2017**, *53*(12), 1330-1334.
[http://dx.doi.org/10.1007/s10593-018-2213-2]

[70] Davodian, T.; Ranjbar-Karimi, R.; Mehrabi, H. Synthesis of diheteroaryl sulfides *via* chemoselective reaction of 4, 6-diaminopyrimidine-2 (1H)-thione with haloheteroaryl compounds. *Chem. Heterocycl. Compd.,* **2017**, *53*(10), 1120-1123.
[http://dx.doi.org/10.1007/s10593-017-2181-y]

[71] Moshchitskii, S.; Zalesskii, G.; Pavlenko, A.; Ivashchenko, Y.N. Some reactions of diethyl 2, 3, 5, 6-tetrachloropyridin-4-ylmalonate. *Chem. Heterocycl. Compd.,* **1970**, *6*(6), 731-734.
[http://dx.doi.org/10.1007/BF00470529]

[72] Moshchitskii, S.; Pavlenko, A.; Zalesskii, G. Reaction of pent achloropyridine with sodioacetoacetic ester. *Chem. Heterocycl. Compd.,* **1978**, *14*(7), 765-769.
[http://dx.doi.org/10.1007/BF00471647]

[73] Suschitzky, H.; Wakefield, B.J.; Walocha, K.; Hughes, N.; Nelson, A.J. Polyhalogenoaromatic compounds. Part 49. Synthesis of carbolines by the reaction of enamines with tetrachloro--cyanopyridine. *J. Chem. Soc., Perkin Trans. 1,* **1983**, 637-641.

[http://dx.doi.org/10.1039/p19830000637]

[74]　Fairlamb, I.J. Regioselective (site-selective) functionalization of unsaturated halogenated nitrogen, oxygen and sulfur heterocycles by Pd-catalysed cross-couplings and direct arylation processes. *Chem. Soc. Rev.,* **2007**, *36*(7), 1036-1045.
[http://dx.doi.org/10.1039/b611177g] [PMID: 17576472]

[75]　Rossi, R.; Bellina, F.; Lessi, M. Selective Palladium-Catalyzed Suzuki–Miyaura Reactions of Polyhalogenated Heteroarenes. *Adv. Synth. Catal.,* **2012**, *354*(7), 1181-1255.
[http://dx.doi.org/10.1002/adsc.201100942]

[76]　Hussain, M.; Hung, N.T.; Khera, R.A.; Malik, I.; Zinad, D.S.; Langer, P. Synthesis of Aryl-substituted pyrimidines by site-selective suzuki–miyura cross-coupling reactions of 2, 4, 5, 6-tetrachloropyrimidine. *Adv. Synth. Catal.,* **2010**, *352*(9), 1429-1433.
[http://dx.doi.org/10.1002/adsc.201000020]

[77]　Mitsudo, K.; Shimohara, S.; Mizoguchi, J.; Mandai, H.; Suga, S. Synthesis of nitrogen-bridged terthiophenes by tandem Buchwald-Hartwig coupling and their properties. *Org. Lett.,* **2012**, *14*(11), 2702-2705.
[http://dx.doi.org/10.1021/ol300887t] [PMID: 22594835]

[78]　Ehlers, P.; Hakobyan, A.; Neubauer, A.; Lochbrunner, S.; Langer, P. Tetraalkynylated and tetraalkenylated benzenes and pyridines: synthesis and photophysical properties. *Adv. Synth. Catal.,* **2013**, *355*(9), 1849-1858.
[http://dx.doi.org/10.1002/adsc.201300201]

[79]　Reimann, S.; Ehlers, P.; Petrosyan, A.; Kohse, S.; Spannenberg, A.; Surkus, A.E.; Ghochikyan, T.V.; Saghyan, A.S.; Lochbrunner, S.; Kühn, O.; Ludwig, R.; Langer, P. Site selective synthesis of pentaarylpyridines *via* multiple suzuki–miyaura cross-coupling reactions. *Adv. Synth. Catal.,* **2014**, *356*(9), 1987-2008.
[http://dx.doi.org/10.1002/adsc.201400164]

[80]　Ehlers, P.; Neubauer, A.; Lochbrunner, S.; Villinger, A.; Langer, P. Multiple sonogashira reactions of polychlorinated molecules. Synthesis and photophysical properties of the first pentaalkynylpyridines. *Org. Lett.,* **2011**, *13*(7), 1618-1621.
[http://dx.doi.org/10.1021/ol2000183] [PMID: 21355569]

[81]　Ehlers, P.; Petrosyan, A.; Neubauer, A.; Bröse, T.; Lochbrunner, S.; Ghochikyan, T.V.; Saghyan, A.S.; Langer, P. Synthesis of fluorescent 2,3,5,6-tetraalkynylpyridines by site-selective Sonogashira-reactions of 2,3,5,6-tetrachloropyridines. *Org. Biomol. Chem.,* **2014**, *12*(43), 8627-8640.
[http://dx.doi.org/10.1039/C4OB01292E] [PMID: 25247374]

[82]　Bratt, J.; Iddon, B.; Mack, A.G.; Suschitzky, H.; Taylor, J.A.; Wakefield, B.J. Polyhalogenoaromatic compounds. Part 41. Photochemical dehalogenation and arylation reactions of polyhalogenoaromatic and polyhalogenoheteroaromatic compounds. *J. Chem. Soc., Perkin Trans. 1,* **1980**, 648-656.
[http://dx.doi.org/10.1039/p19800000648]

[83]　Chivers, G.; Suschitzky, H. A new method of preparing N-oxides from polyhalogenated N-heteroaromatic compounds. *J. Chem. Soc. Chem. Commun.,* **1971**, (1), 28-29.
[http://dx.doi.org/10.1039/c29710000028]

[84]　Iddon, B.; Suschitzky, H.; Thompson, A.W.; Ager, E. Polyhalogeno-aromatic compounds. Part XXXII. Synthesis and some reactions of tetrachloropyridine-2-thiol and related compounds. *J. Chem. Soc., Perkin Trans. 1,* **1974**, 2300-2307.
[http://dx.doi.org/10.1039/p19740002300]

[85]　Suschitzky, H.; Wakefield, B.J.; Whitten, J.P. Reactions of enamines with pentachloropyridine N-oxide; a novel ring contraction. *J. Chem. Soc. Chem. Commun.,* **1979**, (4), 183-184.
[http://dx.doi.org/10.1039/c39790000183]

[86]　Sipyagin, A.; Kolchanov, V.; Pal'tsun, S. Reactions of polyhalopyridines. 2. New substitution reaction of pentachloropyridine N-oxide. *Chem. Heterocycl. Compd.,* **1993**, *29*(9), 1038-1040.

[http://dx.doi.org/10.1007/BF00534388]

[87]   Sutter, P.; Weis, C. The specificity of reductive dechlorination in the polychloropyridine series. Synthesis of 2, 3, 5-trichloro-and of 2, 3, 5, 6-tetrachloropyridine. *J. Heterocycl. Chem.,* **1980**, *17*(3), 493-496.
[http://dx.doi.org/10.1002/jhet.5570170314]

[88]   Binns, F.; Roberts, S.; Suschitzky, H. Polyhalogenoaromatic compounds. Part XIII. The reduction of pentachloropyridine and derivatives with lithium aluminium hydride and other complex metal hydrides. *J. Chem. Soc. C: Organ.,* **1970**, (10), 1375-1380.

[89]   Cook, J.; Wakefield, B. Polychloroaromatic compounds II. Tetrachloropyridyl derivatives of lithium, magnesium and mercury. *J. Organomet. Chem.,* **1968**, *13*(1), 15-23.
[http://dx.doi.org/10.1016/S0022-328X(00)88851-8]

[90]   Edmondson, R.; Jukes, A.; Gilman, H. Some competitive reactions involving polyhaloaryl-metallic reagents. *J. Organomet. Chem.,* **1970**, *25*(2), 273-276.
[http://dx.doi.org/10.1016/S0022-328X(00)87825-0]

[91]   Dua, S.; Gilman, H. Polyhalo-organometallic and-organometalloidal compounds: XIX. Some reactions of pentachloropyridine with organometallic compounds. *J. Organomet. Chem.,* **1968**, *12*(2), 299-303.
[http://dx.doi.org/10.1016/S0022-328X(00)93851-8]

[92]   Dua, S.; Gilman, H. Polyhalo-organometallic and-organometalloidal compounds XVI. Some derivatives of pentachloropyridine. *J. Organomet. Chem.,* **1968**, *12*(1), 234-236.
[http://dx.doi.org/10.1016/S0022-328X(00)90918-5]

[93]   Dua, S.; Edmondson, R.; Gilman, H. 4-silyltetrachloropyridines. *J. Organomet. Chem.,* **1971**, *27*(1), 33-36.
[http://dx.doi.org/10.1016/S0022-328X(00)82989-7]

[94]   Jukes, A.E.; Dua, S.S.; Gilman, H. Reactions of some (polyhaloaryl)copper compounds with acid chlorides and chlorosilanes. *J. Organomet. Chem.,* **1970**, *21*(1), 241-248.
[http://dx.doi.org/10.1016/S0022-328X(00)90617-X]

[95]   Cook, J.; Wakefield, B.; Clayton, C. The reaction of n-butyl-lithium with pentachloropyridine: a solvent effect. *Chem. Commun. (Camb.),* **1967**, (4), 150-151.

[96]   Berry, D.; Cook, J.; Wakefield, B. Reactions of polychloroaryl-lithium compounds with nitriles. *J. Chem. Soc. Chem. Commun.,* **1969**, (21), 1273a-1273a.
[http://dx.doi.org/10.1039/c2969001273a]

[97]   Berry, D.; Cook, J.; Wakefield, B. Polyhalogenoaromatic compounds. Part XXIV. The reaction of chloropyridyl-lithium compounds with nitriles as a route to triazanaphthalenes. *J. Chem. Soc., Perkin Trans. 1,* **1972**, 2190-2192.
[http://dx.doi.org/10.1039/p19720002190]

[98]   Cook, J.; Wakefield, B. Polyhalogenoaromatic compounds. Part VII. Reaction of 4-substituted tetrachloropyridines with n-butyl-lithium, the generation of 2-pyridynes, and their trapping as adducts with furan. *J. Chem. Soc. C: Organ.,* **1969**, (15), 1973-1978.

[99]   Sethi, D.S.; Smith, M.R.; Gilman, H. Carbonation of some perhaloaryllithium compounds. *J. Organomet. Chem.,* **1970**, *24*(3), C41-C42.
[http://dx.doi.org/10.1016/S0022-328X(00)84466-6]

[100] Smith, M.R., Jr; Gilman, H. The cleavage of (perhaloaryl) dimethylsilanes by organolithium compounds. *J. Organomet. Chem.,* **1972**, *37*(1), 35-40.
[http://dx.doi.org/10.1016/S0022-328X(00)89258-X]

[101] Cook, J.; Foulger, N.; Wakefield, B. Polyhalogenoaromatic compounds. Part XXIII. Synthesis and reactions of heptachloro-3-lithio-4, 4'-bipyridyl. *J. Chem. Soc., Perkin Trans. 1,* **1972**, 995-996.
[http://dx.doi.org/10.1039/P19720000995]

[102] Dua, S.; Edmondson, R.; Gilman, H. Polyhaloaryl compounds containing phosphorus. *J. Organomet. Chem.,* **1970**, *24*(3), 703-707.
[http://dx.doi.org/10.1016/S0022-328X(00)84501-5]

[103] Jukes, A.E.; Dua, S.S.; Gilman, H. Reactions of (polyhaloaryl)copper compounds with aryl, alkyl and allyl halides. *J. Organomet. Chem.,* **1970**, *24*(3), 791-796.
[http://dx.doi.org/10.1016/S0022-328X(00)84513-1]

[104] Dua, S.; Jukes, A.; Gilman, H. 2, 3, 5, 6-tetrachloro-4-pyridylcopper and some derivatives. *Organic Preparations and Procedures,* **1969**, *1*(3), 187-191.
[http://dx.doi.org/10.1080/00304946909458378]

[105] Dua, S.S.; Jukes, A.E.; Gilman, H. Polyhalo-organometallic and-organometalloidal compounds: XXIII. Polyhalodiketones from polyhaloarylcopper compounds. *J. Organomet. Chem.,* **1968**, *12*(2), 24-P26.
[http://dx.doi.org/10.1016/S0022-328X(00)93842-7]

[106] Jukes, A.E.; Dua, S.S.; Gilman, H. Polyhalo-organometallic and -organometalloidal compounds XVIII. bis(polyhaloaryl)acetylenes *via* organocopper compounds. *J. Organomet. Chem.,* **1968**, *12*(3), 44-P46.
[http://dx.doi.org/10.1016/S0022-328X(00)88692-1]

[107] Mack, A.G.; Suschitzky, H.; Wakefield, B.J. Polyhalogenoaromatic compounds. Part 43. Inter-and intra-molecular reactions of polychloroaromatic compounds with copper. *J. Chem. Soc., Perkin Trans. 1,* **1980**, 1682-1687.
[http://dx.doi.org/10.1039/p19800001682]

[108] Finger, G.C.; Starr, L.D.; Dickerson, D.; Gutowsky, H.; Hamer, J. Aromatic fluorine compounds. XI. Replacement of chlorine by fluorine in halopyridines. *J. Org. Chem.,* **1963**, *28*(6), 1666-1668.
[http://dx.doi.org/10.1021/jo01041a058]

[109] Berry, D.; Wakefield, B.; Cook, J. Polyhalogenoaromatic compounds. Part XIX. Metal–halogen exchange reactions of n-butyl-lithium with tetrabromo-4-pyridyl and tetrachloro-2-pyridyl derivatives. *J. Chem. Soc. C: Organ.,* **1971**, 1227-1231.

[110] Sell, W.; Dootson, F. I.—The chlorine derivatives of pyridine. Part IV. Constitution of the tetrachloropyridines. *J. Chem. Soc. Trans.,* **1900**, *77*, 1-4.
[http://dx.doi.org/10.1039/CT9007700001]

[111] Kolder, C.; Den Hertog, H. Synthesis and reactivity of 5-chloro-2, 4-dihydroxypyridine. *Recl. Trav. Chim. Pays Bas,* **1953**, *72*(4), 285-295.
[http://dx.doi.org/10.1002/recl.19530720404]

[112] Kolder, C.; Den Hertog, H. Migration of halogen atoms in halogeno-derivatives of 2, 4-dihydroxypyridine (II). *Recl. Trav. Chim. Pays Bas,* **1953**, *72*(10), 853-858.
[http://dx.doi.org/10.1002/recl.19530721005]

[113] Sell, W.; Dootson, F. XLIV.—The chlorine derivatives of pyridine. Part VIII. The interaction of 2: 3: 4: 5-tetrachloropyridine with ethyl sodiomalonate. *J. Chem. Soc. Trans.,* **1903**, *83*, 396-401.
[http://dx.doi.org/10.1039/CT9038300396]

[114] Sell, W.J. CXXVII.—The action of sodium methoxide on 2: 3: 4: 5-tetrachloropyridine. Part I. *J. Chem. Soc. Trans.,* **1912**, *101*, 1193-1196.
[http://dx.doi.org/10.1039/CT9120101193]

[115] Sell, W.J. CCVI.—The action of sodium methoxide on 2: 3: 4: 5-tetrachloropyridine. Part II. *J. Chem. Soc. Trans.,* **1912**, *101*, 1945-1949.
[http://dx.doi.org/10.1039/CT9120101945]

[116] Ager, E.; Chivers, G.; Suschitzky, H. Photolysis of pentachloropyridine and pentachloropyridine 1-oxide. *J. Chem. Soc. Chem. Commun.,* **1972**, (9), 505-506.
[http://dx.doi.org/10.1039/c39720000505]

[117]   Joshi, A.V.; Baidossi, M.; Qafisheh, N.; Chachashvili, E.; Sasson, Y. Mild electrophilic halogenation of chloropyridines using CC_{14} or C_2C_{16} under basic phase transfer conditions. *Tetrahedron Lett.,* **2004**, *45*(26), 5061-5063.
[http://dx.doi.org/10.1016/j.tetlet.2004.04.177]

CHAPTER 4

Perbromopyridines

Abstract: Pentabromopyridine is prepared from 4-hydroxypyridine *via* two pathways. Pentabromopyridine is less active than pentachloro- and pentafluoropyridine toward nucleophilic attack. Its nucleophilic reaction is affected by the hindrance of the bromine atom. Oxidation and methylation of pentabromopyridine give pentabromopyridine-*N*-oxide and *N*-methylbromopyridinium salt. Metal-halogen exchange between pentabromopyridine and *n*-butyl-lithium or magnesium give tetrabromo-4-pyridyl-lithium and tetrabromo-4-pyridylmagnesium bromide. 2,4,6-tribromo-3,5-difluoropyridine is obtained from the bromination of pentafluoropyridine in the reaction with nucleophiles at the C-F bond. Cross-coupling reactions of 2,4,6-tribromo-3,5-difluoropyridine and 3,5-dibromo-2,6-dichloropyridine produced arylated and alkenylpyridines pyridines.

Keywords: 2,3,5,6-Tetrabromo-4-pyridylamidophosphate Esters, 2,3,5,6-Tetrabromo-4-pyridylmethylsulfoxide, 2,4,6-Triazido-3,5-dibromopyridine, 2,4,6-Tribromo-3,5-difluoropyridine, 2,4,6-Tris(triethoxyphosphazenyl)-3,5-dibromopyridine, 2,6-dichloro-3,5-dialkynyl-substituted Pyridines, 2-*N*,N-dialkylaminotetrabromopyridines, 3,5-Dibromo-2,6-dichloropyridine, 3,5-Dibromo-2,6-dichloropyridine, Lithium–bromine Exchange, Nitrotetrabromopyridines, *N*-Methylbromopyridinium Fluorosulphonate, Pentabromopyridine, Pentabromopyridine-*N*-oxide, Suzuki Cross-coupling Reaction, Tetraalkynylpyridines, Tetrabromo-4-pyridyl-lithium, Tetrabromo-4-pyridylmagnesium Bromide, Tetrabromopyridine-4-sulfenyl Chloride, Tetrabromopyridine-4-thiol.

1. SYNTHESIS OF PENTABROMOPYRIDINE

Pentabromopyridine **3** was prepared *via* a two steps method from 4-hydroxypyridine **1** [1]. The reaction of 4-hydroxypyridine with bromine in 80% oleum gives 2,3,5,6-tetrabromo-4-hydroxypyridine **2**, while it converted to pentabromopyridine **3** on treatment with phosphorus oxybromid (Scheme **4-1**). Also, 2,3,5,6-tetrabromo-4-hydroxypyridine was obtained from the reaction of 4-hydroxypyridine with 48% hydrobromic acid, and followed by treatment with bromine in 80% oleum (Scheme **4-1**).

Reza Ranjbar-Karimi & Alireza Poorfreidoni

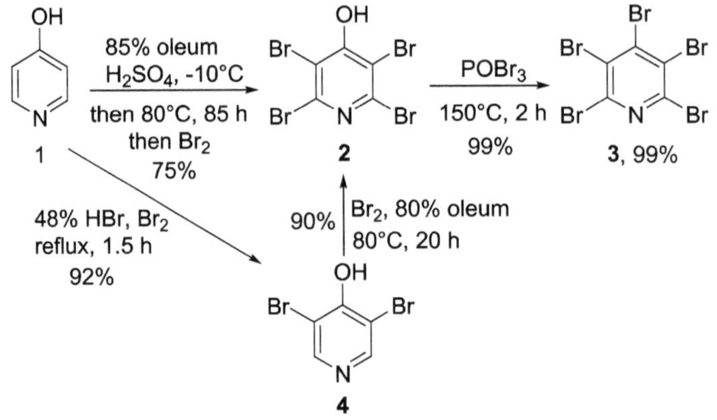

Scheme 4-1. Preparation of pentabromopyridine **3**.

2. NUCLEOPHILIC REACTIONS OF PENTABROMOPYRIDINE

2.1. Reaction of O-centered Nucleophile with Pentabromopyridine

Pentabromopyridine **3** invariably gives a lower proportion of the 4-substituted product with larger nucleophiles [2]. This is due to steric deflection from the 4-position by the larger bromine atoms to the less hindered 2-position, whereas small nucleophiles give 4-substituted products as the major product and 2-substituted products (Scheme **4-2**).

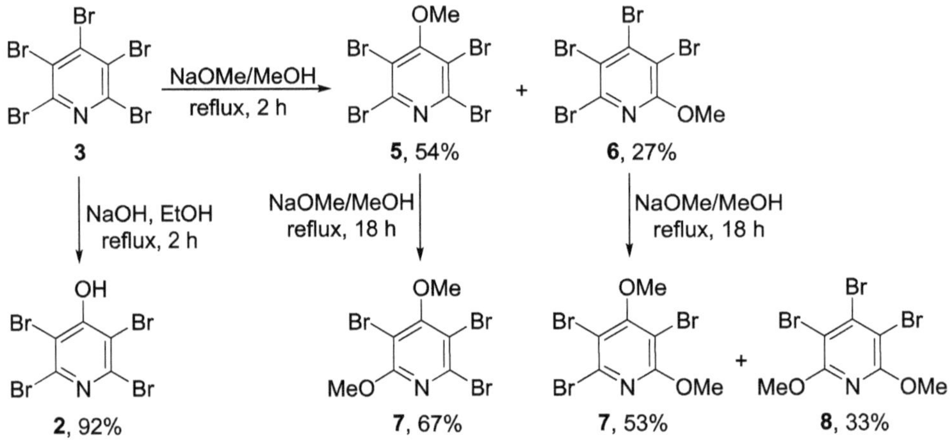

Scheme 4-2. Reaction of pentabromopyridine **3** with sodium methoxide.

2.2. Reaction of N-centered Nucleophile with Pentabromopyridine

Reaction of pentabromopyridine **3** with nitrogen nucleophiles has been carried out at both 2- and 4-positions of pyridine ring depend on the steric hindrance of the nucleophile (Scheme **4-3**) [2].

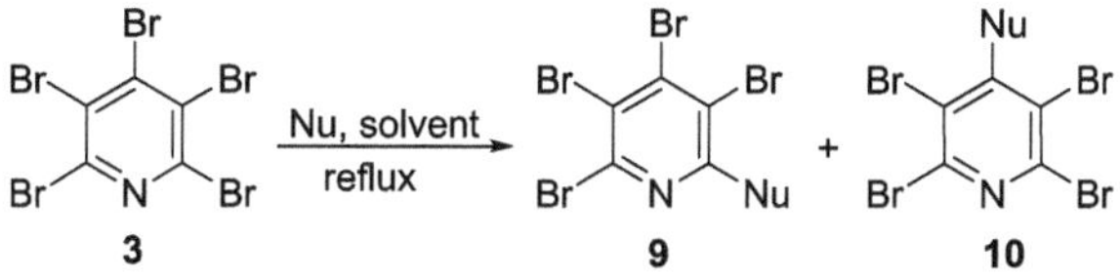

Nu	solvent	reflux		
Me$_2$NH	C$_6$H$_6$	18 h	100%	-
	EtOH	18 h	85%	15%
C$_5$H$_{10}$NH	C$_6$H$_6$	18 h	100%	-
	EtOH	18 h	85%	15%
MeNH$_2$	dioxan	18 h	52%	48%
N$_2$H$_4$.H$_2$O	EtOH	18 h	33%	66%

Scheme 4-3. Reaction of pentabromopyridine **3** with various nucleophiles.

The 2-*N,N*-dialkylaminotetrabromopyridines **9** upon reaction with amines produced the 2,6-bis-(*N,N*-dialkylamino)tribromopyridine **11** as the only product. Whilst sodium hydroxide in reaction with tetrabromo-6-dimethylaminopyridine **9a** was replaced at the 4-position of pyridine ring (Scheme **4-4**) [2]. Piperidine on reaction with tetrabromo-4-methoxy- and 4-piperidinopyridines produced tribromo-4-methoxy-6-piperidinopyridine **13a** and tribromo-4,6-dipiperidinopyridine **13b** *via* replacing at the 2-position of pyridine ring (Scheme **4-5**) [2].

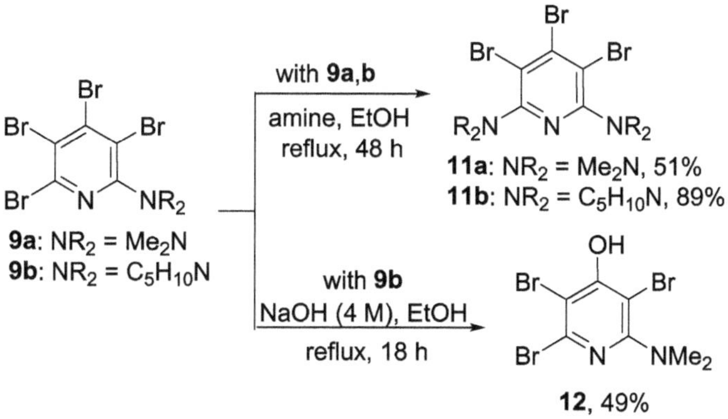

Scheme 4-4. Reaction of 2-alkylaminotetrabromoyridines **9** with various nucleophiles.

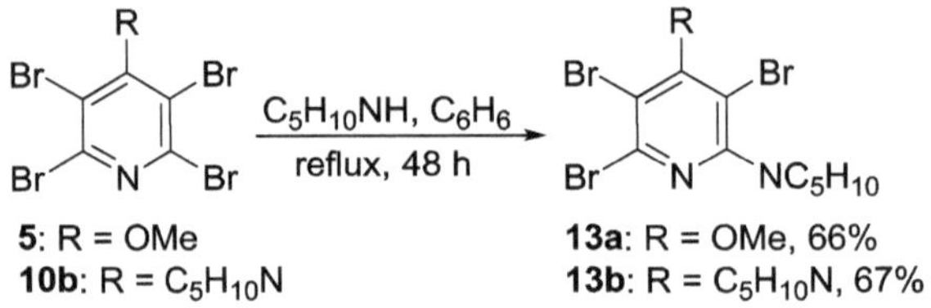

Scheme 4-5. Reaction of tetrabromo-4-methoxy- and -4-piperidinopyridines **5** and **10b** with piperidine.

Amine substituent of 2-*N*,*N*-dialkylaminotetrabromopyridines **9** in the presence of 98% formic acid and 30% hydrogen peroxide underwent oxidation reaction and produced 2-*N*,*N*-dialkylhydroxyaminotetrabromopyridines **14** (Scheme **4-6**) [2]. Oxidation of tetrabromo-4-piperidinopyridine, tetrabromo-4-dimethylamino-pyridine and tetrabromo-6-methylaminopyridine occurred at amine group to give corresponding nitroso and nitro products in the presence of TFA (Schemes **4-7** and **4-8**), while tetrabromo-6-methylaminopyridine using formic acid instead TFA converted to 2-aminotetrabromopyridine (Scheme **4-8**) [2].

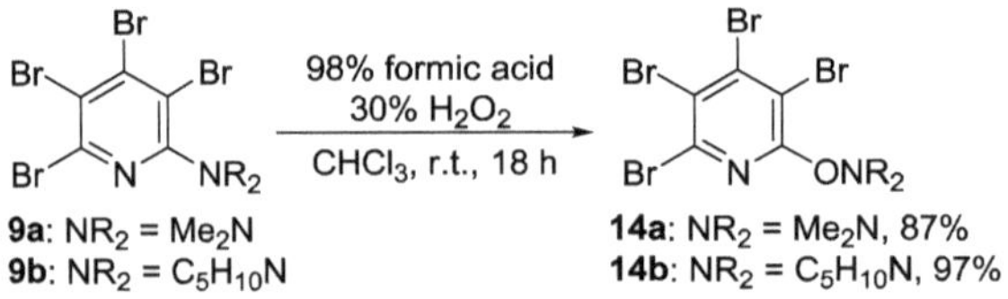

Scheme 4-6. Oxidation of 2-*N*,*N*-dialkylaminopolybromopyridines **9**.

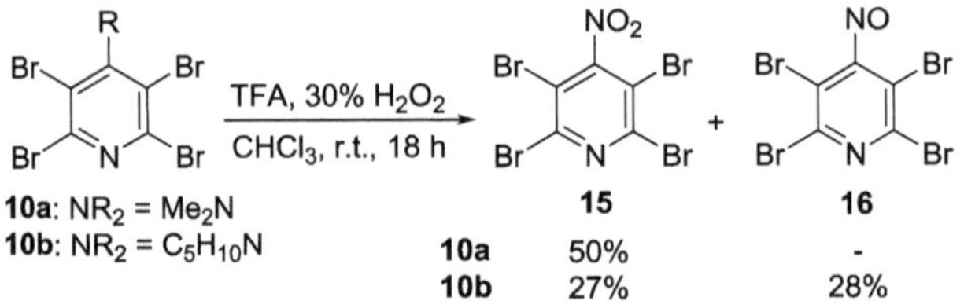

Scheme 4-7. Oxidation of 4-*N*,*N*-dialkylaminopolybromopyridines **10**.

4-nitro and 6-nitrotetrabromopyridine are active toward nucleophilic attack and their reactions with piperidine accomplished with replacement of nitro group with piperidine (Schemes **4-9** and **4-10**) [2].

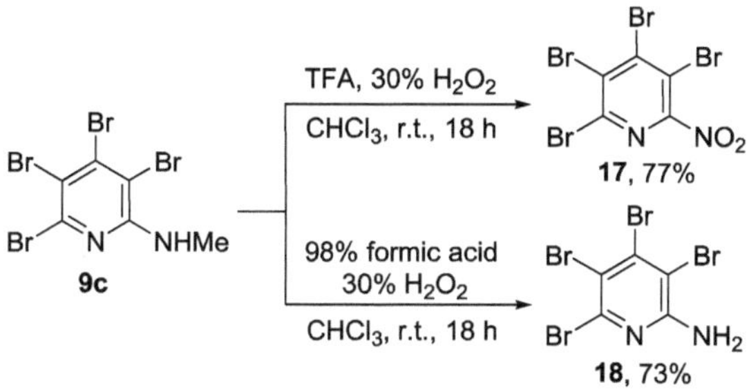

Scheme 4-8. Oxidation of tetrabromo-6-methylaminopyridine **9c**.

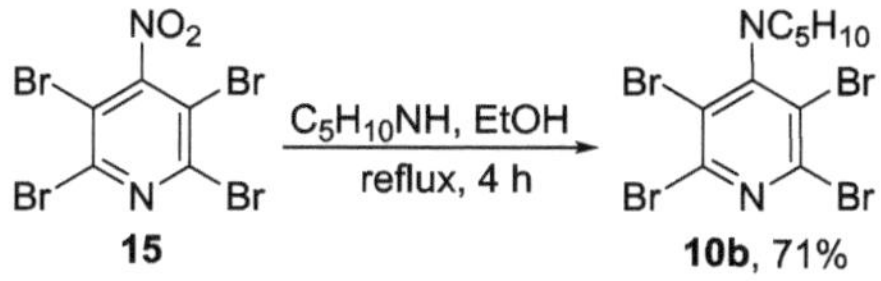

Scheme 4-9. Reaction of piperidine with 4-nitrotetrabromopyridine **15**.

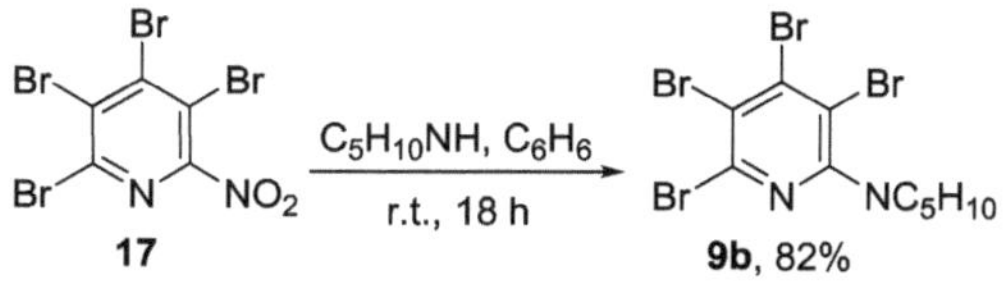

Scheme 4-10. Reaction of piperidine with 6-nitrotetrabromopyridine **17**.

Reaction of pentabromopyridine **3** with sodium azide in DMSO proceeded *via* attack of azide ion at the 4-position to give compound **19** as quantitative (Scheme **4-11**) [3]. Also, it obtained in high yield using 2,3,5,6-tetrabromo-4-pyridyl methylsulfone. Reaction of excess sodium azide with pentabromopyridine gives 2,4,6-triazido-3,5-dibromopyridine **20** (Scheme **4-11**) [3, 4].

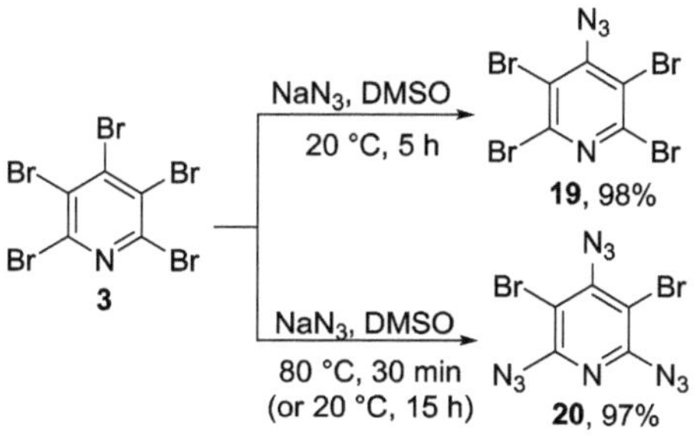

Scheme 4-11. Reaction of pentabromopyridine with sodium azide.

Thermal decomposition of aromatic azides is known to generate nitrenes, which are capable either of conversion to primary amines or of insertion into the C-H bond of hydrocarbons. Reduction of azide **19** with lithium aluminum hydride and its thermolysis with *N,N*-dimethylaniline formed 4-amino-2,3,5,6-tetrabromo-pyridine (Scheme **4-12**) [3]. Reaction of excess cyclohexene with azide **19** produced compound **22** (Scheme **4-12**) *via* the unstable triazoline intermediate **28** (Scheme **4-13**). This azide has been readily carried out the Staudinger reaction with triphenylphosphlne, triethyl phosphite, and triphenyl phosphite (Scheme **4-12**) [3]. The reaction of azide **19** with triphenylphosphine proceeded *via* the relatively stable 4-(triphenylphosphazido)-2,3,5,6-tetrabromopyrldine **24**, which at 118 °C converted to the 4-triphenylphosphazenyl-2,3,5,6-tetrabromopyridine **25** with losing nitrogen (Scheme **4-12**). Treatment of azide **19** with triethyl and triphenyl phosphite has been rapidly performed and hydrolysis of the resulting phosphazenyl compounds with HCl yielded the 2,3,5,6-tetrabromo-4-pyridyl amidophosphate esters **26** and **27** (Scheme **4-12**).

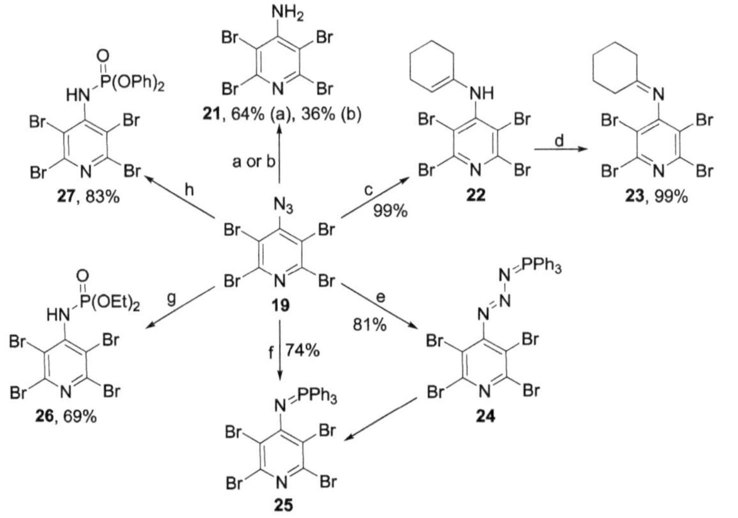

a) LiAlH$_4$, Et$_2$O, reflux, 3 h; b) N,N-dimethylaniline, 165-170°C, 4 h; c) cyclohexene, reflux, 8 h; d) 20°C, 5 h; e) PPh$_3$, Et$_2$O, -10°C, 30 min; f) PPh$_3$, ether, reflux, 4 h; g) P(OEt)$_3$, Et$_2$O; h) P(OPh)$_3$, Et$_2$O.

Scheme 4-12. Various reactions of 4-azidotetrabromopyridine **19**.

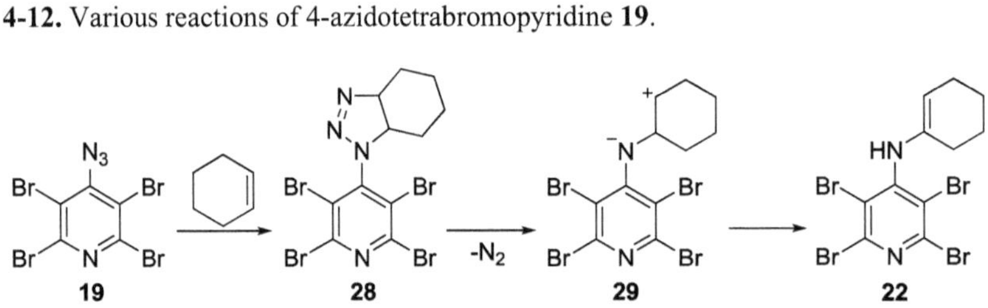

Scheme 4-13. Mechanism of formation compound **22**.

The reaction of triethyl phosphite with azide **20** involved two of the azido groups and gave phosphazenyl compound, which converted to 4-azido-2,6-bis (diethoxyphosphinylamine)-3,5-dibromopyridine **30** by hydrolysis with HCl (Scheme **4-14**). When it is heated, all three azido groups reacted with triethyl phosphite and formed 2,4,6-tris(triethoxyphosphazenyl)-3,5-dibromopyridine **31** (Scheme **4-14**) [3].

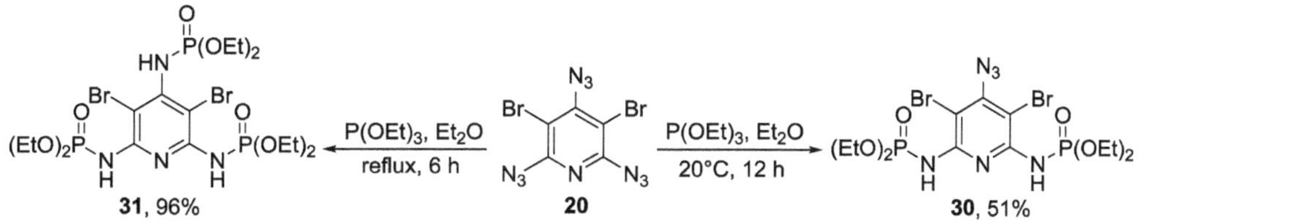

Scheme 4-14. Reaction of 2,4,6-triazido-3,5-dibromopyridine with triethyl phosphite.

In other report, it has been demonstrated that triazide **20** selectively reacted with electron-rich triethyl phosphite at the most electron-deficient azido group of located in the γ-position of the pyridine ring and produced phosphorimidate **32**, which on addition of another molecule of triethyl phosphite gave a mixture of 6-azido-2,4-bis(triethoxyphosphorimino)-3,5-dibromopyridine **33** and its tetrazolo [1,5-*a*] pyridine isomer **34** (Scheme **4-15**) [4]. The mixture on acidic hydrolysis converted to 6-Azido-2,4-bis(diethoxyphosphoramino)-3,5-dibromo-pyridine **35** (Scheme **4-15**).

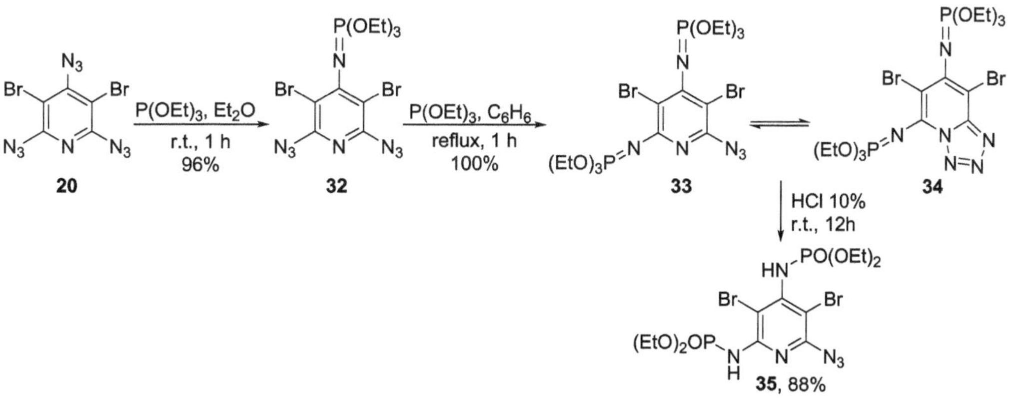

Scheme 4-15. Reaction of 2,4,6-triazido-3,5-dibromopyridine **20** with triethyl phosphite.

2.3. Reaction of S-centered Nucleophile with Pentabromopyridine

2,3,5,6-tetrabromopyridine-4-thiol **36** has been synthesized from the reaction of pentabromopyridine **3** with KSH (Scheme **4-16**). This thiol group has been used as nucleophile in nucleophilic substitution reactions and produced 4-substituted tetrabromopyridines (Schemes **4-17** and **4-18**) [5].

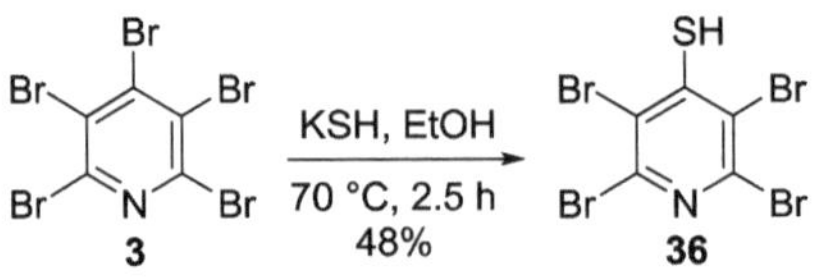

Scheme 4-16. Synthesis of 2,3,5,6-tetrabromopyridine-4-thiol **36**.

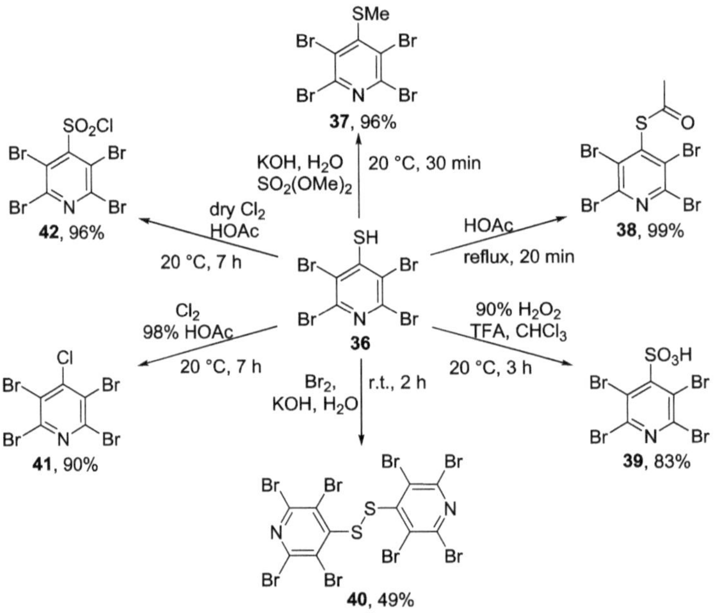

Scheme 4-17. Reactions of 4-mercapto-2,3,5,6-tetrachloropyridine **36**.

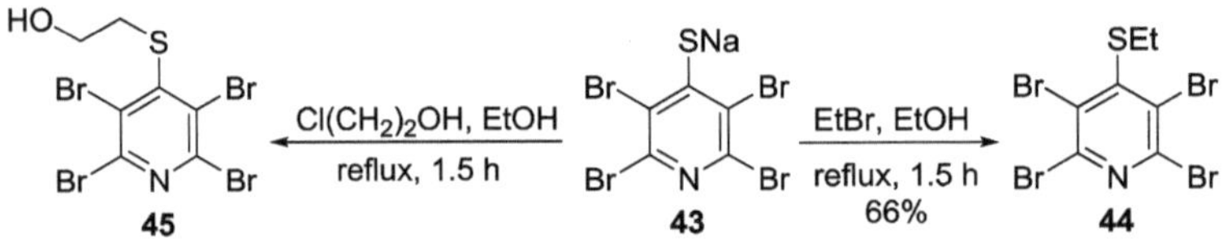

Scheme 4-18. Reactions of sodium 2,3,5,6-tetrabromopyridine-4-thiolate **43**.

Oxidation of 2,3,5,6-tetrabromo-4-pyridyl methyl sulfide **37** with HNO_3 and H_2O_2 gave 2,3,5,6-tetrabromo-4-pyridyl methyl sulfone **46** and 2,3,5,6-tetrabromo-4-pyridyl methyl sulfoxide **47**, respectively (Scheme **4-19**) [5]. Action of dray ammonia gas with 2,3,5,6-tetrabromo-4-pyridyl methyl sulfone **46** gave 4-amin--tetrabromopyridine **21** in 88% yield (Scheme **4-20**) [5].

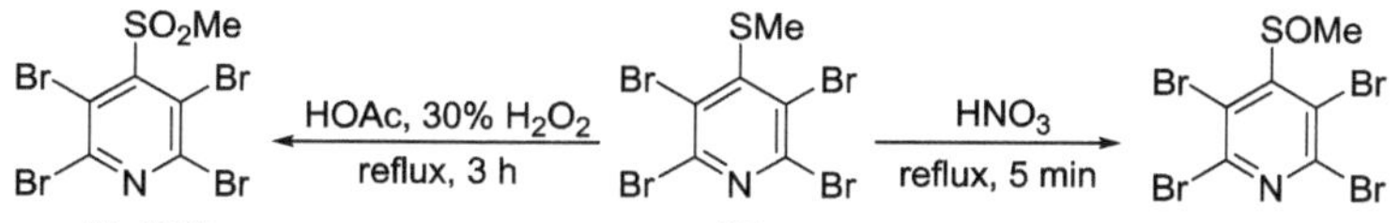

Scheme 4-19. Oxidation of 2,3,5,6-tetrabromo-4-pyridyl methyl sulfide **37**.

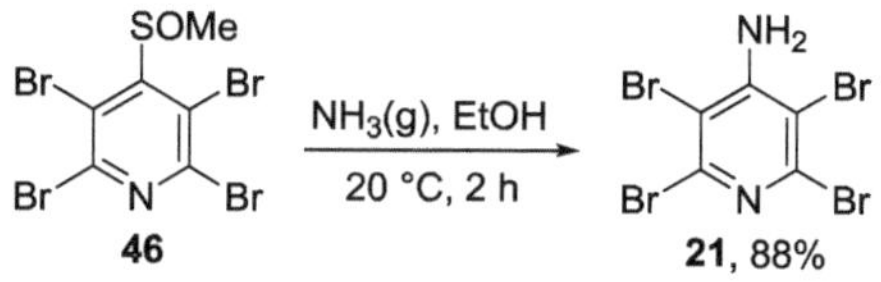

Scheme 4-20. Synthesis of 4-amino-tetrabromopyridine **21**.

2,3,5,6-Tetrabromopyridine-4-sulfenyl chloride **48** has been obtained on treatment of 2,3,5,6-tetrabromopyridine-4-thiol **36** with chlorine (Scheme **4-21**) [5]. This compound reacted with acetone and aniline and formed 2,3,5,6-tetrabromo-4-pyridylthioacetone **49** and 2,3,5,6-tetrabromopyridine-4-sulfenic acid anilide **50** (Scheme **4-21**) [5]. Its reaction with NaCN leads to formation of 2,3,5,6-tetrabromo-4-(thiocyanato) pyridine **51** (Scheme **4-21**) [6].

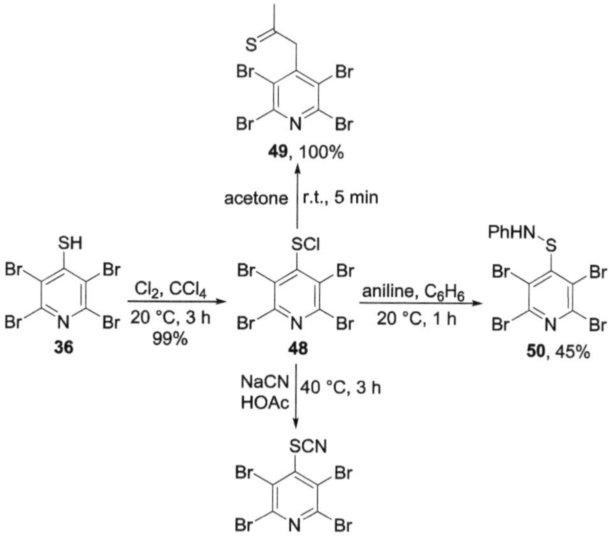

Scheme 4-21. Synthesis and reactions of 2,3,5,6-tetrabromopyridine-4-sulfenyl chloride **48**.

3. ORGANOMETALIC REAGENT OF POLYBROMOPYRIDINES

Metal-halogen exchange between pentabromopyridine **3** and *n*-butyl-lithium or magnesium gave tetrabromo-4-pyridyl-lithium **52** and tetrabromo-4-pyridyl-magnesium bromide **53**, respectively (Scheme **4-22**), which yielded 2,3,5,6-tetrabromopyridine **54** and tetrabromopyridine-4-carboxylic acid **55** on hydrolysis and carboxylation, respectively (Scheme **4-23**) [7]. Thermal elimination of metal halide from the organometallic compounds **52** and **53** lead to formation of tribromo-3-pyridyne intermediate, while trapped as 1,4-adducts in the presence of benzene and p-di-isopropylbenzene (Scheme **4-23**) [7].

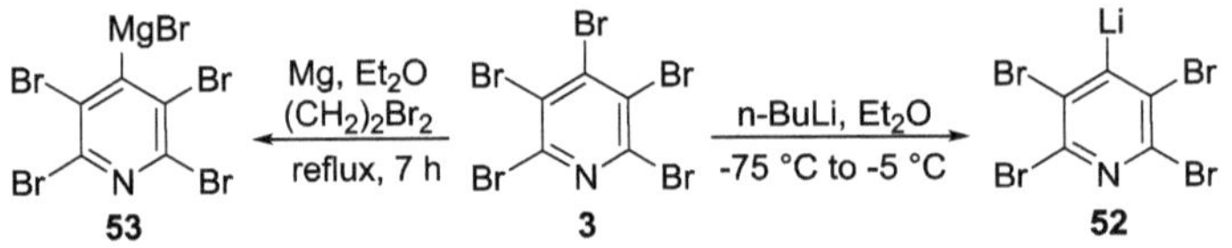

Scheme 4-22. Synthesis of tetrabromo-4-pyridyl-lithium **52** and tetrabromo-4-pyridylmagnesium bromide **53**.

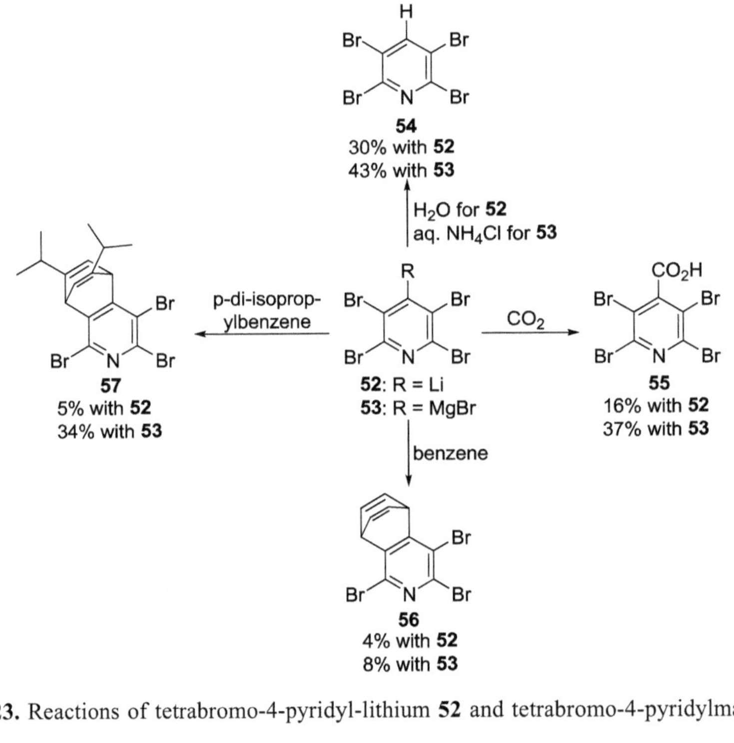

Scheme 4-23. Reactions of tetrabromo-4-pyridyl-lithium **52** and tetrabromo-4-pyridylmagnesium bromide **53**.

4. SALTS OF PENTABROMOPYRIDINE

Pentabromopyridine **3** has been successfully reacted with methyl fluorosulphonate at free solvent condition and gives corresponding *N*-methylated pyridinium fluorosulphonate **59** (Scheme **4-24**) [8, 9]. The strong inductive effect of the positively charged nitrogen atom active the 2(6)-positions of ring toward nucleophilic substitution (Scheme **4-25**) [8].

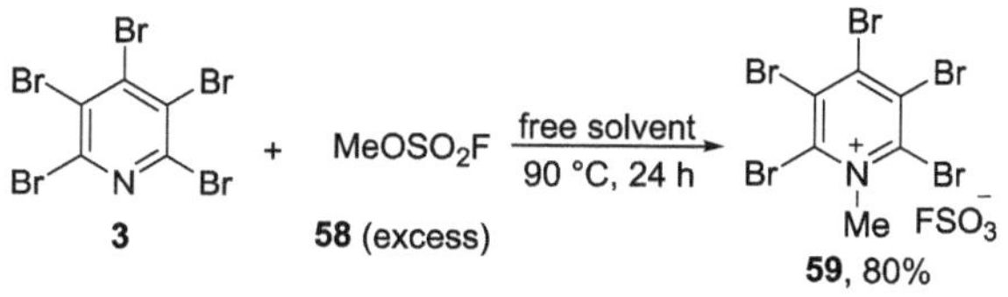

Scheme 4-24. Reactions of pentabromopyridine **3** with methyl fluorosulphonate **58**.

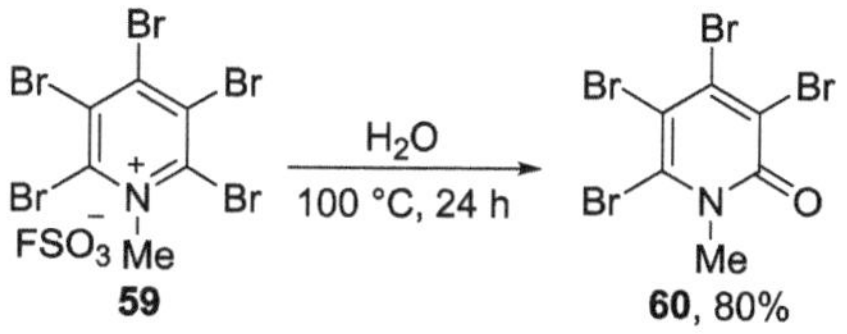

Scheme 4-25. Reactions of *N*-methyl bromopyridinium fluorosulphonate **59** with H_2O.

5. OXIDATION OF PENTABROMOPYRIDINE

N-Oxidation of pentabromopyridine **3** proceeded by its reaction with mixture of trifluoroacetic acid, concentrated sulphuric acid and H_2O_2 90% (Scheme **4-26**) [10].

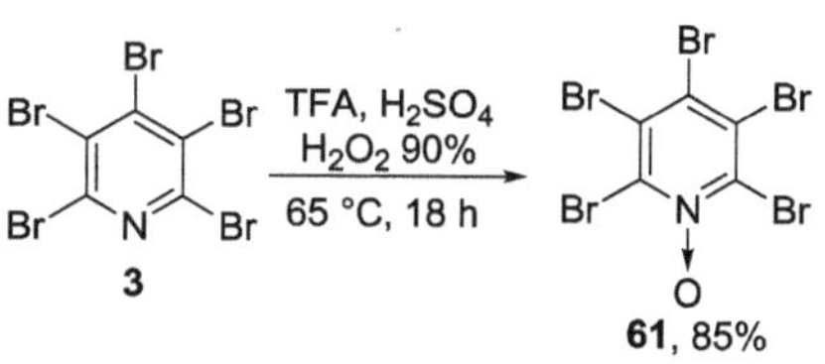

Scheme 4-26. Synthesis of pentabromopyridine-*N*-oxide **61**.

6. PHOTOCHEMICAL REACTIONS OF PENTABROMOPYRIDINE

Pentabromopyridine **3** on photoirradiation gives mainly 2,4,5-tribromopyridine **62** and 2,3,4,6-tetrabromopyridine **63** as side product (Scheme **4-27**) [11].

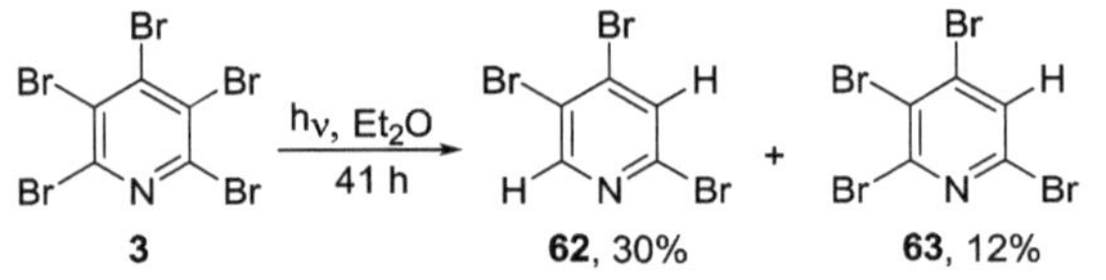

Scheme 4-27. Photolysis of pentabromopyridine **3** in ether.

7. SYNTHESIS AND REACTIONS OF 2,4,6-TRIBROMO-3-5-DIFLUOROPYRIDINE

Reduction of 2,4,6-tribromo-3,5-difluoropyridine **65**, obtained from reaction of pentafluoropyridine **64** with $AlBr_3$/HBr, in the presence of Pd-C/H_2 (Scheme **4-28**) occurred at the α- and γ-position to ring nitrogen and gives 2,5-difluoropyridine **66** (Scheme **4-28**) [12].

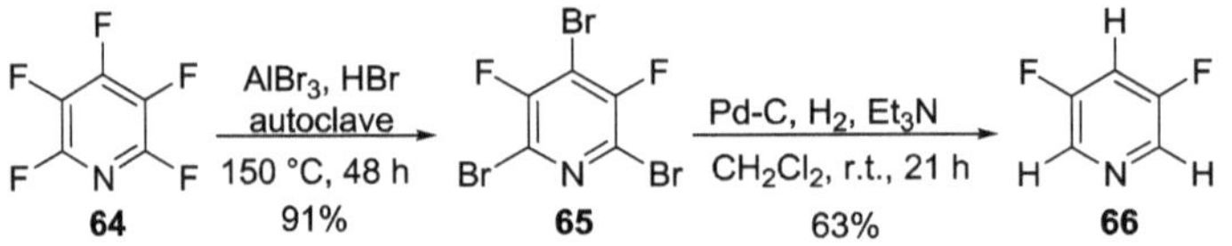

Scheme 4-28. Synthesis and reduction of 2,4,6-tribromo-3,5-difluoropyridine **65**.

Reactions of the tribromo derivative **65** with various nucleophiles depended on nucleophile nature [12], so that harder nucleophiles such as NaOMe and aqueous ammonia replaced displacement of fluorine and softer nucleophiles such as Et_2NH, PhSNa and piperidine replaced of bromine (Scheme **4-29**). Surprisingly, it on reaction with the enolate anion derived from cyclohexanone underwent reduction reactions (Scheme **4-29**).

Compound **65** readily carried out lithium–bromine exchange at 4-position of pyridine ring using *n*-BuLi, which has been produced 4-allyl-2,6-dibromo-3,5-difluoropyridine **77** in reaction with allyl bromide (Scheme **4-30**) [12].

Displacement of bromine in compound **65** has been found to occured readily in palladium-induced processes [12]. Reactions with phenylacetylene or pent-1-yne results in the selective replacement of 2- and 6-bromine atoms, which explained a directing role by the ring nitrogen (Schemes **4-31** and **4-32**).

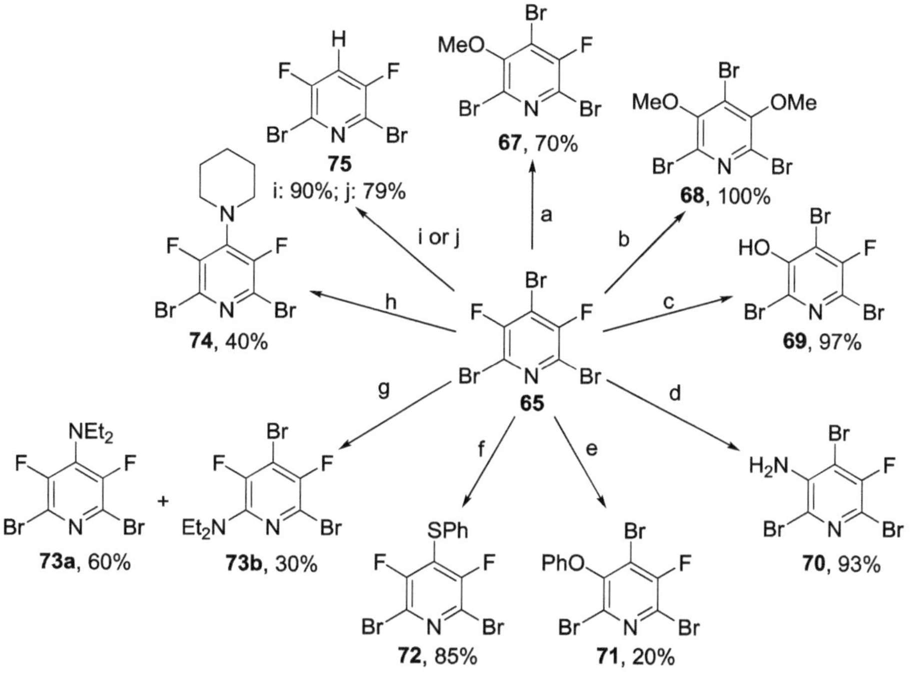

a) NaOMe, MeOH, r.t., 60 h; b) NaOMe (ex.), MeOH, r.t., 48 h; c) KOH, 2-methylpropan-2-ol, reflux, 3 h; d) aq. NH_3, CH_3CN, 75 °C, 72 h; e) NaOPh, Et_2O, N_2, reflux, 23 h; f) PhSH, CH_3CN, Na_2CO_3, reflux, 19 h; g) Et_2NH, 50 C, 95 h; h) piperidine, CH_3CN, reflux, 23 h; i) 2-Trimethylsilyloxypent-2-en-4-one, KF, N_2, CH_3CN,   60°C, 18 h; j) 1-(trimethylsilyloxy)-cyclohexene, KF, N_2, CH_3CN, r.t., 16 h then 60°C, 8 h.

Scheme 4-29. Reaction of various nucleophiles with 2,4,6-tribromo-3,5-difluoropyridine **65**.

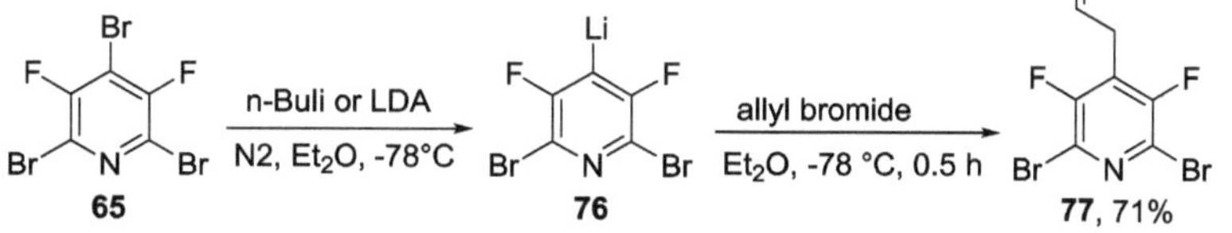

Scheme 4-30. Preparation of 4-allyl-2,6-dibromo-3,5-difuoropyridine **77**.

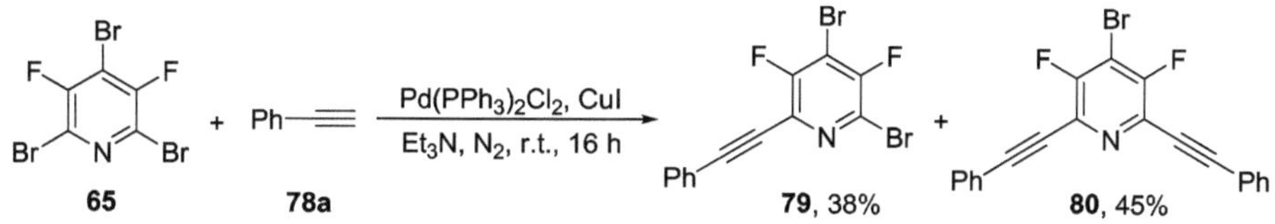

Scheme 4-31. Reaction of 2,4,6-tribromo-3,5-difluoropyridine **65** with phenylacetylene **78a**.

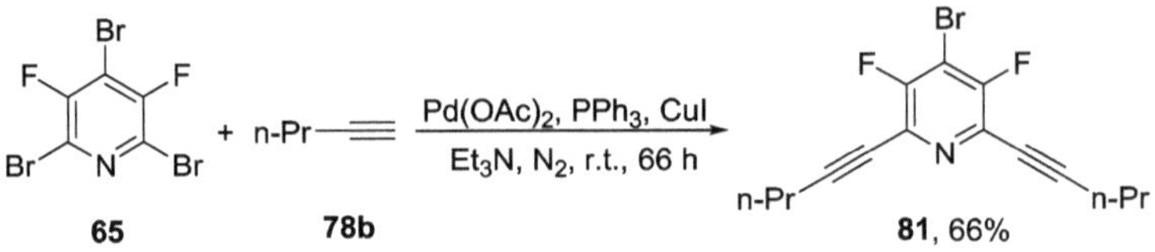

Scheme 4-32. Reaction of 2,4,6-tribromo-3,5-difluoropyridine **65** with n-propylacetylene **78b**.

Suzuki cross-coupling reaction between 2,4,6-tribromo-3,5-difluoropyridine **65** and aromatic boronic acids have been leaded to synthesis of 4-bromo-3-5-difluoro-2,6-diarylpyridines **83** and 3,5-difluoro-2,4,6-triadylpyridines 84 depending on the reaction conditions (Table **4-1**) [13].

Table 4-1. Suzuki reactions of 2,4,6-tribromo-3,5-difluoropyridine 65.

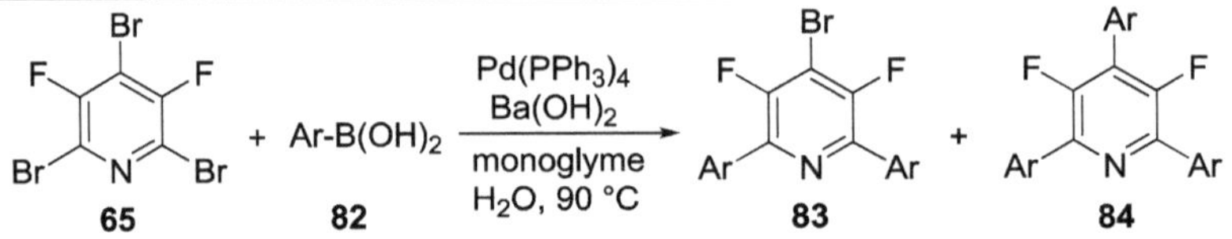

Ar-B(OH)$_2$	83	84
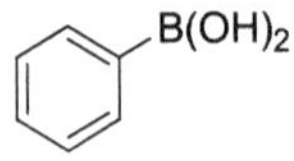 **82a** (3 equiv.)	-	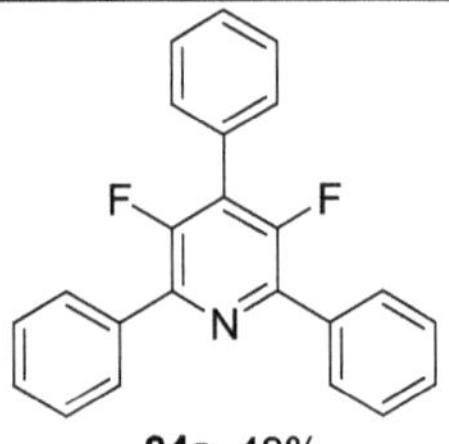 **84a**, 43%
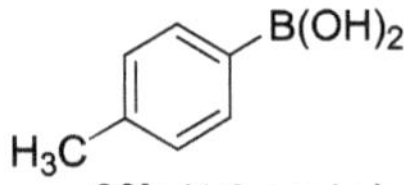 **82b** (1.2 equiv.)	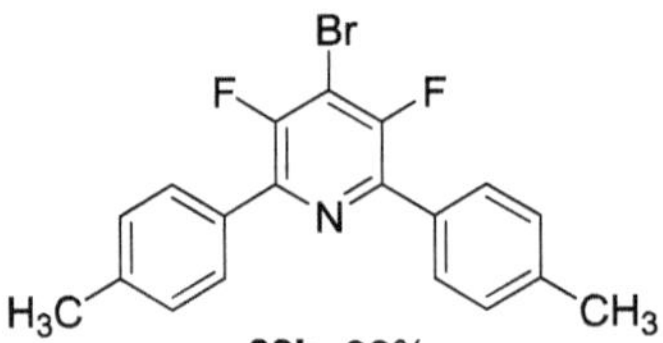 **83b**, 32%	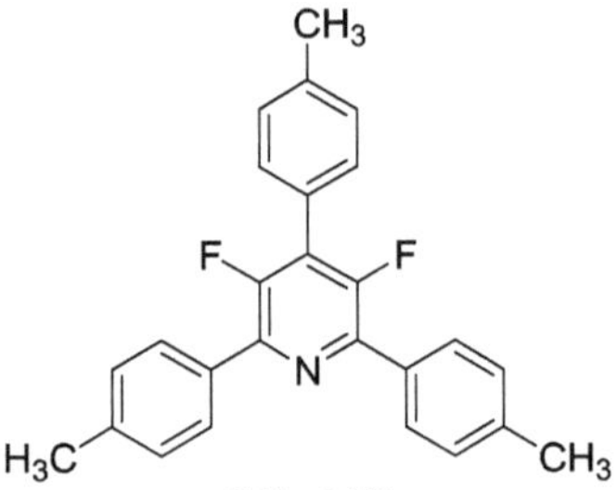 **84b**, 21%
82b (3 equiv.)	-	**84b**, 52%

(Table 4-1) cont.....

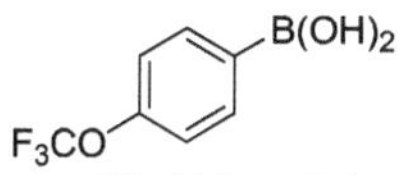

82c (1.2 equiv.) → **83c**, 22% ; **84c**, 8%

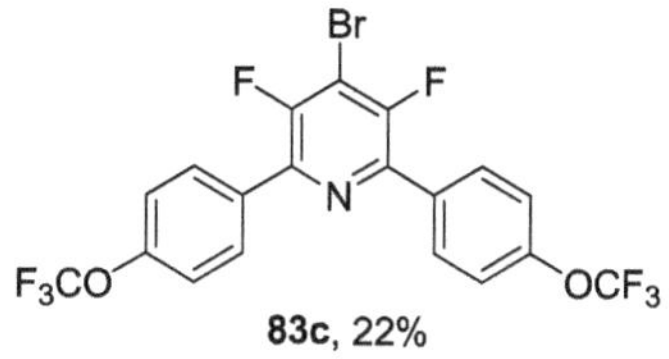

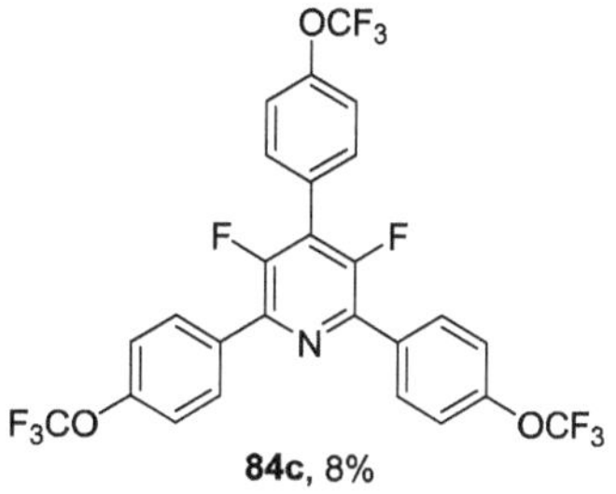

82c, (3 equiv.) → - ; **84c**, 80%

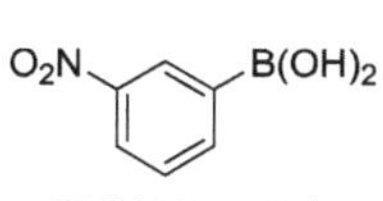

82d (1.2 equiv.) → **83d**, 54% ; -

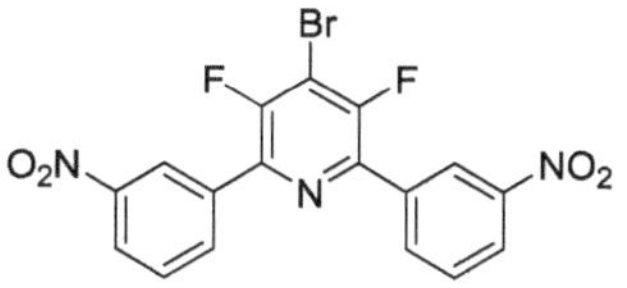

8.　SYNTHESIS　AND　REACTIONS　OF　3,5-DIBROMO-2-6-DICHLOROPYRIDINE

3,5-Dibromo-2,6-dichloropyridine **87** has synthesized in two steps from 2,6-diaminopyridine (Scheme **4-33**) [14]. **87** reacted chemoselectively with various substituted acetylenes to afforded 2,6-dichloro-3,5-dialkynyl-substituted pyridines **88** (Scheme **4-34**) [15]. By employing 8.0 equivalents of acetylenes, corresponding tetraalkynylpyridines **89** are obtained in high yields (Scheme **4-35**). Unsymmetrically tetraalkynylated pyridines **90** produced on reaction of 2,6-dichlor--3,5-dialkynyl-substituted pyridines **88** with substituted acetylenes (Scheme **4-36**).

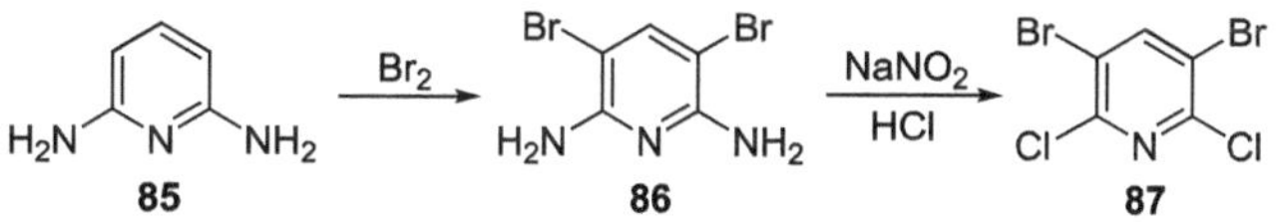

Scheme 4-33. Synthesis of 3,5-Dibromo-2,6-dichloropyridine **87**.

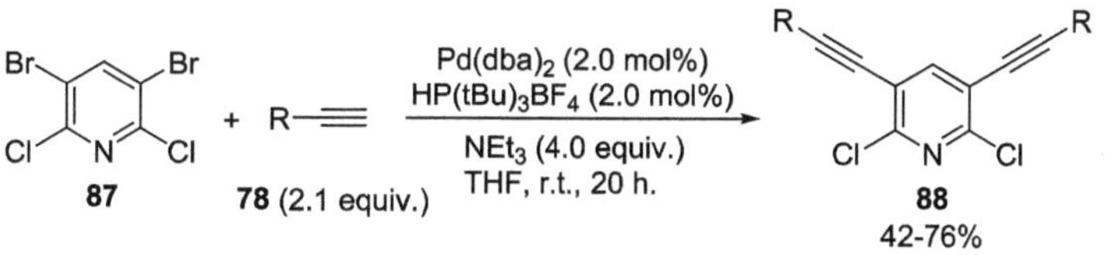

R = Ph, 4-tBuC$_6$H$_4$, 4-OMeC$_6$H$_4$, 4-nHexC$_6$H$_4$, 4-FC$_6$H$_4$, 3-MeC$_6$H$_4$, n-Bu

Scheme 4-34. Synthesis of 2,6-dichloro-3,5-dialkynyl-substituted pyridines **88**.

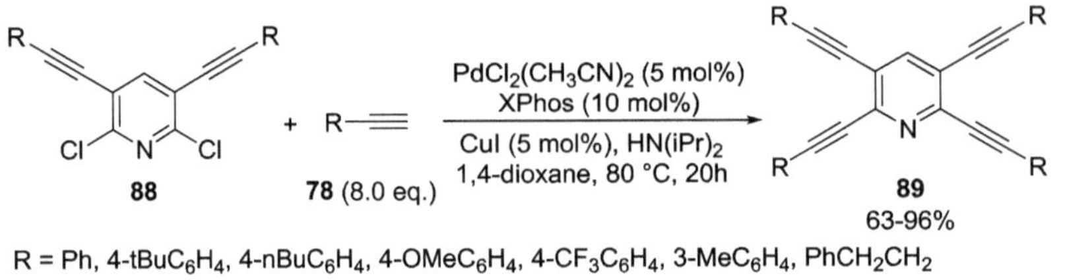

Scheme 4-35. Synthesis of tetraalkynylpyridines **89**.

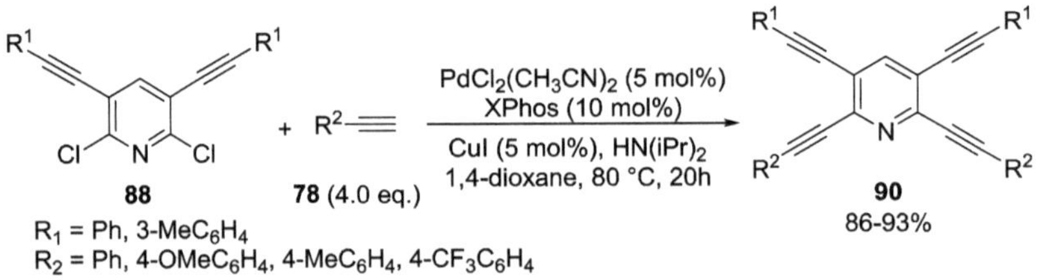

Scheme 4-36. Synthesis of unsymmetrical tetraalkynylpyridines **90**.

REFERENCES

[1]   Moshchitskii, S.; Kisilenko, A. Pentabromopyridine. *Chem. Heterocycl. Compd.,* **1978**, *14*(1), 55-56.
[http://dx.doi.org/10.1007/BF00635943]

[2]   Collins, I.; Suschitzky, H. Polyhalogeno-aromatic compounds. Part XIV. Nucleophilic substitution and peroxy-acid oxidation of pentabromopyridine and some of its NN-dialkylamino- and bis-(NN-dialkylamino)-derivatives. *J. Chem. Soc. C: Organ.,* **1970**, *1*(11), 1523-1530.

[3]   Moshchitskii, S.; Pavlenko, A. Synthesis and reactions of azidopolybromopyridines. *Chem. Heterocycl. Compd.,* **1979**, *15*(11), 1197-1200.
[http://dx.doi.org/10.1007/BF00471431]

[4]   Chapyshev, S.V.; Chernyak, A.V.; Yakushchenko, I.K. Chemoselective Staudinger&-Phosphite Reaction on the Azido Groups of 2, 4, 6&-Triazido&-3, 5&-dibromopyridine. *J. Heterocycl. Chem.,* **2016**, *53*(3), 970-974.
[http://dx.doi.org/10.1002/jhet.2339]

[5]   Moshchitskii, S.; Zeikan', A. Synthesis and properties of 4-mercapto-2, 3, 5, 6-tetrabromopyridine. *Chem. Heterocycl. Compd.,* **1978**, *14*(11), 1232-1236.
[http://dx.doi.org/10.1007/BF00509743]

[6]   Domenico, P. *Halopyridyl thiocyanates*; Google Patents, **1974**.

[7]   Berry, D.; Wakefield, B. Polyhalogeno-aromatic compounds. Part IX. Preparation of pentabromophenyl and tetrabromo-4-pyridyl derivatives of lithium and magnesium, and the generation and trapping of tetrabromobenzyne and tribromo-3-pyridyne. *J. Chem. Soc. C: Organ.,* **1969**, *1*(18), 2342-2346.

[8]   Ager, E.; Suschitzky, H. Reactions of polyhalogenopyridines with methyl fluorosulphonate. *J. Fluor. Chem.,* **1973**, *3*(2), 230-232.
[http://dx.doi.org/10.1016/S0022-1139(00)84167-6]

[9]   Ager, E.; Suschitzky, H. Polyhalogeno-aromatic compounds. Part XXV. Quaternisation of polyhalogenopyridines and reactions of the pyridinium salts. *J. Chem. Soc., Perkin Trans. 1*, **1973**, 2839-2841.
[http://dx.doi.org/10.1039/p19730002839]

[10]   Chivers, G.; Suschitzky, H. A new method of preparing N-oxides from polyhalogenated N-heteroaromatic compounds. *J. Chem. Soc. Chem. Commun.*, **1971**, (1), 28-29.
[http://dx.doi.org/10.1039/c29710000028]

[11]   Bratt, J.; Iddon, B.; Mack, A.G.; Suschitzky, H.; Taylor, J.A.; Wakefield, B.J. Polyhalogenoaromatic compounds. Part 41. Photochemical dehalogenation and arylation reactions of polyhalogenoaromatic and polyhalogenoheteroaromatic compounds. *J. Chem. Soc., Perkin Trans. 1*, **1980**, 648-656.
[http://dx.doi.org/10.1039/p19800000648]

[12]   Chambers, D. R.; W. Hall, C.; Hutchinson, J.; W. Millar, R., Polyhalogenated heterocyclic compounds. Part 42.1 Fluorinated nitrogen heterocycles with unusual substitution patterns. *J. Chem. Soc., Perkin Trans. 1*, **1998**, (10), 1705-1713.
[http://dx.doi.org/10.1039/a709291a]

[13]   Benmansour, H.; Chambers, R.D.; Sandford, G.; Batsanov, A.S.; Howard, J.A. Polyhalogenoheterocyclic compounds: Part 54:[1] Suzuki reactions of 2, 4, 6-tribromo-3, 5-difluoropyridine. *J. Fluor. Chem.*, **2007**, *128*(7), 718-722.
[http://dx.doi.org/10.1016/j.jfluchem.2007.02.012]

[14]   Chen, T.K.; Flowers, W.T. A convenient synthesis of 2, 3, 5, 6-tetrahalogenopyridines and of 3, 5-bis (alkylthio) pyridines from 2, 6-diaminopyridine. *J. Chem. Soc. Chem. Commun.*, **1980**, (23), 1139-1140.
[http://dx.doi.org/10.1039/c39800001139]

[15]   Reimann, S.; Ehlers, P.; Ohlendorf, L.; Langer, P. Sonogashira cross-coupling reactions of 3,5-dibromo-2,6-dichloropyridine. *Org. Biomol. Chem.*, **2017**, *15*(6), 1510-1520.
[http://dx.doi.org/10.1039/C6OB02264B] [PMID: 28116379]

SUBJECT INDEX

A

Absorption 2, 45
  narrow 45
  band 2
Acetamidine 89, 91, 92
  hydrochloride 91, 92
Acetic anhydride 86
Acetic acid 2, 153, 154, 177, 196, 198
  glacial 177
Acetone 19, 61, 181, 199, 227
  oxime 19
Acetylation 85, 86
Acetylcholinesterase 22
Acetylenes 22, 233
  substituted 233
Acid 2, 23, 32, 38, 44, 98, 107, 154, 177, 183,
    188, 190, 196, 198, 205, 206, 219, 222,
    228, 229
  3,4,5,6-tetrachloro-2-pyridylacetic 190
  4-amino-2,5,6-trifluoronicotinic 98
  4-amino-3,5,6-trichloropicolinic 183
  4-amino-3,6-dichloropicolinic 183
  concentrated sulphuric 2, 196, 229
  formic 222
  hydrobromic 219
  hydrofluoric 38
  hydrolysis 188
   peroxytrifluoroacetic 32
  phenylboronic 107
  polyphosphoric 198
  tetrabromopyridine-4-carboxylic 228
  thioacetic 44
  trifluoroacetic 154, 196, 229
  ylacetic 190
Acrylonitrile 153
Activating effect 1, 3, 11, 82
  high 3, 11
Acyclic products 92
Addition 1, 17, 43, 54, 55, 63, 77, 89, 91, 100,
    114, 115, 121, 124, 194
  -elimination mechanism 1
   nucleophilic 63, 124
  oxidative 194

smooth 55
Agrochemical compounds 8
Alkylating ability 31
Alkylation reaction 118
Alkynes 131, 193
  isomeric aryl-tetrafluoropyridyl 31
Allylmagnesium halides 94
Aluminium 28, 170
  tribromide 28
  hydride 170
Alzheimer therapy 132
Amines 34, 35, 40, 63, 72, 81, 111, 156, 165,
    178, 181, 221, 222, 224
  aliphatic 156
  alkyl 34, 35
  benzyl 34, 35
  diallyl 178
  diethyl 165
  primary 81, 224
  secondary 81, 181
  substituent 222
Amino 21, 134
  -functionalized quinolines 134
  -oxylating agents 21
Amino acid derivatives 60, 61
  non-natural fluorinated 60
Ammonia 1, 32, 34, 35, 36, 154, 162, 197,
    227, 230
  aqueous 230
  gas 227
Ammonium 57, 99, 178, 200
  chloride 99, 200
  formate 57
  hydroxide 178
Anion 16, 19, 22, 24, 59, 64, 182
  alkylthiolate 182
  nucleophilic attack oximate 19
  perfluorinated 24
  thiolate 182
  thiophenolate 182
Antibacterial 131, 134
  agents 131
  effects 134
Antimalarial activity 134

Apoptotic activities 134
Arbuzov reaction on reaction 165
Aromatic 35, 39, 40, 64, 156, 157, 179, 185, 195
   aldehyde 163
   amines 35, 39, 40, 156, 157, 179, 195
   azides 169, 224
   boronic acids 232
   character of pentafluoropyridine 2
   N-centered nucleophiles 34
   nucleophilic substitution precess 11
   systems 10
Arylboronic acids 192
Atom, nucleophilic 74

B

Basicity 1, 103, 122, 201
   low 1, 122, 201
   reduced 1
Benzoied compounds 10
Biological 8, 123, 152, 153, 185
   activities 8, 152, 153, 185
   properties 123
Bispyridineproduced 25
Bispyridine systems 25
   multifunctional 25
Bis-silane derivatives 125
Bond activation 30, 100, 102, 117
   products 102

C

Carbanions, produced 22
Carbanion stability 11
Carbonate 1, 66
   potassium 66
Catalysts 3, 8, 32, 57, 94, 96, 101, 102, 123, 132
   cobalt 102
   cross-coupling 96
   metallic 3
   nickel 57
   transfer hydrogenation 101
Catalytic 101, 102, 105, 107, 108
   cross-coupling reactions 107, 108
   formation 105
   hydrodefluorination 101, 102
   reaction 105

Catalyzed coupling reaction 96
Chemical 1, 2, 45
   shifts 1, 2
   stability 45
Chemistry 8, 10, 15, 41, 48, 123, 129, 133, 152
   medicinal 8, 48, 129, 133
   metal 99
   organic 8, 41, 123
Competition 155, 176
   hydrogen bonding 155
Complexes 29, 103, 105, 106, 107, 108
   cationic 103
   nickel tetrafluoropyridyl 108
   produced 106
Complex VII/TF factor inhibitors 130
Compounds 13, 15, 22, 52, 53, 56, 57, 58, 69, 71, 73, 84, 85, 94, 116, 117, 119, 129, 133, 152, 153, 157, 191, 193, 207, 224, 228
   3,5-difluoro-triaryloxypyridine 129
   3,5-difluoro-triaryloxypyrine 129
   bioactive 133
   cyclohexene 191
   decacationic 157
   electrophilic 207
   host 153
   organomagnesium 184
   organometallic 94, 152, 228
   phosphazenyl 224
   produced 116
   tetraalkenylpyridine 193
Computed transition state 105
Copolymerization 121
Copolymers 8, 121
   novel 121
Copper 33, 95, 152, 168, 196, 207, 208
   tetrachloro-4-pyridyl 152, 207, 208
   powder 33
   reagent 95
   sulfate 168
Cross-coupling reactions 53, 54, 107, 152, 192, 193, 194, 219
   catalysed 194
   palladium-catalyzed 193
   selective 192
Curtius reaction on treatment 98
Cyclic products 80
Cyclization 46, 61, 119, 169, 177, 186, 204
   intermolecular 186

photochemical 119
   radical ipso 46
   reactions 169
Cycloaddition reactions 114

D

Decarboxylation 61, 63
   thermal 61
Decomposition 122, 176
   of salt 122
Density 1, 2, 10, 11
   heron electron 11
Drugs 8, 111, 130
   anti-clotting 130
   total commercial 8

E

Effect 1, 2, 11, 31, 129
   dominant 11
   inactivating 11
   induced withdrawing 11
   medium inhibitory 129
   protecting 31
   shielding 1, 2
Electrochemical reduction 183
Electrophilic 36, 37, 108
   fluorinating agent 37
     site-selective 36
Electroreduction 15

F

Fluorinated 8, 9, 22, 76
   medicinal 8
   pyridine aldoximes 22
   ring-fused heterocyles 76
   synthetic blocks 9
Fluorinated compounds 8, 42
   produced 42
Formation 14, 47, 48, 57, 58, 65, 66, 67, 70, 118, 119, 120, 156, 163, 169, 186, 190
   bromotetrachloropyridines 169
   photochemical 118
Functionalization of 3-chlorotrifluoropyridine 112
Functionalized fluorinated organic compounds 96

G

Grignard reagent 34, 95, 205
Guanidine 69

H

Haloacetic acids 174
Halogenating reagents 51
Halogen 1, 3, 8, 9, 10, 122, 123
   atoms 1, 3, 8, 122, 123
   exchange 9
   substitution act 10
Heating 177, 184, 190
   mixture 184
   of acid 177
   of ester 190
Herbicides 153, 183
   plant growth regulator 183
Heteroarenium 157, 159
   molecules 157
   salt 159
Heterocyclic compounds 8, 157, 185
   fluorinated 8
   multifunctional 157
   novel 185
Heterocyclic systems 8, 123, 191
   fluorinated 8
   ring-fused 191
Human melanoma cell growth, inhibited 31
Hydrazine 58, 59, 197
   hydrate 197
   monohydrate 58, 59
Hydrodefluorination 8, 57, 101, 102, 110, 111
   catalytic homogeneous 57
   selective 102
   reactions 101
Hydrogen fluoride (HF) 64
Hydrolysis 63, 115, 116, 188, 224, 225, 228
   acidic 225

I

Imidazopyridine, produced 89
Iminothionyl chlorides 162
Inhibitory 129, 130, 133
   activity 133
   property 130
Irradiation 67, 68, 116

ultrasonic 67, 68

L

Lithium 52, 53, 55, 85, 94, 95
  diethylamide 85
  exchange 55
  organometallic compounds 94
  reagents 52, 53, 95

M

Macrocycles 8, 123, 124, 125, 126, 127, 128, 133
  synthesis of 123, 124, 125, 126, 127, 128, 133
Macrocyclic 8, 123, 125, 127, 128
  compounds 8, 123
  systems 123, 127
   produced 125, 128
Mechanism 3, 10, 20, 44, 47, 48, 65, 70, 73, 89, 91, 118, 119, 120, 173, 179, 182, 185, 190, 224
  addition nucleophile 10
  amidation 44, 190
  bimolecular addition-elimination 3, 10
  elimination-addition 10
  free-radical 120
  irradiation of pentafluoropyridine 120
  of photocycloaddition 118, 119
  plausible 48
  postulated 70, 89, 91, 118
  steps addition-elimination 3
  suggested radical 182
Meldrum's acid 63
Metal-halogen exchange 206, 219, 228
  reaction 206
Methanethiolate 14, 15
  sodium 14
Method 25, 40, 9
  electrochemical 9
  halogen exchange 9
  selective 40
  synthetic 25
Methyl ester 71, 73, 200
  ammonium methylphosphonic acid 200
  mono-protected L-threonine 73
  perfluorinated dehydrobutyrine 73
Microreactor technology 40

Miyaura cross-coupling 152, 192
Molecules 44, 70, 74, 111, 114, 176, 225
  asymmetric 111
  form amide 44
  heteroaromatic 114
  multiagent 74
Multifunctional puridines, produced 161
Multisubstituted 25, 77
  bicyclic N-heterocycles 77
  heteroaromatics 25

N

Nature 1, 3, 8, 64, 88, 152, 185
  electron-withdrawing 1
  withdrawing 8
Necleophiles 12
Nickel compounds 108
Nitrogen 44, 64, 67, 68, 171, 185, 221, 224
  bidentate nucleophiles 67
  gas 44
  losing 224
  Nitrogen nucleophiles 68, 221
  monodentate 171
Nitro products 222
Nucleophiles 3, 4, 10, 11, 25, 52, 59, 66, 68, 76, 82, 88, 152, 155, 156, 161, 180, 181, 220, 221, 230
  ambident 68, 188
  attacking 88
  hard 59
  heteroaromatic 161
  hindrance 152
  less-hindered 172
  multidentate 59, 76
  nature 230
  primary 181
Nucleophilic 3, 8, 10, 11, 60, 63, 64, 65, 123, 185, 186, 188, 191, 219, 222
  addition-elimination reactions 123
  attack 3, 8, 10, 11, 60, 63, 64, 123, 185, 186, 188, 191, 219, 222
Nucleophilic reactions 19, 25, 26, 40, 74, 152, 155, 162, 165, 179, 180, 209, 219, 220
  of bi-perfluoropyridine 26
  of pentabromopyridine 220
  of pentachloropyridine 155
  of perchloropyridines 155
Nucleophilic substitution 1, 8, 11, 12, 108, 122, 123, 185, 195, 198, 202, 229

of 4-bromotetrachloropyridine 195
   of sodium dimethyldithiocarbamate 198
   of sodium dimethyldithiocarbamate on
      pentachloropyridine-N-oxide 198
   intramolecular 185
Nucleophilic substitution reactions 1, 3, 10,
      82, 84, 88, 152, 155, 208, 226
   in *N*-heterocyclic systems 10
Nucleoplilicity, high 76

O

One-step synthesis of pentaalkynylpyridines
      193
Organic 3, 29, 48, 96
   oxidants 157
   solar cells 29
   synthesis 3, 48, 96
Organofluorine compounds 36
Organometalic 8, 228
   reagent of polybromopyridines 228
   reactions 8
Organophosphorus nerve-agent poisoning 22
Oxazolone enolates 60
Oxidation 14, 152, 167, 168, 169, 175, 176,
      196, 198, 219, 222, 223, 229
   and methylation of pentabromopyridine
      219
   of 4-aryl and 4-alkylthio tetrachloropyrine
      derivatives 175
   of pentabromopyridine 229
   of pentachloropyridine 152, 196
   of polychloropyridines 196
   of tetrabromo-6-methylaminopyridine 223
   of tetrabromo-4-piperidinopyridine 222
   of tetrachloro-4-dimethylaminopyridine
      167, 168
   of tetrachloro-2-hydrazinopyridine 169
   of tetrachloro-4-hydrazinopyridine 168,
      169
   of tetrachloro-4-methoxypyridine 198
   of tetrachloro-4-methoxypyririne 198
   of tetrachloropyridine-4-thiol 176
   reaction 222
   -reduction process 14

P

Pentaalkynylpyridine

Pentachloropyridine 1, 2, 3, 5, 152, 153, 154,
      155, 156, 157, 166, 167, 168, 172, 173,
      180, 182, 183, 184, 185, 187, 195, 201,
      205, 208, 229
   optimum reaction condition 180
   persulfuration of 182
   preparation of 152, 153, 154, 208
   produced 153, 154
   reactions 5, 229
    reduced 201
   synthesis of 153, 154
Pentafluoropyridine 1, 2, 8, 9, 10, 12, 15, 17,
      18, 19, 20, 32, 40, 64, 66, 88, 89, 100,
      101, 102, 103, 104, 106, 111, 115, 116,
      122, 124
   bond of 100, 101, 102, 104, 111
   cation 8
    protonate 1
    leades 106
    salt 122
Pentakis 15, 16, 30
   produced 16, 30
Perfluorinated
   dehydrobutyrine-containing amino acids
      24, 56, 59, 73, 123
   heteroaromatics 24
   heterocycles 123
   Heterocyles 59
   Pyridines 56
Perfluoroalkylation 13, 25, 124, 176
   of perchloropyridine-4-thiols 176
Perfluoroheteroaromatics 8, 94
   organometallic 8, 94
Perfluoropyridyl 75, 104, 105
   boronate ester 104, 105
   ether 75
Perhalogenated heteroaromatic compounds 41
Perhalogenated heterocycles 123
Peronosporu fungi 153
Persulfurated pyridine derivatives 15
Phosphorimidate, produced 225
Phosphorus 153, 154, 162, 197, 219
   oxybromid 219
   pentachloride 153, 154, 162
   pentasulfide 197
   trichloride 197
Photocatalytic 109, 110, 111, 112, 113, 114
   alkylation 110
   arylation 111
   coupling 111

E-alkenylation 114
hydrodefluorination 112
Z-alkenylation 113, 114
Photochemical 114, 115, 116, 119, 120
  addition 114, 115, 116
  products 120
` transformations 114, 119
Photochemical reactions 8, 109, 117, 118,
    152, 153, 203, 229
  self-condensing 153
  of pentabromopyridine 229
Photocycloaddition 116, 118, 119
  of m-amido isomer 118
  of o-amido isomer 118
  of p-amido isomer 118
Photoinduced electron transfer (PET) 119
Photolysis 102, 169, 203, 204, 205, 230
  of 2-aryloxy and
    arylaminotetrachloropyridines 205
  of 4-aryl and
    heteroarylthiotetrachloropyridines 204
  of 4-aryloxy and
    arylaminotetrachloropyridines 204
  of 4-bromotetrachloropyridine 203
  of pentabromopyridine 230
  of pentachloropyridine 203
  of tachloropyridines 203
  of tetrachloro-2-iodopyridine 203
  of tetrachloro-3-iodopyridine 204
  of tetrachloro-4-iodopyridine 203
Polychlorinated heterocycles 153
Polychloroheteroaromatic compounds 153
Polyethylene glycol 123
Polyfluorinated heteroaromatic compounds 25
Polyfluoroaromatic compounds 10, 18
Polyfunctional 30, 77, 86, 192
  analogues 77
  pyridines 192
Polyhalogenated 122, 194
  pyridines 122
  substrates 194
Polymeric material 69
Preparation 122, 200, 220
  of pentabromopyridine 220
  of pentafluoropyridine salt 122
  problem 200
Primary 117, 179
  aliphatic amines 179
  hydroxy alkane solutions 117
Produced 26, 38, 127

4-alkoxytetrafluoropyridine derivatives 127
multisubstituted perfluoropyridine
    derivatives 26
perfluorinated azoxy-compounds 38
Pyridine 1, 2, 3, 8, 10, 11, 15, 16, 30, 39, 59,
    77, 82, 106, 109, 117, 153, 157, 179,
    180, 184, 188, 194, 221, 233
  bond 30
  fluorinated 109, 117
  polyfluorinated 59
  polysubstituted 157
  tetraalkynylated 194, 233
Pyridine derivatives 25, 41, 67, 123, 134
  fluorinated 134
  multifunctional 67
  produced multisubstituted 41
Pyrolysis 38, 169
Pyrrolic squaraine dye 45

Q

Quinazolines 152
Quinoline nucleus 134
Quinoxaline scaffolds 89

R

Radical Addition 8, 48, 51
  initiated 48
Raman analysis 1, 2
Reaction 14, 26, 34, 35, 43, 44, 45, 59, 67, 71,
    79, 87, 90, 128, 155, 156, 157, 159, 162,
    163, 167, 168, 169, 181, 172, 173, 181,
    182, 184, 185, 189, 191, 195, 196, 197,
    199, 200, 208, 220, 221, 223, 229
  4-phenylsulphonyltetrafluoropyridine 87
  of 2-aminotetrachloropyridine 163
  of 4-aminotetrachloropyridine 163
  of 4-bromotetrachloropyridine 195, 196
  of 4-bromotetrafluoropyridine 35
  of 4-phenylsulfonyl-tetrachloropyridine
    181
  of 4-phenylsulphonyltetraflouropyridine 85
  of 4-phenylsulphonyl tetrafluoropyridine
    90
  of aromatic N-centered nucleophiles 34
  of excess sodium azide 223
  of heteroarenium salt 159
  of morpholine and piperidine 159

of nitrogen bidentate nucleophiles 67
of pentabromopyridine 220, 221, 223
of pentachloropyridine 128, 155, 156, 157,
　　162, 167, 168, 169, 172, 173, 181, 182,
　　184, 185, 189
of pentachloropyridine *N*-oxide 199
of pentacloropyridine 208
of pentafluororpyridine 71
of perfluorinated compounds 59
of piperidine 223
of sodium salt 173
of tetrachloro-4-cyanopyridine 171, 182,
　　191
of tetrafluoro-4-isopropyl pyridine 26
of 4-azidotetrafluoropyridine 43, 44, 45
of 4-thioalkyltetrafluoropyridines 14
of bromofluoropyridine 52
of grignard reagent of 4-
　　bromotetrafluoropyridine 34
of imidazopyridines 79
of N-methyl bromopyridinium
　　fluorosulphonate 229
of pentachloropyridine-N-oxide 197, 200
Reagents 8, 75, 95, 100, 103, 155, 156, 205
　nucleophilic 103
　organolithium 205
　organometallic 8, 205
　perfluoroarylcopper 95
　preferred organometallic 205
Reduction 30, 36, 56, 57, 58, 157, 200, 201,
　　224, 230
　　of 3-chlorotetrafluoropyridine 57
　　of azide 224
　　of nitroamines 36
　　of pentachloropyridine by lithium
　　　aluminum hydride 201
　　of pentachloropyridine by lithium
　　　borohydride 201
　　of pentafluoropyridine 56, 58
　　of Perfluorinated Pyridines 56
　　of polychloropyridines 200
Refluxing 103, 199
　mixture 103
Reflux temperature 166
Ring-fused 76, 204
　heterocyles 76
　products 204
Ring-fused systems 8, 77, 79, 80, 81, 86, 91,
　　152, 204
　fluorinated 77

Route 77, 95, 124, 128
　synthetic 77

S

Salts 11, 17, 36, 41, 42, 62, 63, 73, 81, 122,
　　152, 157, 158, 159, 160, 161, 162, 178,
　　200, 202, 229
　ammonium enolate 63
　bisheteroaromatic 161, 162
　formate 101
　heteronium 152, 157, 158, 161
　keto-oxime 11
　monosodium 36
　of pentabromopyridine 229
　　of perfluoropyridine 122
　　produced 178, 200
　produced ammonium enolate 62
　produced pyridinum 41
　pyridinum 41, 42
　reaction of 157, 159, 160
　sulfonate 17
　tricationic pyridinium 159
Selective electrophilic fluorinating agents 36
Selective reduction 112, 113
　　of 4-acetamidotetrafluoropyridines 112
　　of 4-arylaminotetrafluoropyridines 112
Singlet oxygen scavengers 31
Sites 3, 29, 59, 62, 64, 68, 76, 81, 85, 186,
　　187, 188, 192
　activated 3
　carbon 81
　nucleophilic 68
　oxygen 59, 68
SNAr reactions 71, 72
Sodium 1, 19, 28, 34, 35, 36, 54, 88, 157, 172,
　　176, 177, 180, 183, 188, 195, 197, 198,
　　199, 220, 221
　acetate 197
　benzenesulphinate 88, 180
　borohydride 157
　bromide 195
　cation 19
　cyanide 172
　dimethyldithiocarbamate 198, 199
　formate 102
　hydrogensulfide 176
　hydrohide 172
　hydroxide 1, 34, 35, 172, 177, 183, 188,
　　197, 221

iodide 54
  methoxide 28, 36, 172, 220
Sodium nitrite 38, 180
  phenylsulfnate 180
Solution 64, 77, 173
  aqueous sodium bicarbonate 173
  concentrated acetonitrile 64
  diluted acetonitrile 77
Solvents 45, 94, 155, 199, 206
  etheric 94
  hydrocarbon 206
  low polarity 45
  protic 155
Spectrum of pentafluoropyridine 2
Stabilizing 3, 11, 41, 157
  influence 3
  properties 41
Stable perfluoropyridyl carbanion 24
Staphylococcus aureus 134
Staudinger reaction 43, 224
Steric 1, 4, 100
  deflection 220
  factors 1, 4
Steric hindrance 180
  cases 180
  nucleophiles 180
Stoichiometric coupling reaction 105
Substituents 25, 31, 64, 86, 88, 89, 103, 119,
    152, 157, 185, 192
  amidine 89
  electron-withdrawing tetrafluoropyridine
    119
  high chlorine 152
  hydrogen 86
  lysine 31
  ring 64, 185
Substituted 30, 31, 62, 64, 92
  acetylene amino acid conjugates 30, 31
  imidamide systems 64
  imidazopyridines 92
  Meldrum's acids 62
Substitution 4, 10, 11, 16, 20, 28, 56, 60, 71,
    77, 88, 117, 180, 182
  active aromatic electrophilic 10
  nucleophilic aromatic 60, 71
  regiospecific 117
Substitution reactions 3, 24, 55, 68, 82, 123,
    155, 208
  aromatic nucleophilic 3, 123
  nucleophilic aromatic 82

of perfluorinated heteroaromatics 24
  susceptible nucleophilic 208
Sulfuric acid 153, 189, 196, 198
  concentrated 198
  concerted 153
Sulfur nucleophiles 12, 13
Suzuki 219, 232
  Cross-coupling Reaction 219, 232
  reactions 232
Synthesis 15, 23, 24, 33, 38, 41, 43, 46, 59,
    67, 68, 76, 86, 117, 123, 157, 186, 192,
    195, 197, 200, 219, 227, 234
  and reactions of salt 200
  efficient 86
  heterocyclic compounds 186
  of 2-alkoxy-4-aminotrifluoropyridine
    derivatives 41
  of 2-alkoxy-4-dialkylamino
    trifluoropyridine derivatives 41
  of 4-amino-tetrabromopyridine 227
  of 4-aminotetrafluoropyridine 33
  of 4-azidotetrafluoropyridine 43
  of 4-bromotetrachloropyridine 195
  of 4-substitued tetrafluoropyridines 67
  of bis-perfluoropyridines 68
  of fluorinated ring-fused heterocyles 76
  of macrocycles by aromatic nucleophilic
    substitutions 123
  of pentabromopyridine 219
    of pentachloropyridine-n-oxide 197
  of perflouropyridinum salts 41
  of perfluorinated azo dyes 38
  of perfluorinated heterocyles 59
  of perfluoropyridine-pyrrolic squaraine dye
    46
  of persulfurated pyridine derivatives 15
  of polyfunctional pyridines 192
  of tetrafluoropyridine-2-aldoxime 23
  of tetrafluoropyridine-4-aldoxime 23
  of tetrafluoropyridine-4-carboxylic acid 24
  of unsymmetrical tetraalkynylpyridines 234
  regiospecific 117
  selective 157, 192
Systems 1, 2, 3, 9, 25, 40, 64, 76, 77, 84, 88,
    89, 94, 116, 123, 124, 129, 157, 186
  activated 3
  bis-perfluoropyridyl 76
  bis-perfuoropyridylimidamide 64
  bridged bispyridyl 88
  chelating 81

continuous flow reactor 40
efficient perfluorinated structural 25
fluorinatetd 9
fused ring 77
macrocycls 129
macrocylic 124
multifunctional heteroaromatic 25
perchlorinated 9
perfluoropyeidineimidamide 64
polycationic 157
polysubstituted 25
pyrazine 84, 88
pyridooxadiazine 77
quinazoline 186
triazine 94
tricyclic 89, 116

T

Tetracloropyyridine sulfonamides 178
TFA salt 71
Therapeutic agents 131
Thermal 95, 102, 224, 228
    decomposition 224
    elimination 228
    reaction 102
    stability 95
Thermolysis 224
Treatment 2, 8, 21, 22, 23, 98, 103, 106, 107,
        108, 152, 153, 169, 177, 188, 189, 195,
        219, 224
    acetic anhydride 177
    of azide 224
    of tetrachlorohydrazinopyridine 169
    medical 8
    seed 153
Triethyl phosphite 38, 165, 225
    electron-rich 225
Trifluorobenzo, produced 88
Trifluoroperoxyacetic acid 167

U

Ultrasonic irradiation conditions 81
UV-Vis Spectrum 1, 2

W

Well-documented photoconducting
        capabilities 45

X

Xanthates 45, 47, 48, 156, 182
    DMF 156
        potassium 182
Xenone 176
        bisperfluoroalkane carboxylate 176
        difluoride 176

Z

Zinc 28, 29, 94, 95, 200
        acetate 29
        complexes 29
        perfluoroheteroaromatics 94
        powder 94, 95, 200
Z-isomer 73, 113
        single elimination product 73